# Emergency Imaging of At-Risk Patients

# Emergency Imaging of At-Risk Patients

## General Principles

**Michael N. Patlas, MD, FRCPC**
Professor of Radiology
Director, Division of Trauma/Emergency Radiology
McMaster University, Hamilton
Ontario, Canada

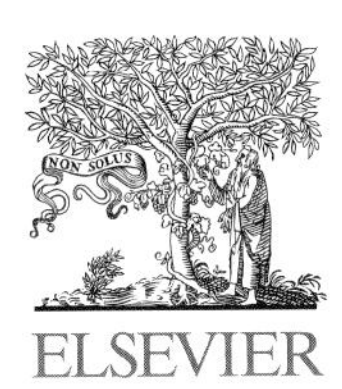


ELSEVIER

Elsevier
1600 John F. Kennedy Blvd.
Ste 1800
Philadelphia, PA 19103-2899

EMERGENCY IMAGING OF AT-RISK PATIENTS: GENERAL PRINCIPLES ISBN: 978-0-323-87661-2



Senior *Content Development Manager*: Somodatta Roy Choudhury
*Senior Acquisitions Editor*: Melanie Tucker
*Senior Content Development Specialist*: Shilpa Kumar
*Publishing Services Manager*: Shereen Jameel
*Project Manager*: Vishnu T. Jiji
*Design Direction*: Ryan Cook

Printed in India

Last digit is the print number: 9 8 7 6 5 4 3 2 1

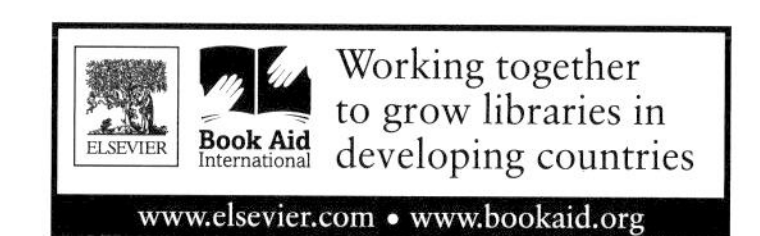

# Contributors

**Abdullah Alabousi, MD, FRCPC**
Department of Radiology
McMaster University, St. Joseph's Healthcare, Hamilton
Ontario, Canada

**Omar Alwahbi, MD**
Department of Radiology
McMaster University, Hamilton
Ontario, Canada

**Sanjeev Bhalla, MD**
Professor
Mallinckrodt Institute of Radiology
Missouri, United States

**Maria J. Borja, MD**
Assistant Professor
Division of Neuroradiology, Department of Radiology
New York University Grossman School of Medicine
New York, United States

**Mauricio Castillo, MD, FACR**
Professor of Radiology
Division of Neuroradiology, Department of Radiology
University of North Carolina School of Medicine, Chapel Hill
North Carolina, United States

**Melissa A. Davis, MD, MBA**
Assistant Professor
Department of Radiology and Biomedical Imaging
Yale University School of Medicine, New Haven
Connecticut, United States

**Richard Duszak, MD, FACR, FSIR, FRBMA**
Professor and Chair
Department of Radiology
University of Mississippi Medical Center, Jackson
Mississippi, United States

**Daniel D. Friedman, MD**
Resident
Department of Radiology
Mallinckrodt Institute of Radiology
Washington University School of Medicine, Saint Louis
Missouri, United States

**Anahi Goransky, MD**
Staff, Radiologist
Department of Radiology
Cimac Center
San Juan, Argentina

**Joshua Gu, MD**
Resident
Department of Radiology
University of Texas Health (University of Texas Health Science Center at Houston) – McGovern Medical School
Texas, United States

**Angela Guarnizo, MD**
Division of Neuroradiology
Department of Radiology
Hospital Universitario Fundación Santa Fe de Bogota
Bogota, Colombia

**Neetika Gupta, MBBS, MD**
Pediatric Radiology Fellow
Department of Medical Imaging
Children's Hospital of Eastern Ontario (CHEO)
University of Ottawa, Ottawa
Ontario, Canada

**Ehsan A. Haider, ChB, MB, FRCPC**
Associate Professor
Department of Radiology
McMaster University, St Joseph's Healthcare, Hamilton
Ontario, Canada

**Kathleen Hames, PhD, MD, FRCPC**
Assistant Professor
Department of Radiology
McMaster University, Hamilton
Ontario, Canada

**Malak Itani, MD**
Assistant Professor
Mallinckrodt Institute of Radiology
Washington University School of Medicine
Missouri, United States

**Iain D.C. Kirkpatrick, MD**
Professor
Department of Radiology
University of Manitoba, Winnipeg
Manitoba, Canada

**Manickam Kumaravel, MD**
Professor
Diagnostic and Interventional Imaging
University of Texas Health, Houston
Texas, United States

**Neeraj Lalwani, MD, FSAR, DABR**
Associate Professor
Department of Radiology
Virginia Commonwealth University, Richmond
Virginia, United States

**Daniel R. Ludwig, MD**
Assistant Professor
Mallinckrodt Institute of Radiology
Washington University School of Medicine, Saint Louis
Missouri, United States

**Elizabeth S. Lustrin, MD**
Associate Professor
Division of Neuroradiology
Department of Radiology
New York University Langone Hospital – Long Island Division
New York, United States

**Joseph Mansour, MD**
Cardiothoracic Imaging Fellow
Mallinckrodt Institute of Radiology
Missouri, United States

**Thomas Mehuron, MD**
Resident
Department of Radiology
New York University Grossman School of Medicine
New York, United States

**Vincent M. Mellnick, MD**
Mallinckrodt Institute of Radiology
Washington University School of Medicine, Saint Louis
Missouri, United States

**Elka Miller, MD, FRCPC**
Professor
Department of Medical Imaging
Children's Hospital of Eastern Ontario (CHEO)
Chief and Research Director
University of Ottawa
Ontario, Canada

**Gina Nirula, MD**
Lecturer
Department of Diagnostic Imaging
Children's Hospital of Winnipeg, Health Science Center
University of Manitoba, Winnipeg
Manitoba, Canada

**Saagar Patel, MD, MBA**
Resident
Department of Radiology
University of Texas Health (UTHealth) – McGovern Medical School
Texas, United States

**Michael N. Patlas, MD, FRCPC**
Professor of Radiology
Director, Division of Trauma/Emergency Radiology
McMaster University, Hamilton
Ontario, Canada

**Paulo Puac-Polanco, MD, MSc**
Assistant Professor
Department of Radiology
McMaster University, St. Joseph's Healthcare
Hamilton
Ontario, Canada

**Demetrios A. Raptis, MD**
Assistant Professor
Department of Radiology
Mallinckrodt Institute of Radiology, Saint Louis
Missouri, United States

**Katya Rozovsky, MD**
Associate Professor
Department of Diagnostic Imaging
Children's Hospital of Winnipeg
Health Science Center
University of Manitoba, Winnipeg
Manitoba, Canada

**Reza Salari, MD, PhD**
Mallinckrodt Institute of Radiology
Washington University School of Medicine
Saint Louis, United States

**Steven Sapozhnikov, DO, MS**
Resident
Department of Radiology
New York University Langone Hospital – Long Island
New York, United States

**Rahul Sarkar, MD, MSc, FRCPC**
Assistant Professor
Department of Radiology
McMaster University, Hamilton
Ontario, Canada
Staff Radiologist
Department of Diagnostic Imaging
Juravinski Hospital and Cancer Centre, Hamilton Health Sciences, Hamilton
Ontario, Canada

**Gali Shapira-Zaltsberg, MD**
Department of Medical Imaging
Children's Hospital of Eastern Ontario (CHEO), University of Ottawa, Ottawa
Ontario, Canada

**Carlos Torres, MD, FRCPC**
Professor of Radiology
Department of Radiology, Radiation Oncology and Medical Physics. Faculty of Medicine, University of Ottawa
Neuroradiologist and CME Director, Department of Medical Imaging, The Ottawa Hospital
Clinician Investigator, Ottawa Hospital Research Institute OHRI and Ottawa Brain and Mind Research Institute
Ontario, Canada

**Amar Udare, MD**
Clinical Fellow
Department of Diagnostic Imaging
Juravinski Hospital and Cancer Centre, Hamilton Health Sciences
McMaster University, Hamilton
Ontario, Canada

**Christian B. van der Pol, MD**
Assistant Professor
Department of Radiology
McMaster University, Hamilton
Ontario, Canada

**Nader Zakhari, MD, FRCPC**
Assistant Professor
Department of Radiology, Division of Neuroradiology, Department of Diagnostic Imaging
University of Ottawa, The Ottawa Hospital Civic and General Campus, Ottawa
Ontario, Canada

**Carlos Zamora, MD**
Associate Professor of Radiology
Division of Neuroradiology, Department of Radiology
University of North Carolina School of Medicine, Chapel Hill
North Carolina, United States

**Brian Zhu, MD**
Resident
Department of Radiology
New York University Langone Hospital – Long Island
New York, United States

# Preface

The goal of *Emergency Imaging of At-Risk Patients* is to bring together in one book emergency findings in at-risk patient populations with unique clinical and imaging presentations. We elected to focus on emergency conditions in a diverse group of vulnerable patients. It is challenging to assess at-risk patients due to a myriad of factors, including atypical clinical pictures, normal physiological changes, delays in seeking medical care, comorbidities, and blunted inflammatory responses. History and physical examination can be misleading in at-risk patients, and imaging plays a crucial role in effective triage of vulnerable patients.

The emergency radiologist is expected to be comfortable with the interpretation of imaging studies covering all anatomic areas and to be at ease with different imaging modalities, including radiography, fluoroscopy, and cross-sectional imaging. The editor of this book spent two decades teaching emergency and trauma imaging and noted that his trainees excel in interpretation of cross-sectional examinations but can find it quite challenging to deal with radiographs, especially with the high volume of abnormal x-rays typical of the multitrauma patient. Therefore, numerous adult and pediatric radiographs have been included. Multidetector computed tomography (MDCT) is a workhorse in the emergency department. The book extensively discusses emergency indications for MDCT, with specific exploration of MDCT protocol adaptation and adjustment of contrast injection techniques in vulnerable patients. However, emergency imagers should be cognizant of the effects of ionizing radiation related to computed tomography. These considerations are of paramount importance in emergency and trauma imaging of pediatric and pregnant patients. Hence, the role of ultrasound and magnetic resonance imaging (MRI) in the emergency evaluation of vulnerable patients is discussed. *Emergency Imaging of At-Risk Patients* contains multiple MRI cases with a thorough discussion of the intelligent use of MRI not only for the evaluation of brain, spine, and musculoskeletal emergencies but also for assessment of acute chest, abdominal, and pelvic conditions.

The book starts with an overview of social determinants of health, which disproportionately affect diverse, marginalized, and vulnerable populations. We discuss health disparities that exist within acute diagnostic imaging. This overview is followed by two chapters describing neurological emergencies in geriatric, cancer, and immunocompromised patients. The following chapters cover traumatic and nontraumatic chest, abdominal, and pelvic emergencies encountered in pregnant patients. Then, abdominal emergencies in postoperative bariatric patients and geriatric patients are discussed. It is unusual to have a subspecialty pediatric imaging emergency coverage 24/7/365 outside of major children's hospitals. Instead, imaging examinations of acutely ill children admitted to the emergency department are typically performed by emergency radiologists. Therefore, this book contains two dedicated chapters describing imaging pitfalls in the assessment of common pediatric neurological, chest, and abdominal entities seen in the emergency setting, including an in-depth discussion of imaging of foreign bodies and complications related to malposition of central lines and gastrointestinal tubes. Both pediatric chapters cover different aspects of imaging in victims of nonaccidental trauma and provide practical tips for the evaluation of imaging studies in this extremely vulnerable population. In the editor's opinion, there is one additional group of patients with special imaging presentations justifying a dedicated chapter: recreational drug users.

The book draws on the vast clinical experience of emergency and trauma radiologists from the largest academic medical centers across North America. The authors present basic and advanced emergency imaging concepts and discuss subtle imaging findings that will be useful for radiologists in training and more seasoned imagers, as well as emergency physicians, general, trauma and orthopedic surgeons, pediatricians, obstetricians and gynecologists, and critical care physicians looking for an update on this difficult topic.

# Foreword

When most people think about vulnerability, they typically consider the concept in the first-person emotional context of being harmed or exposed to harm by another person or entity—whether intended or not.[1–3] For physicians, who are tasked with ensuring the best outcomes for some of society's most vulnerable populations, the concept of vulnerability (and associated duty) becomes much more complex. Sadly, even the most modern health care delivery systems leave gaps in care that result in significant disparities for the people most in need.

To understand how to best approach the care of vulnerable patients requires a nuanced understanding of what vulnerability means in the context of health care. This ultimately requires a deliberate willingness to fully appreciate the situation, context, and environment that have placed patients in a position in which they are not able to fully protect and care for themselves. These drivers are complex and often interconnected, and include socioeconomic status, language barriers, age, mental status, mental health, racial bias, and physical ability. The risks of vulnerability are both serious and real and range from falls to delayed diagnosis, neglect, abuse, and, in some cases, death.[2,3] Increasingly, research and recent events have highlighted links between patient vulnerability and health care disparities. The COVID-19 pandemic, of note, caused a significant strain on health care delivery systems worldwide, disproportionately impacting Indigenous, Black, and Hispanic populations and catalyzing important conversations about the vulnerability of patients due to race, socioeconomic status, and class.[4] Examples of such disparities include Indigenous and Black mothers who are two to three times more likely to die from pregnancy-related causes than White women, a number that increases to four and five times over the age of 30 years.[5,6] Similarly, rural populations that have historically had inadequate access to preventative, specialized, and emergent health care now increasingly struggle, as a significant number of rural hospitals and health systems have closed.[7–9]

Radiology and imaging are increasingly used, particularly in acute care settings, and thus often play a central role in health access. Like other health care service lines, imaging is not immune to the health disparity issues that disproportionately impact vulnerable populations.[10] Screening mammography has received considerable attention, with ample evidence linking underutilization to socioeconomic status, race, ethnicity, age, and location. For example, less than 40% of newly immigrated women report having a mammogram in the past 2 years, compared with over 70% of women who were born in or have long resided in the United States.[11–13] Similar work has highlighted how race and location (rural vs. urban) are often differentiators in access to imaging for lung cancer screening. Of note, such vulnerable patients may be additionally vulnerable because of prior exposure to toxins like asbestos, making adequate lung cancer screening imaging even more critical.[14–17]

In busy emergency department settings, radiologists may be the first physicians to identify vulnerable patients. This is particularly important for victims of child abuse and intimate partner violence. Recent work by Khurana et al., for example, demonstrated that an isolated ulnar fracture may be a marker for intimate partner violence in up to one-third of adult women with this finding.[18] Such work highlights the historically hidden but critical contributions that radiologists can make to the care of such patients. Recent advances in machine learning have now led to algorithms that can leverage imaging findings to identify victims of intimate partner violence up to 3 years before known victims have historically entered violence prevention programs.[19] Although such work is relatively new, it could be highly generalizable and impactful. Radiologists have long been trained to identify healing and new fractures in children as potential signs of violence. They are often critical initiators of conversations of potential abuse in children (and now intimate partners) with important legal and social implications for patients, their families, and consulting providers.

As imaging leaders, radiologists have a unique role in improving the health of vulnerable populations.[10,20] The criticality of that role in the emergency department is highlighted for several groups of vulnerable populations. As the leaders in emergency imaging, radiologists must recognize their role in improving imaging access for these groups. Progress within the radiology community will require several steps: (1) understanding the barriers to hospital access and how these can be lessened through imaging; (2) participating in and leading collaborative conversations with emergency medicine colleagues to first identify vulnerable patient groups and existing disparities in imaging, so as to close such gaps; (3) ensuring that vulnerable patients receive the proper imaging, care, and timely communication of their results; and (4) facilitating and ensuring access to appropriate imaging follow-up.

Readers of this book will gain a depth of knowledge regarding imaging in a breadth of vulnerable populations, with a focus on the emergency department, where many of these patients disproportionately receive their care. Our hope is that, through reading this text, radiologists will better identify the value of their impact in ensuring that all populations receive the care they need, and hopefully they will then lead their radiology practices, departments, hospitals, and communities with a lens of health equity and a focus on lifting up vulnerable populations. Engaged imaging experts looking at the entire continuum of care can make a difference!

**Melissa A. Davis, MD, MBA**
**Richard Duszak, MD, FACR, FSIR, FRBMA**

## BIBLIOGRAPHY


1. Adler NE, Rehkopf DH. U.S. disparities in health: descriptions, causes, and mechanisms. *Annu Rev Public Health*. 2008;29:235–252.
2. Waisel DB. Vulnerable populations in healthcare. *Curr Opin Anaesthesiol*. 2013;26(2):186–192.
3. Am J. Vulnerable populations: who are they? *Manag Care*. 2006;12(13 Suppl):S348–S352.
4. Rogers TN, Rogers CR, VanSant-Webb E, Gu LY, Yan B, Qeadan F. Racial disparities in COVID-19 mortality among essential workers in the United States. *World Med Health Policy*. 2020; https://doi.org/10.1002/wmh3.358.
5. Howell EA. Reducing disparities in severe maternal morbidity and mortality. *Clin Obstet Gynecol*. 2018;61(2):387–399.
6. Heaman MI, Sword W, Elliott L, Moffatt M, Helewa ME, Morris H, et al. Barriers and facilitators related to use of prenatal care by inner-city women: perceptions of health care providers. *BMC Pregnancy Childbirth*. 2015;15:2.
7. Cyr ME, Etchin AG, Guthrie BJ, Benneyan JC. Access to specialty healthcare in urban versus rural US populations: a systematic literature review. *BMC Health Serv Res*. 2019;19(1):974.
8. Institute of Medicine (U.S.). *Committee on Monitoring Access to Personal Health Care Services. Access to health care in America*. In: Millman M, ed. Washington, DC: National Academies Press; 1993.
9. Hartley D. Rural health disparities, population health, and rural culture. *Am J Public Health*. 2004;94(10):1675–1678.
10. Waite S, Scott J, Colombo D. Narrowing the gap: imaging disparities in radiology. *Radiology*. 2021;299(1):27–35.
11. Peek ME, Han JH. Disparities in screening mammography. Current status, interventions and implications. *J Gen Intern Med*. 2004;19(2):184–194.
12. Ahmed AT, Welch BT, Brinjikji W, Farah WH, Henrichsen TL, Murad MH, et al. Racial disparities in screening mammography in the United States: a systematic review and meta-analysis. *J Am Coll Radiol*. 2017;14(2):157–165.e9.
13. Rauscher GH, Allgood KL, Whitman S, Conant E. Disparities in screening mammography services by race/ethnicity and health insurance. *J Womens Health (Larchmt)*. 2012;21(2):154–160.
14. Haddad DN, Sandler KL, Henderson LM, Rivera MP, Aldrich MC. Disparities in lung cancer screening: a review. *Annals of the American Thoracic Society*. 2020;17(4):399–405.
15. Borondy Kitts AK. The patient perspective on lung cancer screening and health disparities. *J Am Coll Radiol*. 2019;16(4 Pt B):601–606.
16. Odahowski CL, Zahnd WE, Eberth JM. Challenges and opportunities for lung cancer screening in rural America. *J Am Coll Radiol*. 2019;16(4 Pt B):590–595.
17. Prosper A, Brown K, Schussel B, Aberle D. Lung cancer screening in African Americans: the time to act is now. *Radiol Imaging Cancer*. 2020;2(5):e200107.
18. Khurana B, Sing D, Gujrathi R, Keraliya A, Bay CP, Chen I, et al. Recognizing isolated ulnar fracture as a potential marker for intimate partner violence. *J Am Coll Radiol*. 2021;18(8):1108–1117.
19. Chen IY, Alsentzer E, Park H, Thomas R, Gosangi B, Gujrathi R, et al. Intimate partner violence and injury prediction from radiology reports. Biocomputing 2021. *World Scientific*. 2020;26:55–66.
20. Safdar NM. An introduction to health disparities for the practicing radiologist. *J Am Coll Radiol*. 2019;16(4 Pt B):542–546.

# Contents

Chapter 1

# Emergency Imaging of At-Risk Patients: General Principles

Kathleen Hames and Michael N. Patlas

## Outline



## Introduction

Emergency departments (EDs) comprise a major source of medical care for patients in the United States, accounting for approximately 47.7% of the total number of medical care contacts.[1] In 2018, there were over 143 million ED visits, of which over 123 million ended in release.[2] Patients seek care in the ED for a variety of reasons, including having limited access to other appropriate health care services. The patients most vulnerable to health inequity and the compounding effects of inadequate health care are those who face systemic barriers to care due to a complex network of social, economic, and environmental factors that contribute to social determinants of health.

Structural and systemic racism, discrimination based on sex, gender, and sexual orientation, implicit weight bias against people with obesity, bias against patients with substance use disorder, and ableist language and barriers to accessibility (to name but a few) all create barriers to care. Implicit racial bias among clinicians in particular has been found to be a determining factor in patient access to quality care and has been associated with poorer doctor-patient interactions, treatment decisions, and patient health outcomes.[3] Radiology is not exempt from these issues, as health disparities related to imaging have been widely reported in the literature.[4–6] For example, many studies have demonstrated significant racial and socioeconomic disparities in cancer screening, diagnostic imaging, and procedures such as mammography,[7,8] lung cancer,[9] and colorectal cancer screening.[10,11]

Disparities in diagnostic imaging also exist within the ED both from an ordering standpoint as well as within the department itself, as this chapter will discuss. Radiologists and members of the diagnostic imaging team are not exempt from harboring bias against particular patient populations. For example, in a 2016 Medscape Lifestyle Report survey, 22% of radiologists admitted to being biased against specific types or groups of patients, while 62% of emergency medicine physicians admitted the same biases.[12] Patients presenting for care in the ED are not only medically vulnerable but may also face numerous obstacles to care based on complex socioeconomic and structural conditions that foster health disparity and contribute to worse health outcomes for individuals and communities.

A multitude of factors both within and beyond the health care system drive disparities in population health and access to quality health care. The US federal government's Healthy People 2030 initiative defines health disparity as "a particular type of health difference that is closely linked with social, economic, and/or environmental disadvantage."[13] Disparities affect groups that "have experienced barriers due to their racial or ethnic group; religion; socioeconomic status; gender; age; mental health; cognitive, sensory, or physical disability; sexual orientation or gender identity; geographic location; or other characteristics historically linked to discrimination or exclusion."[13] Health disparities disproportionately affect at-risk, vulnerable populations whose health conditions may be exacerbated by a complex network of factors that contribute to social determinants of health and create barriers to health care.

Addressing the social determinants of health is essential to understanding the systemic and structural factors at every level of society that contribute to health disparities. Social determinants of health comprise the material and social conditions in which people are born, grow, live, work, and age, as well as the complex, interrelated economic systems and social structures that fundamentally shape these conditions.[14] According to the Centers for Disease Control and Prevention (CDC), social determinants have been found to influence health outcomes more than lifestyle choices or health care. Studies have found that social determinants of health account for between 30% and 55% of health outcomes, with some estimates showing that the contribution of sectors outside health to population health outcomes exceeds the contribution from the health sector.[14] To achieve health equity requires addressing obstacles to health such as poverty, discrimination, lack of access to quality education and housing, good jobs with fair pay, and safe environments, as well as access to quality health care.[15] Appropriately addressing social determinants of health is therefore "fundamental for improving health and reducing longstanding inequities in health, which requires action by all sectors and civil society."[14]

Some of the most vulnerable and at-risk patient populations addressed in this book include geriatric patients, pediatric patients, pregnant patients, patients with obesity, patients with cancer and compromised immune systems, and patients with substance use disorder. Each of these patient populations presents particular challenges to care in the ED while also facing various barriers to care that cut across race, class, gender, and socioeconomic factors that contribute to health disparities. As many of these patients are considered high-risk both medically and socially, it is incumbent upon the entire health care team, including radiology, to work together to address the explicit and implicit biases and structural issues that create barriers to care and lead to worse health outcomes for individuals and communities.

## Geriatric Patients

In 2018, approximately 29 million US adults over the age of 65 years, 16 million of whom were over the age of 75 years, sought ED care.[16] Studies have shown that older adults suffer higher rates of morbidity and mortality in the ED despite receiving intensified resource use, including more physician time, more diagnostic testing, longer lengths of stay in the ED, and higher admission rates.[17] In a 2014 study, nearly half (49.8%) of all elderly patients presenting to the ED across the United States underwent diagnostic imaging, 42.8% of whom were evaluated with X-ray and 12.6% with computed tomography (CT).[18] There are many unique challenges to imaging elderly patients, including limited mobility and increased falls risk, potential decreased cognitive abilities, inability to hold still due to voluntary or involuntary motion, and increased anxiety and disorientation in the ED setting. To obtain proper imaging and maintain safety, it may be necessary to use soft immobilization techniques, adjust patient positioning, and assist with transfers.

Elderly patients are also more vulnerable to social isolation, socioeconomic instability, and abuse and neglect, which increase their likelihood of presenting to the ED.[19] For example, seniors with lower incomes or those who rely on Medicaid insurance may have unmet health care needs, prompting them to seek out emergency services to meet these needs.[20] Isolation and lack of social support have also been found to be significant indicators of increased frequency of ED visits by older adults.[21] In particular, individuals with dementia have been shown to have consistently higher rates of ED visits.[22] Dementia is also a well-documented risk factor for elder abuse,[23] which may be overlooked in the fast-paced environment of the ED.

Elder abuse is common, but unfortunately frequently underrecognized and underreported. As many as 10% of older adults in the United States are victims of elder abuse each year, with fewer than 1 in 24 cases identified and reported.[24] Surprisingly, physicians account for only 2% of all reported cases of elder abuse.[23] Because many elderly patients who present to the ED undergo some form of diagnostic imaging, the radiologist is optimally positioned to identify potential signs of abuse and communicate these concerns with the health care team.

Due to an overall increased risk of falls, osteoporosis, and age-related brain atrophy, it can be difficult to distinguish accidental from nonaccidental injury in elderly patients.[24,25] While there is substantial evidence-based literature regarding radiologic findings of nonaccidental trauma in children, less literature is available on the subject of elder abuse. However, imaging correlates do exist, particularly regarding fracture patterns[24] and "mechanism mismatch," whereby the fracture pattern is discordant with the mechanism of injury described by the patient or caregiver.[25] Additionally, screening tools such as the Elder Abuse Index and Elder Abuse Suspicion Index that incorporate physical findings and social factors have been developed and validated for use in the community and in busy clinics or EDs to assist in detection of elder abuse.[23,26]

Elderly patients not only have more comorbidities and complex medical needs but also are more vulnerable to socioeconomic instability, decreased access to care, and abuse and neglect. As many elderly patients in the ED undergo diagnostic imaging, radiologists have the potential to play an important role in the detection of elder physical abuse and advocacy for the health and safety of their patients.

## Cancer and Immunocompromised Patients

Immunocompromised patients represent a growing population in the United States and account for an increasing number of emergency room visits annually.[27–29] Among cancer patients, more than 650,000 individuals per year receive cytotoxic chemotherapy,[28] the side effects of which frequently require ED visits and hospitalization for management.[29,30] The number of patients undergoing solid organ transplants has tripled over the last 30 years with advancements in immunosuppressive drugs,[28,31] and currently more than 1.2 million people in the United States are living with human immunodeficiency virus.[32] Treatment-associated toxicity, opportunistic infections, and direct and indirect complications related to cancer present significant challenges in the ED. Immunocompromised patients are often sicker, present with atypical infections, and have more complex medical needs compared with the general population.

Many patients may also be first diagnosed with cancer during an ED visit.[33,34] Patients of lower socioeconomic status are often more dependent on ED services for health care and are therefore more likely to present emergently with undiagnosed cancer.[33,35] Many studies have demonstrated significant racial and socioeconomic disparities in cancer screening imaging and procedures such as mammography,[7] lung cancer screening,[9] and colorectal cancer screening.[10] For example, Black Americans have the highest incidence and mortality rates of colorectal cancer, with many of the disparities arising from access to care and screening, as well as other socioeconomic factors.[10,11] Emergency cancer presentations have also been associated with lower curative rates when compared with cancers diagnosed on an elective or screening basis, even when the cancer is at the same stage.[33]

Patients with cancer constitute a significant percentage of ED visits in the United States, with nearly 4 million visits per year.[36] Common oncology-related presentations include abdominal pain, nausea and vomiting, fever, infection, and systemic reactions to therapeutic agents.[27,37] Over 65% of patient with cancer presenting to the ED undergo radiological imaging,[27] highlighting the central role diagnostic imaging plays in the diagnosis and management of acutely ill oncology patients in the ED. Hsu et al. found that patients with cancer were nearly twice as likely to undergo head, chest, and abdomen pelvis CT scans and 30% more likely to receive X-ray imaging than patients without cancer presenting to the ED.[36]

Some of the most common ED presentations in immunocompromised patients include acute abdomen and central nervous system (CNS) infections. Acute abdomen accounts for nearly 40% of ED presentations of cancer patients.[38] Patients may present with treatment-induced enteritis; complications related to a primary tumor; or treatment-related complications from surgery, chemotherapy, or radiotherapy.[38] Prompt radiological diagnosis of life-threatening complications such as bowel perforation, obstruction, hemoperitoneum, or graft-versus-host disease is necessary to ensure timely and appropriate surgical and medical management. Immunocompromised patients are also at higher risk of CNS infections.[28] Although many image findings may be nonspecific, the radiologist must be alert to both overt and subtle findings of a wide range of bacterial, fungal, parasitic, viral, and neoplastic pathologies. Prompt identification of meningitis, encephalopathy, abscesses, and mass-like lesions with or without herniation is key to directing appropriate emergent medical and neurosurgical treatment.

Immunocompromised patients presenting to the ED for acute care represent a highly vulnerable population at risk of numerous life-threatening infections, malignancy-related complications, and treatment-related complications. Diagnostic imaging plays a central role in the detection and diagnosis of such complications, as well as identifying the extent of disease and its local and systemic affects. Timely clinical management requires prompt and accurate diagnosis in order to decrease morbidity and mortality in this at-risk population. It is incumbent upon the radiologist to work closely with referring clinicians to ensure patients receive appropriate medical and surgical management.

## Pregnant Patients

Pregnant patients presenting to the ED represent a highly vulnerable population. Studies have found that 30% of pregnant women in the United States presenting to the ED for care had one or more comorbidities (such as obesity, asthma, diabetes, and hypertension), compared with 21% of pregnant women who did not seek ED care.[39] Pregnant women seeking ED care are also more likely to be at higher risk of socioeconomic disparity, have delayed entry to prenatal care, be of a minority race, be on Medicaid insurance, and have experienced domestic abuse.[39,40] For example, many studies have shown that pregnant women of racial or ethnic minority are at higher risk of pregnancy-related morbidity and mortality due in large part to disparities in care driven by implicit racial bias.[40] Pregnant women are also at higher risk of domestic abuse, and may present to the ED with a variety of complex injuries that endanger both the mother and the fetus.[40,41]

Managing pregnant women in the ED poses many unique challenges. The anatomical changes that occur during pregnancy make physical examinations difficult, while physiological changes can complicate airway management and interpretation of vital signs. These changes may result in diagnostic uncertainty and delay in care, which in turn increases the risk of complications both for the mother and for the fetus. The radiologist, therefore, plays a crucial role in obtaining timely and accurate imaging in order to make a correct diagnosis and direct appropriate care. The radiologist is also responsible for ensuring diagnostic imaging quality while balancing the risks of ionizing radiation to the fetus and the mother.

The first-line modality in imaging pregnant patients is ultrasound, which avoids ionizing radiation and allows for assessment of both the mother and the fetus. When ultrasound in inconclusive, magnetic resonance imaging (MRI) is the preferred second-line modality, particularly in the assessment of acute abdominal pain.[42,43] In the setting of trauma, or when other modalities are nondiagnostic, CT is the modality of choice,[42,43] although the benefits need to be weighed against the risk of exposing the fetus to radiation. In the setting of acute trauma, the American College of Radiology (ACR) recommends CT of the abdomen and pelvis with contrast, and when serious injury is suspected, CT is the proven modality for full evaluation.[43]

The most common nonobstetric nontraumatic emergency presentations in pregnant patients include acute appendicitis, cholecystitis, and bowel obstruction.[42,43] Studies have found that abdominal emergencies during pregnancy complicate approximately one in 500 to 700 pregnancies, and up to 2% of cases require surgical intervention.[42] The need for timely diagnosis is key, as delays in treatment increase the risk of complication. For example, in the setting of acute appendicitis, diagnostic delay is associated with a higher risk of perforation, which is associated with a 20% to 35% rate of fetal loss.[42]

Acute trauma also poses a significant risk to the pregnant patient and the fetus and is the leading cause of nonobstetric maternal death in the United States, affecting 5% to 8% of all pregnancies.[43–45] Studies have found that, in cases of severe trauma, the rate of fetal loss is as high as 50% to 90%.[43,44] The most common cause of injury is motor vehicle collisions, followed by falls, assault, accidents, and suicide.[44] Blunt abdominal trauma accounts for 69% of all traumas[45] and is a leading cause of adverse fetal outcomes, including preterm labor, abruption, uterine rupture, and fetal demise.[41,44] Radiology, therefore, plays a critical role in the rapid and accurate diagnosis of potentially life-threatening injuries in both the mother and the fetus.

Although the majority of traumas are nonviolent, pregnant women are nearly twice as likely to experience violent trauma as nonpregnant women.[44] Studies have shown that the reported prevalence of interpersonal violence ranges between 1% and 20% of all pregnant women, although this is likely grossly underestimated due to the underreporting of domestic violence.[45] As there is an increased risk of abuse among pregnant patients seeking emergency care, health care providers are in a unique position to help identify and assist patients in finding safe and accessible resources. The radiology department in particular offers a uniquely private space away from the potential abuser in which patients may feel safe disclosing abuse and requesting help.

Radiology plays a critical role in the timely and accurate diagnosis of nontraumatic and trauma-related emergencies in pregnant patients in the ED. The diagnostic imaging team may also play an important role in assisting victims of abuse, as well as advocating for all patients to have equal access to high-quality health care regardless of race, ethnicity, or socioeconomic status.

## Bariatric Patients

The prevalence of obesity has steadily increased over the past three decades and has become a major public health issue. According to the CDC and the National Center for Health Statistics, the prevalence of obesity across the United States has risen to 42.2%, with severe obesity reaching highs of 9.2%.[46] There are significant health issues related to obesity, including heart disease, stroke, type II diabetes, hypertension, hyperlipidemia, and obstructive sleep apnea, to name a few. The cost of obesity-related health care is significant, with an estimated annual cost of $147 billion[46] and a 41.5% increase in per capita medical spending compared with nonobese adults.[47] Prior studies have also shown that patients with obesity have a greater use of hospital services with greater hospital costs than do nonobese patients.[48]

Evaluation of patients with obesity in the ED poses unique challenges both to the clinical care team as well as to the diagnostic imaging team. Studies have reported increased difficulty in cardiopulmonary auscultation, abdominal palpation, venous cannulation, sedation, intubation, and patient positioning.[49] Obesity also creates significant challenges for diagnostic imaging. For example, limited mobility may result in suboptimal patient positioning; the aperture diameter of CT and MRI scanners and maximum table load limits may exclude some patients from receiving more advanced imaging; CT images may have more truncation artifact and photon starvation, which decrease imaging quality[50]; increased body mass and thickness result in increased photon scatter and reduced contrast resolution in radiography[50]; and the thickness of subcutaneous tissue and sound-attenuating properties of fat limit the use of ultrasound in larger patients.[51] Additionally, studies performed in phantoms indicate that patients with obesity receive higher radiation doses during CT and radiography than do nonobese patients.[52]

As the rates of obesity have risen, so too has the use of bariatric surgery, as it remains the most effective long-term treatment for severe obesity and associated comorbidities.[53,54] Although bariatric surgery has a low complication profile, studies have shown that up to 10% to 12% of patients visit the ED within 30 days of surgery.[53] The most common postoperative complications include surgical site infection,[55] cholelithiasis,[56] bowel obstruction,[54,55] and anastomotic leaks.[57] As diagnostic imaging, particularly the use of abdominal CT, is central to the diagnosis of many postbariatric surgery complications, it is imperative that appropriate patient positioning and modified protocols be used to optimize image quality and ensure a timely and accurate diagnosis.

Patients with obesity not only face obstacles to care based on particular physical and technological limitations but are also subject to pervasive stigmatization and weight bias, which has been shown to contribute (independent of weight or body mass index) to increased morbidity and mortality.[58,59] Weight bias is defined as the negative beliefs and attitudes attributed to an individual based on their weight, and stems from perceptions that obesity is caused by an individual's failure to control their diet and exercise. The stigmatization of people with obesity has contributed not only to health and social inequalities but also to inequities in obesity treatment with respect to both access and quality of care.[60,61] The perceived message of shame and blame perpetuated by health care professionals and public health officials may be at least partly responsible for health care avoidance and decreased adherence to medical advice.[60] Therefore, it is important that health care professionals and policy makers advocate for and support people living with obesity, including supporting policy action to prevent weight bias and weight-based discrimination.[22,28]

Radiology plays a key role in the management of patients with obesity in the ED, particularly in postbariatric surgery patients. In order to provide high-quality care, it is important that the radiology team possess a thorough understanding of the limits of imaging equipment, how to reduce image artifacts, and how to implement specific techniques and protocols to ensure high-quality imaging. The entire radiology department should also work to ensure their clinical environment is accessible, safe, and respectful to all patients regardless of their weight or size.[58]

## Patients With Drug Abuse

Recreational abuse of both pharmaceutical and illicit drugs has risen sharply in the United States over the past two decades. According to the CDC, the number of deaths related to drug overdose increased by nearly 5% from 2018 to 2019 and has quadrupled since 1999.[62] Opioid abuse in particular has risen to epidemic proportions, prompting the US Department of Health and Human Services to declare a public health emergency in 2017.[63,64] Of all the drug-related deaths in 2019, over 70% involved an opioid, while deaths related to synthetic opioids (excluding methadone) increased by over 15% in 2019.[62] Drug "misuse" and "abuse" account for approximately 2.5 million visits to the ED per year, nearly half of which are due to illicit drugs.[65,66] The most common drug-related deaths from pharmaceuticals are due to opioids and benzodiazepines, while the most common illicit drugs encountered in the ED include cocaine, marijuana, methamphetamines, and hallucinogens.[65,66]

Managing drug and alcohol abuse in the ED poses a number of challenges. Patients with substance abuse may present not only with life-threatening physiological symptoms related to neurologic, pulmonary, or cardiovascular failure but also with complications secondary to infection, trauma, and behavioral/psychosocial changes, as well as altered mental status. Patients suffering from substance abuse and addiction also face the added burden of stigma within the medical community, which has been associated with a higher rate of diagnostic errors and adverse effects on health outcomes.[67,68]

Substance abuse results in a wide variety of medical complications affecting nearly every organ system in the body.[69] Diagnostic imaging plays a critical role in the diagnosis and guidance of treatment for many drug abuse–related complications, which can be associated with significant morbidity and mortality.[70] As patients may be unconscious or otherwise unable to describe their symptoms, many drug-related complications may only be detected by imaging, and it is incumbent upon the radiologist to provide timely and accurate diagnoses to help direct care. Patients presenting with altered mental status due to substance abuse may also make it difficult to obtain high-quality imaging. Patients may be unable to lie still or follow directions related to positioning or breath-holding, or may in some cases be combative toward health care workers. As such, patients may require physical or chemical restraints for the safety of both themselves and the imaging team in order to obtain quality images to aid in a correct diagnosis.

For the radiologist, awareness of the imaging features associated with recreational drug abuse is key, as the complications from many drugs, particularly intravenous drugs, often affect multiple body systems.[71] For example, CNS manifestations may include posterior reversible encephalopathy syndrome, spongiform leukoencephalopathy, infarct, hemorrhage, and vasoconstriction[72]; respiratory complications include pneumonitis, pulmonary edema, pneumothorax, and alveolar hemorrhage[73]; cardiovascular injury may present as aortic dissection, mycotic aneurisms, and septic thrombophlebitis; gastrointestinal manifestations include decreased motility and constipation resulting in pressure-associated ischemia,[69] as well as body packing of drugs within the bowel, resulting in obstruction or perforation[74]; and musculoskeletal complications may occur from infection, trauma, thrombosis, foreign bodies, compartment syndrome, and osteomyelitis.[69,75] However, many of these imaging features are nonspecific, and clinical history may be lacking. As such, the radiologist should maintain a high index of suspicion, particularly in patients with unexplained symptoms or clinical presentations, and should communicate directly with referring physicians to ensure patients receive timely and appropriate care.

All members of the health care team should also be aware of the internal bias and stigmatizing attitudes toward patients who suffer from substance abuse. Studies have found that negative attitudes of health professionals toward patients with addiction lead to poor communication, poor therapeutic alliance, and increased diagnostic errors.[67,76] In addition to the ethical implications of stigmatizing patients with addiction, studies have also shown that patients who felt discriminated against by health professionals were less likely to complete their treatment.[76] As the radiologist plays a key role in the detection and diagnosis of complications related to substance abuse, it is imperative that the diagnostic imaging team work together to ensure patients not only receive timely and accurate imaging but also feel safe, supported, and respected within the health care environment.

## Pediatric Patients

Pediatric ED visits constitute nearly 20% of all ED visits. In 2018, there were approximately 29 million ED visits in the United States for children under the age of 18 years, with a rate of 388.2 per 1000 population.[16] Although patient presentations vary by age, some of the most common conditions include wounds, sprains, strains, fractures, viral and respiratory infections, fever, cough, nausea and vomiting, and abdominal pain.[77] Pediatric trauma more specifically is one of the leading causes of ED presentations and a leading cause of morbidity and mortality.[78,79]

Radiological imaging is commonly used for pediatric patients in the ED setting, with approximately one-third of all visits including at least one imaging study.[3,80] Pediatric imaging poses a number of challenges in the ED setting. Injured and sick children presenting to the ED are often frightened, irritable, wary of strangers, and intimidated by the ED environment. These factors make it difficult to obtain diagnostic-quality imaging, especially if the child is unable to hold still or otherwise cooperate.[81] Pediatric imaging also requires specific protocols across all modalities, as well as strict adherence to the As Low As Reasonably Achievable (ALARA) principle in order to minimize radiation. As such, it is important that all radiology personnel involved work to gain the child's trust and cooperation prior to and throughout the entirety of the exam.[81]

Children are also highly vulnerable to abuse, exploitation, and discrimination, and it is the duty of all health care professionals to be alert to signs of maltreatment at both the domestic and the societal level. Radiology technologists, and the reporting radiologist in particular, play an important role in the identification, evaluation, intervention, and prevention of child abuse by being attentive to signs of nonaccidental trauma (NAT).[82] In 2019, approximately 3.5 million children were subject to investigation due to suspicion for NAT, with 656,000 determined to be victims of maltreatment. Additionally, there were 877 victims of sex trafficking identified in the 29 states for which these reporting data are available.[83] As radiology technologists have direct physical contact with the child, particularly during sonographic imaging, this presents a valuable opportunity to evaluate the child for any signs of potential abuse. The radiologist in turn is doubly responsible for being alert to signs of NAT, as well as communicating any concerns to the health care team.

As the appropriate use of diagnostic testing in children is an essential determinant of health care quality, it is important to understand the ways in which health care disparities may manifest in the use of diagnostic imaging in the pediatric emergency setting. Many studies have identified disparities in both access to and quality of health care for children of different races, ethnicities, and income levels regardless of presenting complaint.[3,79,84] For example, a 2021 study found that ED imaging was performed in 33.5% of non-Hispanic White children compared with 24.1% of non-Hispanic Black children and 26.1% of Hispanic children.[3] A 2016 study similarly found that Black and other minority patients and patients without private insurance had lower odds of receiving advanced imaging for abdominal pain compared with

White patients.[84] In the trauma setting, Black patients with blunt abdominal trauma were 20% less likely to receive an abdominal CT exam compared with White patients.[85]

These racial disparities arise from a variety of confounding factors encompassing a wide range of individual, structural, and systemic issues surrounding racial inequality. Such factors include parent/guardian preferences, physicians' implicit racial biases, and pervasive structural factors rooted in the health care system.[3] Implicit racial bias among clinicians in particular has been found to be a determining factor in patient access to quality care and has been associated with doctor-patient interactions, treatment decisions, and patient health outcomes.[3]

Such biases have also been found to play a role in the racial disparity surrounding reporting of suspected child abuse. For example, a 2002 study found that minority children aged 12 months to 3 years who sustained a skull or long bone fracture were significantly more likely to undergo a skeletal survey than non-Hispanic White children and also more likely to be reported to Child Protective Services.[86] However, after the implementation of abuse-screening guidelines, other studies found that racial disparities in reporting significantly decreased, resulting in no statistically significant difference by race.[87]

Radiology plays an important role in the diagnosis and management of pediatric patients in the ED. The diagnostic imaging team may help identify and prevent not only child maltreatment but also potential racial disparities in access to imaging. Through clear communication with the referring care team, the radiologist can work to ensure appropriate imaging and timely and accurate diagnoses, and promote equitable access to high quality care.

## Conclusion

There are many ways in which radiologists can participate in reducing health care disparities and improve access to high-quality care for all patients. However, as radiologists typically have less direct patient interaction than many other medical specialists, it may feel daunting to know where to begin to help advocate for change. One of the most important first steps is through education. In 2017, the Accreditation Council for Graduate Medical Education updated the Common Program Requirements for residency training programs and specifically included health care disparities as a key component of quality health care.[88,89] There are a number of resources designed to help provide basic introductions to cultural competency and social determinants of health, all of which are applicable to radiology.[4,89,90] A departmental and profession-wide commitment to education is key to developing a professional community that is capable of discussing and addressing health disparities at all levels of society.

Improving diversity within the workforce is also fundamental to improving care for diverse populations. Despite more recent efforts to improve diversity within radiology, women as well as racial and ethnic minorities remain significantly underrepresented in diagnostic imaging.[91,92] The ACR Commission for Women and General Diversity emphasizes that the benefits of a diverse specialty are not limited only to physicians, but that patients also receive better care in an inclusive, diverse health care system.[93] Participating in research related to health disparities is also a valuable way to interrogate inequities in diagnostic imaging while also providing a road map for actionable change. Radiologists may also choose to participate in various forms of advocacy at the local and national level as a means to promote the specialty and improve access to imaging services for all patient populations. Through education, commitment to diversity and inclusion, research, and advocacy, radiologists can work to address health care disparities and improve care for diverse, marginalized, and vulnerable populations.

## REFERENCES


1. Marcozzi D, Carr B, Liferidge A, Baehr N, Browne B. Trends in the contribution of emergency departments to the provision of hospital-associated health care in the USA. *Int J Health Serv*. 2018;48(2):267–288.
2. Trends in the Utilization of Emergency Department Services, 2009-2018 [Internet]. ASPE. Updated 2021. Accessed May 24, 2021. https://aspe.hhs.gov/pdf-report/utilization-emergency-department-services
3. Marin JR, Rodean J, Hall M, et al. Racial and ethnic differences in emergency department diagnostic imaging at US children's hospitals, 2016-2019. *JAMA Netw Open*. 2021;4(1):e2033710. https://doi:10.1001/jamanetworkopen.2020.33710.
4. Safdar NM. An introduction to health disparities for the practicing radiologist. *J Am Coll Radiol*. 2019;16(4):542–546.
5. Perry H, Eisenberg RL, Swedeen ST, Snell AM, Siewert B, Kruskal JB. Improving imaging care for diverse, marginalized, and vulnerable patient populations. *RadioGraphics*. 2018;38(6):1833–1844.

6. Betancourt JR, Tan-McGrory A, Flores E, López D. Racial and ethnic disparities in radiology: a call to action. *J Am Coll Radiol*. 2019;16(4 Pt B):547–553.
7. Ahmed AT, Welch BT, Brinjikji W, et al. Racial disparities in screening mammography in the United States: a systematic review and meta-analysis. *J Am Coll Radiol*. 2017;14(2):157–165.e9.
8. Zha N, Alabousi M, Patel BK, Patlas MN. Beyond universal health care: barriers to breast cancer screening participation in Canada. *J Am Coll Radiol*. 2019;16(4 Pt B):570–579.
9. Pasquinelli MM, Kovitz KL, Koshy M, et al. Outcomes from a minority-based lung cancer screening program vs the national lung screening trial. *JAMA Oncol*. 2018;4(9):1291.
10. Augustus GJ, Ellis NA. Colorectal cancer disparity in African Americans. *Am J Pathol*. 2018;188(2):291–303.
11. Warren Andersen S, Blot WJ, Lipworth L, Steinwandel M, Murff HJ, Zheng W. Association of race and socioeconomic status with colorectal cancer screening, colorectal cancer risk, and mortality in southern US adults. *JAMA Netw Open*. 2019;2(12):e1917995 https://doi:10.1001/jamanetworkopen.2019.17995.
12. Medscape Lifestyle Report 2016: Bias and Burnout [Internet]. Medscape. Accessed: May 26, 2021. https://www.medscape.com/slideshow/lifestyle-2016-overview-6007335
13. Healthy People 2030 | health.gov [Internet]. Accessed May 26, 2021. https://health.gov/healthypeople
14. Social Determinants of Health | NCHHSTP | CDC [Internet]. Updated 2021. Accessed May 24, 2021. https://www.cdc.gov/nchhstp/socialdeterminants/index.html
15. What is Health Equity? [Internet]. RWJF. Updated 2017. Accessed May 24, 2021. https://www.rwjf.org/en/library/research/2017/05/what-is-health-equity-.html
16. Trends in Emergency Department Visits - HCUP Fast Stats [Internet]. Accessed Apr 28, 2021. https://www.hcup-us.ahrq.gov/faststats/NationalTrendsEDServlet?measure1=04&characteristic1=12&measure2=&characteristic2=11&expansionInfoState=hide&dataTablesState=show&definitionsState=hide&exportState=hide
17. Schumacher JG, Hirshon JM, Magidson P, Chrisman M, Hogan T. Tracking the rise of geriatric emergency departments in the United States. *J Applied Gerontol*. 2020;39(8):871–879.
18. Latham LP, Ackroyd-Stolarz S. Emergency department utilization by older adults: a descriptive study. *Can Geriatr J*. 2014;17(4):118–125.
19. Atenstaedt R, Gregory J, Price-Jones C, Newman J, Roberts L, Turner J. Why do patients with nonurgent conditions present to the Emergency Department despite the availability of alternative services? *Eur J Emerg Med*. 2015;22(5):370–373.
20. Dufour I, Chouinard M-C, Dubuc N, Beaudin J, Lafontaine S, Hudon C. Factors associated with frequent use of emergency-department services in a geriatric population: a systematic review. *BMC Geriatrics*. 2019;19(1):185.
21. Naughton C, Drennan J, Treacy P, et al. The role of health and non-health-related factors in repeat emergency department visits in an elderly urban population. *Emerg Med J*. 2010;27(9):683–687.
22. Hunt LJ, Coombs LA, Stephens CE. Emergency department use by community-dwelling individuals with dementia in the United States: an integrative review. *J Gerontol Nurs*. 2018;44(3):23–30.
23. Murphy K, Waa S, Jaffer H, Sauter A, Chan A. A literature review of findings in physical elder abuse. *Can Assoc Radiol J*. 2013;64(1):10–14.
24. Wong NZ, Rosen T, Sanchez AM, et al. Imaging findings in elder abuse: a role for radiologists in detection. *Can Assoc Radiol J*. 2017;68(1):16–20.
25. Lee M. Expanding the role of radiology in the detection of physical elder abuse. Updated May 15, 2018. Accessed Mar 22, 2021. https://dash.harvard.edu/handle/1/37006478
26. Fulmer T, Strauss S, Russell SL, et al. Screening for elder mistreatment in dental and medical clinics. *Gerodontol*. 2012;29(2):96–105.
27. Hsu J, Donnelly JP, Xavier Moore J, Meneses K, Williams G, Wang HE. National characteristics of emergency department visits by patients with cancer in the United States. *Am J Emerg Med*. 2018;36(11):2038–2043.
28. Stephens RJ, Liang SY. Central nervous system infections in the immunocompromised adult presenting to the emergency department. *Emerg Med Clin*. 2021;39(1):101–121.
29. Prince RM, Powis M, Zer A, Atenafu EG, Krzyzanowska MK. Hospitalisations and emergency department visits in cancer patients receiving systemic therapy: Systematic review and meta-analysis. *Euro J Cancer Care*. 2019;28(1):e12909.
30. Charshafian S, Liang SY. Infectious disease emergencies in the cancer patient: rapid fire. *Emerg Med Clin North Am*. 2018;36(3):493–516.
31. Fishman JA. Infection in organ transplantation. *Am J Transplant*. 2017;17(4):856–879.
32. March 17 CSH gov U.S. Statistics [Internet]. HIV.gov. Updated 2021. Accessed May 25, 2021. https://www.hiv.gov/hiv-basics/overview/data-and-trends/statistics
33. Pettit N, Sarmiento E, Kline J. Disparities in outcomes among patients diagnosed with cancer associated with emergency department visits. medRxiv. 2021;2021.03.03.21252826.
34. Zhou Y, Abel GA, Hamilton W, et al. Diagnosis of cancer as an emergency: a critical review of current evidence. *Nat Rev Clin Oncol*. 2017;14(1):45–56.
35. Wachelder JJH, Drunen I, van, Stassen PM, et al. Association of socioeconomic status with outcomes in older adult community-dwelling patients after visiting the emergency department: a retrospective cohort study. *BMJ Open*. 2017;7(12):e019318.
36. Hsu J, Donnelly JP, Moore JX, Meneses K, Williams G, Wang HE. National characteristics of Emergency Department visits by patients with cancer in the United States. *Am J Emerg Med*. 2018;36(11):2038–2043.
37. Rivera DR, Gallicchio L, Brown J, Liu B, Kyriacou DN, Shelburne N. Trends in adult cancer–related emergency department utilization: an analysis of data from the nationwide emergency department sample. *JAMA Oncology*. 2017;3(10):e172450–e172450.
38. Morani AC, Hanafy AK, Marcal LP, et al. Imaging of acute abdomen in cancer patients. *Abdom Radiol*. 2020;45(8):2287–2304.
39. Cunningham SD, Magriples U, Thomas JL, et al. Association between maternal comorbidities and emergency department use among a national sample of commercially insured pregnant women. *Acad Emerg Med*. 2017;24(8):940–947.
40. Wang E, Glazer KB, Howell EA, Janevic TM. Social determinants of pregnancy-related mortality and morbidity in the United States: a systematic review. *Obstet Gynecol*. 2020;135(4):896–915.
41. Malik S, Kothari C, MacCallum C, Liepman M, Tareen S, Rhodes KV. Emergency department use in the perinatal period: an opportunity for early intervention. *Ann Emerg Med*. 2017;70(6):835–839.
42. Bouyou J, Gaujoux S, Marcellin L, et al. Abdominal emergencies during pregnancy. *J Visceral Surg*. 2015;152(6, Supplement):S105–S115.

43. Ahluwalia A, Moshiri M, Baheti A, Saboo S, Bhargava P, Katz DS. MRI of acute abdominal and pelvic non-obstetric conditions in pregnancy. *Curr Radiol Rep*. 2018;6(8):25.
44. Deshpande NA, Kucirka LM, Smith RN, Oxford CM. Pregnant trauma victims experience nearly 2-fold higher mortality compared to their nonpregnant counterparts. *Am J Obstet Gynecol*. 2017;217(5):590.e1-590.e9.
45. Petrone P, Jiménez-Morillas P, Axelrad A, Marini CP. Traumatic injuries to the pregnant patient: a critical literature review. *Eur J Trauma Emerg Surg*. 2019;45(3):383–392.
46. CDC. Obesity is a Common, Serious, and Costly Disease [Internet]. Centers for Disease Control and Prevention. Updated 2021. Accesssed May 2, 2021. https://www.cdc.gov/obesity/data/adult.html
47. Finkelstein EA, Trogdon JG, Cohen JW, Dietz W. Annual medical spending attributable to obesity: payer-and service-specific estimates. *Health Affairs*. 2009;28(Supplement 1):w822–w831.
48. Folmann NB, Bossen KS, Willaing I, et al. Obesity, hospital services use and costs. *Adv Health Econ Health Serv Res*. 2007;17:319–332.
49. Ngui B, Taylor D, Shill J. Effects of obesity on patient experience in the emergency department. *EMA*. 2013;25:227–232.
50. Modica MJ, Kanal KM, Gunn ML. The obese emergency patient: imaging challenges and solutions. *Radiograph*. 2011;31(3):811–823.
51. Paladini D. Sonography in obese and overweight pregnant women: clinical, medicolegal and technical issues. *Ultrasound Obstet Gynecol*. 2009;33(6):720–729.
52. Yanch JC, Behrman RH, Hendricks MJ, McCall JH. Increased radiation dose to overweight and obese patients from radiographic examinations. *Radiology*. 2009;252(1):128–139.
53. Khouri A, Alvarez R, Matusko N, Varban O. Characterizing the preventable emergency department visit after bariatric surgery. *Surg Obes Relat Dis*. 2020;16(1):48–55.
54. Wernick B, Jansen M, Noria S, Stawicki SP, El Chaar M. Essential bariatric emergencies for the acute care surgeon. *Eur J Trauma Emerg Surg*. 2016;42(5):571–584.
55. Lewis KD, Takenaka KY, Luber SD. Acute abdominal pain in the bariatric surgery patient. *Emerg Med Clin*. 2016;34(2):387–407.
56. Coupaye M, Castel B, Sami O, Tuyeras G, Msika S, Ledoux S. Comparison of the incidence of cholelithiasis after sleeve gastrectomy and Roux-en-Y gastric bypass in obese patients: a prospective study. *Surg Obes Relat Dis*. 2015;11(4):779–784.
57. Jacobsen HJ, Nergard BJ, Leifsson BG, et al. Management of suspected anastomotic leak after bariatric laparoscopic Roux-en-y gastric bypass. *Br J Surg*. 2014;101(4):417–423.
58. Wharton S, Lau DCW, Vallis M, et al. Obesity in adults: a clinical practice guideline. *CMAJ*. 2020;192(31):E875–E891.
59. Sutin AR, Stephan Y, Terracciano A. Weight discrimination and risk of mortality. *Psychol Sci*. 2015;26(11):1803–1811.
60. Forhan M, Salas XR. Inequities in healthcare: a review of bias and discrimination in obesity treatment. *Can J Diabetes*. 2013;37(3):205–209.
61. Mold F, Forbes A. Patients' and professionals' experiences and perspectives of obesity in health-care settings: a synthesis of current research. *Health Expect*. 2013;16(2):119–142.
62. Understanding the Epidemic | Drug Overdose | CDC Injury Center [Internet]. Updated 2021. Accessed May 16, 2021. https://www.cdc.gov/drugoverdose/epidemic/index.html
63. Lovegrove MC, Dowell D, Geller AI, et al. US emergency department visits for acute harms from prescription opioid use, 2016–2017. *Am J Public Health*. 2019;109(5):784–791.
64. Smith HJ. Ethics, public health, and addressing the opioid crisis. *AMA J Ethics*. 2020;22(8):647–650.
65. Data Overview | Drug Overdose | CDC Injury Center [Internet]. Updated 2021. Accessed May 25, 2021. https://www.cdc.gov/drugoverdose/data/index.html
66. Drug Abuse Warning Network | CBHSQ Data [Internet]. Accessed May 25, 2021. https://www.samhsa.gov/data/data-we-collect/dawn-drug-abuse-warning-network
67. Mendiola CK, Galetto G, Fingerhood M. An exploration of emergency physicians' attitudes toward patients with substance use disorder. *J Addict Med*. 2018;12(2):132–135.
68. Mamede S, Van Gog T, Schuit SCE, et al. Why patients' disruptive behaviours impair diagnostic reasoning: a randomised experiment. *BMJ Qual Saf*. 2017;26(1):13–18.
69. Chaudhry AA, Gul M, Baker KS, Gould ES. Radiologic manifestations of recreational drug abuse. *Contemp Diagnos Radiol*. 2016;39(4):1–8.
70. Almeida RR, Glover M, Mercaldo SF, et al. Temporal trends in imaging utilization for suspected substance use disorder in an academic emergency radiology department. *J Am Coll Radiol*. 2019;16(10):1440–1446.
71. Hsu DJ, McCarthy EP, Stevens JP, Mukamal KJ. Hospitalizations, costs and outcomes associated with heroin and prescription opioid overdoses in the United States 2001-12. *Addiction*. 2017;112(9):1558–1564.
72. Offiah C, Hall E. Heroin-induced leukoencephalopathy: characterization using MRI, diffusion-weighted imaging, and MR spectroscopy. *Clin Radiol*. 2008;63(2):146–152.
73. Venkatanarasimha N, Rock B, Riordan RD, Roobottom CA, Adams WM. Imaging of illicit drug use. *Clin Radiol*. 2010;65(12):1021–1030.
74. Hagan IG, Burney K. Radiology of recreational drug abuse. *Radiographics*. 2007;27(4):919–940.
75. Pineda C, Espinosa R, Pena A. Radiographic imaging in osteomyelitis: the role of plain radiography, computed tomography, ultrasonography, magnetic resonance imaging, and scintigraphy. *Semin Plast Surg*. 2009;23(2):80–89.
76. van Boekel LC, Brouwers EPM, van Weeghel J, Garretsen HFL. Stigma among health professionals towards patients with substance use disorders and its consequences for healthcare delivery: systematic review. *Drug Alcohol Depend*. 2013;131(1–2):23–35.
77. Wier LM, Yu H, Owens PL, Washington R. *Overview of Children in the Emergency Department, 2010: Statistical Brief #157. In: Healthcare Cost and Utilization Project (HCUP) Statistical Briefs [Internet]*. Rockville (MD): Agency for Healthcare Research and Quality (US). Updated 2006. Accessed Apr 28, 2021. http://www.ncbi.nlm.nih.gov/books/NBK154386/.
78. Avraham JB, Bhandari M, Frangos SG, Levine DA, Tunik MG, DiMaggio CJ. Epidemiology of paediatric trauma presenting to US emergency departments: 2006–2012. *Injury Prevent*. 2019;25(2):136–143.
79. LaPlant MB, Hess DJ. A review of racial/ethnic disparities in pediatric trauma care, treatment, and outcomes. *J Trauma Acute Care Surg*. 2019;86(3):540–550.
80. Zhang X, Bellolio MF, Medrano-Gracia P, Werys K, Yang S, Mahajan P. Use of natural language processing to improve predictive models for imaging utilization in children presenting to the emergency department. *BMC Medical Informatics and Decision Making*. 2019;19(1):287.
81. Thukral BB. Problems and preferences in pediatric imaging. *Indian J Radiol Imaging*. 2015;25(4):359–364.

82. Bloemen EM, Rosen T, Lindberg DM, Krugman RD. How experiences of child abuse pediatricians and lessons learned may inform health care providers focused on improving elder abuse geriatrics clinical practice and research. *J Fam Viol*. 2021;36(3):389–398.
83. Child abuse, neglect data released [Internet]. Accessed Apr 26, 2021. https://www.acf.hhs.gov/media/press/2021/child-abuse-neglect-data-released
84. Horner KB, Jones A, Wang L, Winger DG, Marin JR. Variation in advanced imaging for pediatric patients with abdominal pain discharged from the ED. *Am J Emerg Med*. 2016;34(12):2320–2325.
85. Natale JE, Joseph JG, Rogers AJ, et al. Relationship of physician-identified patient race and ethnicity to use of computed tomography in pediatric blunt torso trauma. *Acad Emerg Med*. 2016;23(5):584–590.
86. Lane WG, Rubin DM, Monteith R, Christian CW. Racial differences in the evaluation of pediatric fractures for physical abuse. *JAMA*. 2002;288(13):1603–1609.
87. Higginbotham N, Lawson KA, Gettig K, et al. Utility of a child abuse screening guideline in an urban pediatric emergency department. *J Trauma Acute Care Surg*. 2014;76(3):871–877.
88. Common Program Requirements [Internet]. Accessed May 30, 2021. https://www.acgme.org/What-We-Do/Accreditation/Common-Program-Requirements/
89. Americo L, Ramjit A, Wu M, et al. Health care disparities in radiology: a primer for resident education. *Curr Prob Diagnos Radiol*. 2019;48(2):108–110.
90. ASRT Patient-Centered Care for Diverse Populations - Credit [Internet]. Accessed May 30, 2021. https://www.asrt.org/main/continuing-education/earn-ce/featured-ce/patient-centered-care-for-diverse-populations-credit
91. Lebel K, Hillier E, Spalluto LB, et al. The status of diversity in Canadian radiology-where we stand and what can we do about it. *Can Assoc Radiol J*. 2020;846537120978258.
92. Kubik-Huch RA, Vilgrain V, Krestin GP, et al. Women in radiology: gender diversity is not a metric—it is a tool for excellence. *Eur Radiol*. 2020;30(3):1644–1652.
93. Commission for Women and Diversity [Internet]. Accessed May 30, 2021. https://www.acr.org/Member-Resources/Commissions-Committees/Women-Diversity

# Chapter 2

# Neurological Emergencies in Geriatric Patients

Maria J. Borja, Angela Guarnizo, Elizabeth S. Lustrin, Thomas Mehuron, Brian Zhu, Steven Sapozhnikov, Nader Zakhari, and Carlos Torres

## Outline



## Key Points

- Geriatric patients tend to have atypical presentation of diseases, and the signs and symptoms may be nonspecific, contributing to delayed diagnoses.
- The incidence of intracerebral hemorrhage increases with age.
- Advanced age has been identified as the strongest independent risk factor for cerebrovascular disease, and older adults tend to have worse outcome after stroke, with more stroke-related death, disability, and subsequent increased rates of dementia compared with younger stroke patients.
- Epilepsy is most common in the elderly population due to increased risk factors such as prior stroke, trauma, and neurodegenerative disorders.
- In cases of acute or progressively worsening mental status change, computed tomography of the head is an appropriate study, with follow-up magnetic resonance imaging of the brain in cases of identified pathology or suspected occult pathology, or to confirm a suspected clinical diagnosis.
- In all patients with suspected central vertigo, imaging is a necessity, as the patient should be assumed to have an acute ischemic stroke until proven otherwise.
- In patients with syncope, any suspicion for neurological injury based on the history and physical examination should prompt neuroimaging.

## Introduction

The elderly population is the fastest-growing population group in the world, with an estimate of 71 million adults older than 65 years in the United States and 1 billion worldwide by the year 2030.[1] Elderly patients are more likely to require emergency care, and the number of visits to the emergency departments continues to rise.[2,3] Clinical evaluation in geriatric patients tends to be challenging, as signs and symptoms have low specificity and are less reliable than in younger patients. Furthermore, multiple comorbidities found in older patients may confound diagnoses. Elderly patients are prone to serious neurologic problems, with higher incidence of neurologic conditions such as stroke, hemorrhage, and epilepsy. The increased number of elderly patients, the higher incidence of neurologic conditions, and the clinical challenges faced with this population underscore the importance of neuroimaging in older patients. This chapter will discuss imaging findings of neurological emergencies in geriatric patients.

## Intracranial Hemorrhage

Intracranial hemorrhage (ICH) is a growing cause of death and disability worldwide due to the increasing population of elderly people in the developed world. The incidence of intracerebral hemorrhage is 5.9 per 100,000 in ages 35 to 54 years, 37.2 per 100,000 in ages 55 to 74 years, and 176.3 per 100,000 in ages 75 to 94 years.[4] Risk factors include falls, amyloid angiopathy, hypertension, and greater use of anticoagulant or antiplatelet therapy, with mortality rates as high as 50%.[5,6]

ICH can be subdivided by location, either within the brain parenchyma or in the surrounding compartments, including the subdural, epidural, subarachnoid, and intraventricular spaces. ICH most commonly occurs in the setting of trauma in the elderly population, with falls accounting for 84% of trauma incidents in patients aged 65 years or older, and motor vehicle–related trauma being the second most common mechanism of injury.[7]

Noncontrast computed tomography (NCCT) is the imaging modality of choice in the acute setting due to speed and high sensitivity for detecting ICH. NCCT helps guide the clinician to the etiology of the hemorrhage, assesses ICH evolution, evaluates for the presence of mass effect and shift of midline structures and hydrocephalus, and assesses bony integrity. Computed tomography (CT) angiography (CTA) and CT venography may be useful in the acute setting for the evaluation of arterial and venous vasculature when vascular lesions or vascular injury are suspected.

Although typically not the first imaging modality, magnetic resonance imaging (MRI) can also be used in the evaluation of ICH and has high sensitivity for intraparenchymal microbleeds. The presence of microbleeds may be a marker for underlying pathologies, including hypertension, amyloid angiopathy, vascular malformations, posttreatment changes, and diffuse axonal injury, and can help predict the risk of future bleeding events.[8]

The appearance of blood on CT and MRI varies depending on the staging of blood products and the chemical state of hemoglobin (Table 2.1 and Fig. 2.1).

**TABLE 2.1 Hemorrhage Phases and Appearance on Computed Tomography and Magnetic Resonance Imaging**

| Hemorrhage Phase | Time | Computed Tomography Density[a] | Hemoglobin | Magnetic Resonance Imaging Signal[A] | |
|---|---|---|---|---|---|
| | | | | T1 | T2 |
| Hyperacute | <12 hours | Isodense <1 hour, then hyperdense | Oxyhemoglobin | Isointense | Iso- to hyperintense |
| Acute | 12 hours–3 days | Hyperdense | Deoxyhemoglobin | Iso- to hypointense | Hypointense |
| Early Subacute | 3–7 days | Hyper- to isodense | Intracellular methemoglobin | Hyperintense | Hypointense |
| Late Subacute | 1–3 weeks | Iso- to hypodense | Extracellular methemoglobin | Hyperintense | Hyperintense |
| Chronic | >3 weeks | Hypodense | Hemosiderin | Hypointense | Hypointense in parenchyma, Hyperintense (equivalent to CSF) if extraaxial |

[a]Relative to grey matter.
*CSF*, Cerebrospinal fluid.

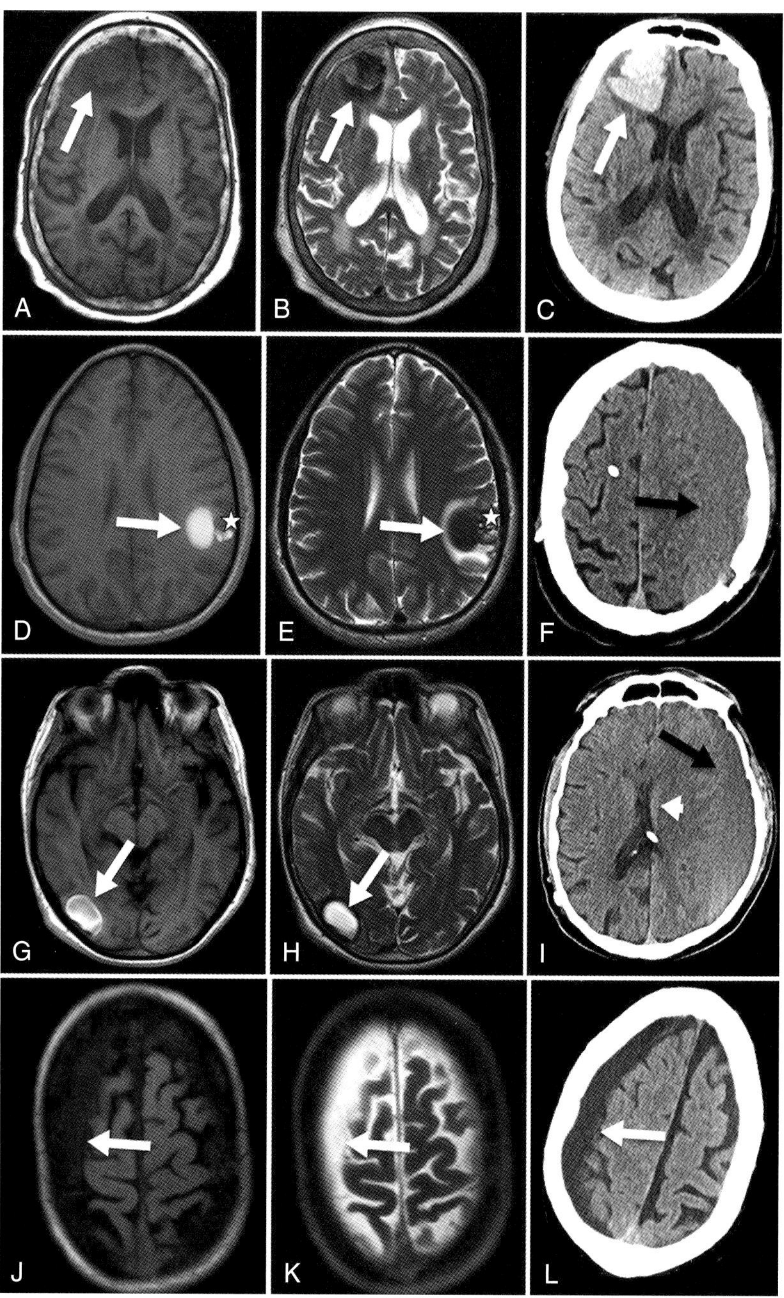


**Fig. 2.1** Magnetic resonance imaging and noncontrast computed tomography (NCCT) images of hemorrhages at different stages. The first row (A–C) shows acute intraparenchymal hemorrhage in the right frontal lobe (arrows). Note isointense signal on T1-weighted imaging (WI) (A), hypointense signal on T2WI (B), and corresponding hyperdensity on NCCT (C). The second row (D–F) shows early subacute hemorrhage. Note hyperintense signal on T1WI (D) and hypointense signal on T2WI (E) in the left parietal lobe (white arrows), consistent with early subacute hemorrhage, with associated cavernous malformation (star). NCCT (F) on a different patient shows isodense attenuation along the left frontoparietal convexity, consistent with early subacute subdural hematoma (black arrow). The third row (G–I) shows late subacute hemorrhage. Note hyperintense signal on both T1WI (G) and T2WI (H) in the right occipital lobe (white arrows) consistent with late subacute intraparenchymal hemorrhage. Iso- to hypodense attenuation along the left convexity on NCCT (I) of a different patient is consistent with late subacute subdural hematoma (black arrow). There is associated midline shift (arrowhead). Fourth row (J–L) shows chronic subdural hematoma along the right frontoparietal convexity (arrows). Note hypointense signal on T1WI (J), hyperintense signal on T2WI following the signal of cerebrospinal fluid (K), and corresponding hypodensity on NCCT (L).

## SUBDURAL HEMATOMA

Subdural hematomas (SDHs) are the most common ICH in the elderly, most of them posttraumatic, with a reported annual incidence of 46.7 per 100,000 in ages 65 to 74 years. The relative risk for SDH is 5 times higher in the 75 to 84–year-old age group, and 13 times higher in those older than 85 years.[9] Minor trauma can produce asymptomatic acute subdural hemorrhage, which then results in chronic SDH. These patients are also predisposed to acute bleeding within the chronic collection, resulting in acute on chronic SDH.[9]

On imaging, SDHs are seen along the falx or tentorium, or appear as crescentic collections along the convexities within the subdural space, typically crossing suture lines (Fig. 2.2).

## EPIDURAL HEMATOMA

Epidural hematomas are relatively uncommon in the elderly population. Most epidural hematomas occur secondary to direct impact, with 80% to 95% of patients having a concomitant skull fracture. Some 90% of epidurals are arterial in nature, often involving trauma to the middle meningeal artery. The remaining 10% are venous in nature, resulting from trauma to a dural sinus.[10]

On imaging, epidural hematomas have a classic hyperdense and biconvex appearance (Fig. 2.3) and

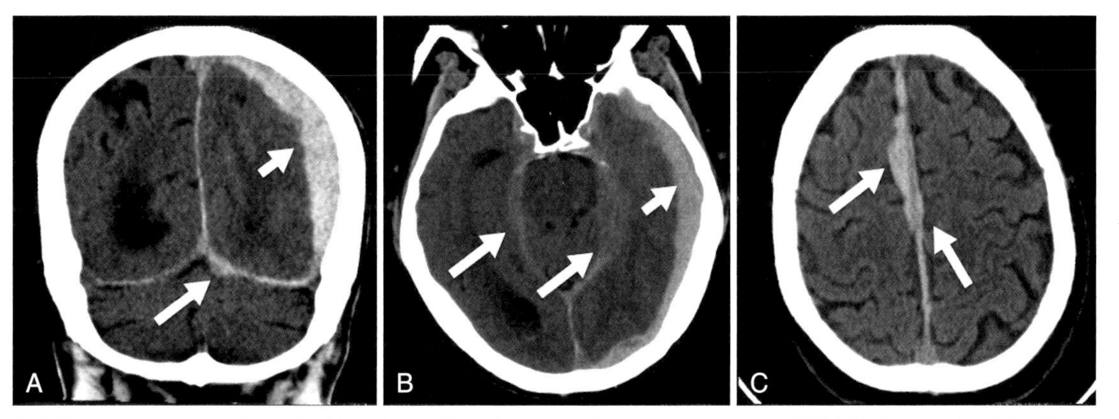


**Fig. 2.2** Different locations of acute subdural hematomas. Coronal noncontrast computed tomography (NCCT) (A) shows acute subdural hematoma along the left tentorial leaflet (long arrow) and left convexity (short arrow). Axial NCCT (B) shows subdural hematoma along the bilateral tentorial leaflets (long arrows) and the left temporo-occipital convexity (short arrow). Axial NCCT through the high frontal and parietal lobes (C) shows acute subdural hematoma along the falx bilaterally (arrows).

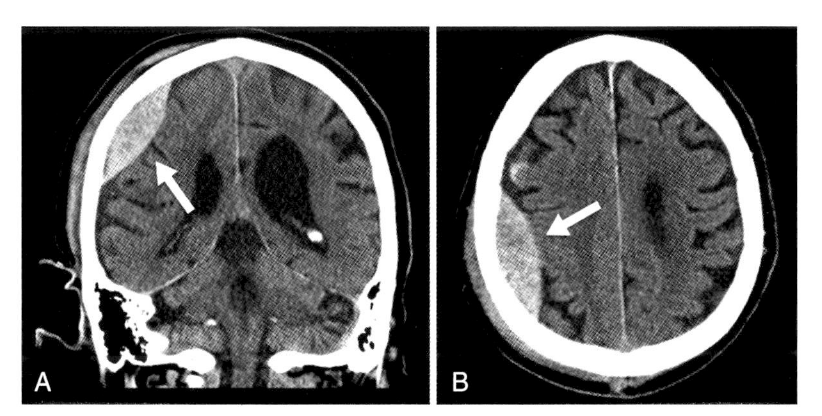


**Fig. 2.3** Epidural hematoma. Coronal (A) and axial (B) noncontrast computed tomography of the brain in a 77-year-old male after a fall demonstrate a biconvex hyperdense lesion centered along the right parietal convexity (arrows in A and B), consistent with epidural hematoma.

do not typically cross suture lines, unless there is a concomitant sutural diastasis. Compression of the adjacent brain parenchyma is often present.

## SUBARACHNOID HEMORRHAGE

Subarachnoid hemorrhage (SAH) is the most encountered type of traumatic ICH,[11] and is typically seen in the cerebral sulci along the convexities and vertex of the head. Although MRI is less commonly used for initial evaluation of head trauma, the combination of fluid attenuation inversion recovery (FLAIR) and susceptibility-weighted imaging (SWI) sequences has excellent sensitivity for acute ICH and has been shown to be superior to CT in detecting acute SAH. Acute traumatic SAH is identified by hyperintense signal abnormality within the cerebral sulci on FLAIR sequences and hypointense blooming on SWI[12] (Fig. 2.4).

Some 80% to 85% of spontaneous (i.e., nontraumatic) SAHs are caused by rupture of saccular aneurysms. Most saccular aneurysms occur at the circle of Willis and bifurcation of the middle cerebral arteries (MCAs); thus, most aneurysmal hemorrhages involve the basal cisterns and sylvian fissures (Fig. 2.5). Once an acute SAH with a basal aneurysmal pattern is identified on initial NCCT, CTA is the indicated next step for identification of aneurysms. Aneurysmal hemorrhages

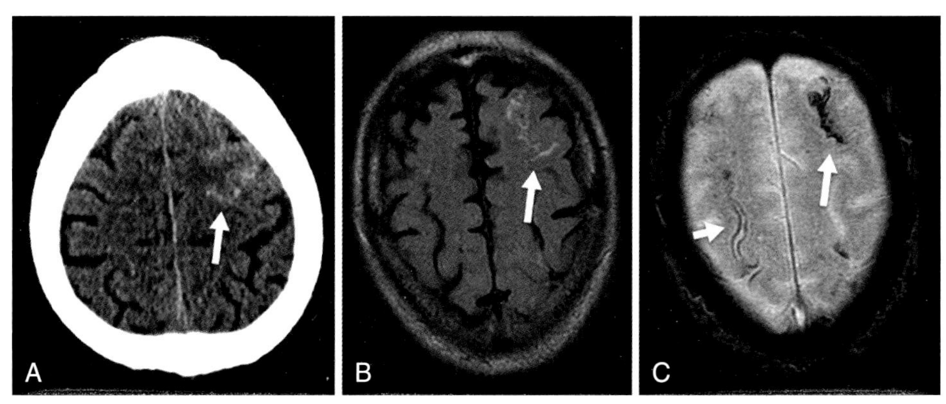


**Fig. 2.4** Acute subarachnoid hemorrhage (SAH). Hyperdensity along the left frontal sulci on noncontrast computed tomography (A), with corresponding hyperintense signal on fluid attenuation inversion recovery (B) and susceptibility on susceptibility-weighted imaging (SWI) (C), is consistent with acute SAH (long arrows). Siderosis from chronic SAH (short arrow) is seen in the right frontal sulci on SWI (C).

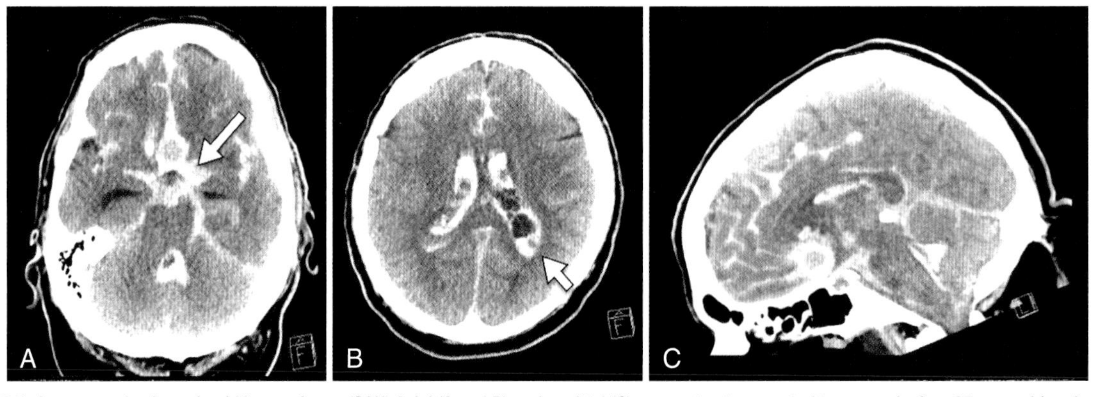


**Fig. 2.5** Aneurysmal subarachnoid hemorrhage. (SAH) Axial (A and B) and sagittal (C) noncontrast computed tomography in a 67-year-old male with acute "worst headache of life" from ruptured anterior communicating artery aneurysm. Extensive SAH centered at the basal cisterns and adjacent sulci (long arrow). Note intraventricular hemorrhage with mild hydrocephalus (short arrow).

commonly result in hydrocephalus and are associated with considerable morbidity and mortality. Although risk is not necessarily associated with increasing age, poor outcomes are associated with advanced age. Mortality from aneurysmal SAH approaches 35%, with 10% to 25% of patients dying before arrival at the hospital. Approximately one-third survive, but with disabling neurologic deficits, and only 30% return to independent living.[13]

## INTRAPARENCHYMAL HEMORRHAGE

### Traumatic

Acceleration and deceleration injury can result in cerebral contusions, which may be hemorrhagic or nonhemorrhagic. These commonly occur in areas closer to the skull base, including the anteroinferior frontal and temporal lobes. Contusions can occur at the site of impact and in a location directly opposite to the point of initial impact secondary to brain recoil, termed coup/contrecoup injury[14] (Fig. 2.6).

### Hypertensive

Hypertension is the most common cause of nontraumatic intraparenchymal hemorrhage among the elderly, and accounts for 40% to 50% of nontraumatic intraparenchymal hemorrhage.[15] Hypertensive hemorrhages occur in typical locations, including the basal ganglia, thalami, pons, and cerebellum. The putamen/external capsule is the most common location and accounts for approximately two-thirds of all hypertensive intraparenchymal hemorrhages[16] (Fig. 2.7).

### Amyloid Angiopathy

Amyloid angiopathy is the second most common cause of nontraumatic intraparenchymal hemorrhage among the elderly, and accounts for 15% to 20% of nontraumatic intracranial bleeds in patients over 60 years of age.[17] Risk for cerebral amyloid angiopathy strongly correlates with age, being uncommon among individuals younger than 65 years. The deposition of amyloid-beta peptides typically involves cortical vessels; thus, hemorrhages typically involve the cerebral hemispheres, often at the grey-white matter junction of the parietal and occipital lobes. Subarachnoid extension of the intraparenchymal hematoma strongly indicates a nonhypertensive cause and suggests vascular etiologies such as amyloid angiopathy[18] (Fig. 2.8).

### Cerebral Venous Thrombosis

Cerebral venous sinus thrombosis (CVST) or cortical vein thromboses are uncommon causes of intracerebral hemorrhage in the elderly. The major risk factor for CVST in the elderly is malignancy. More recently, CVST has been seen in patients with COVID-19 with elevated D dimers.[19] Other, less common, risk factors include hereditary thrombophilia, prior intracranial infection, and dehydration.[20] The most prevalent type of CVST is dural sinus thrombosis, most commonly in the superior sagittal sinus and transverse sinuses (Fig. 2.9).

### Malignancies and Metastases

Intraparenchymal, subarachnoid, and intraventricular hemorrhages can occur secondary to intracranial

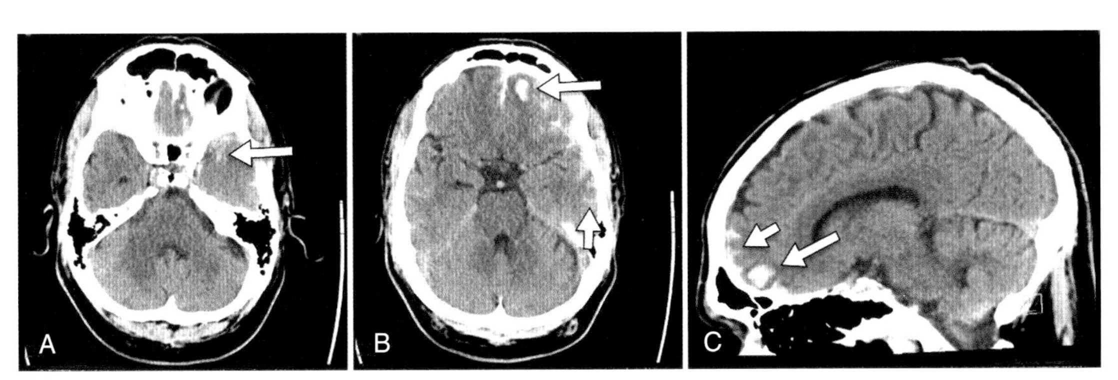


**Fig. 2.6** Intraparenchymal hemorrhagic contusions in a 68-year-old male postfall. Axial (A and B) and sagittal (C) noncontrast computed tomography shows multiple cerebral contusions in the left temporal lobe and inferior left frontal lobe (long arrows) associated with scattered adjacent subarachnoid hemorrhage (short arrows).

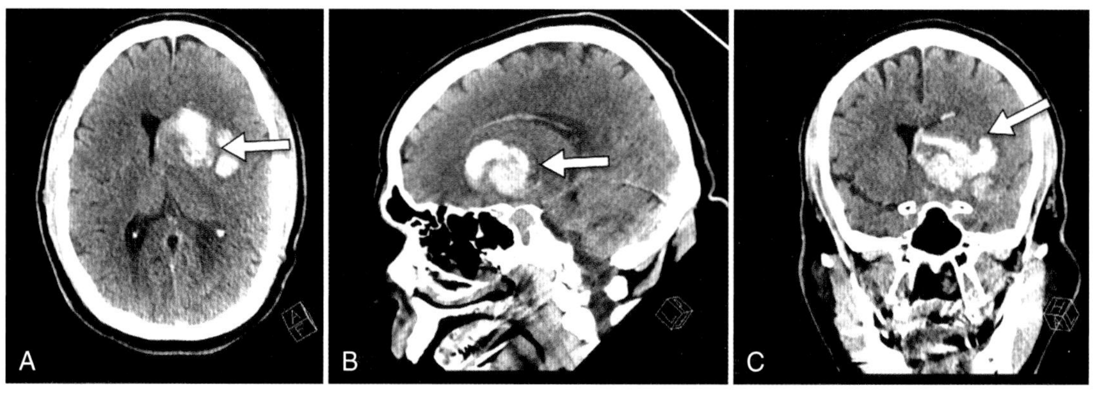


**Fig. 2.7** Hypertensive intraparenchymal hemorrhage. Noncontrast computed tomography with axial (A), sagittal (B), and coronal (C) reconstructions shows a hypertensive intraparenchymal hemorrhage (long arrows) in the region of the left basal ganglia.

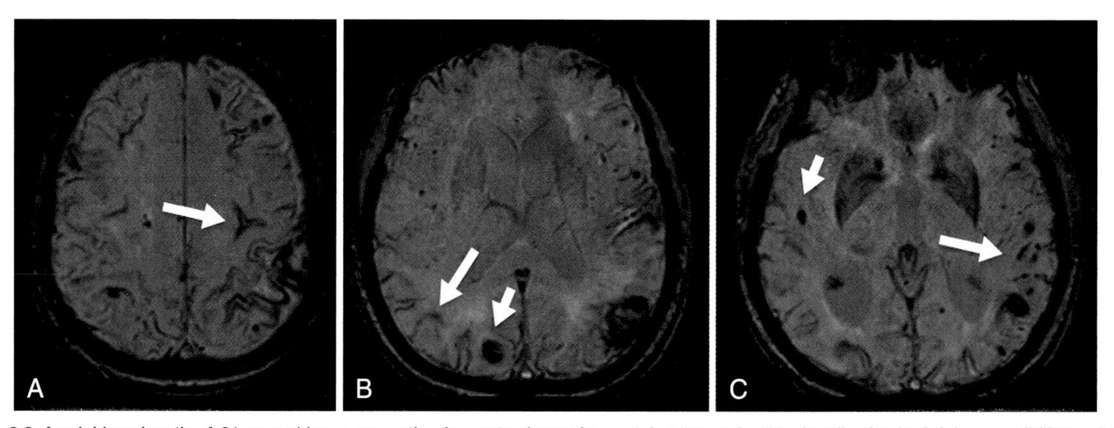


**Fig. 2.8** Amyloid angiopathy. A 91-year-old man presenting for acute change in mental status and a "blackout" episode. Axial susceptibility-weighted imaging magnetic resonance images (A–C) demonstrate hemosiderosis from chronic subarachnoid hemorrhage (long arrows) and extensive parenchymal hemorrhages (short arrows), consistent with amyloid angiopathy.

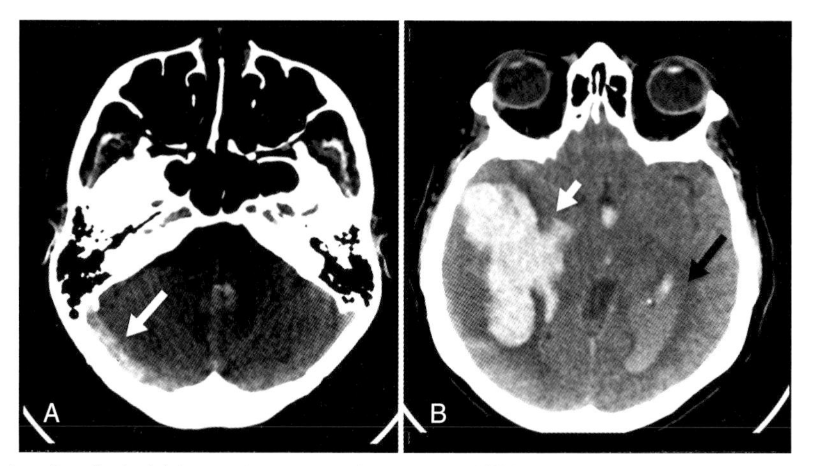


**Fig. 2.9** Dural venous sinus thrombosis. Axial noncontrast computed tomography (NCCT) through the posterior fossa (A) showing hyperdense acute thrombosis within the right transverse sinus (long arrow). Axial NCCT through the temporal lobes showing a large hemorrhagic venous infarct in the right temporal lobe (short arrow). Note intraventricular extension of hemorrhage (black arrow).

malignancies and metastases.[21] Metastatic disease is associated with a higher risk of ICH and dural venous sinus thrombosis compared with primary brain tumors. Metastases of choriocarcinoma, melanoma, and non–small cell lung cancer are most prone to massive bleeding.[22] Although acute hemorrhage can be assessed with NCCT, follow-up imaging with MRI is necessary to characterize intracranial tumors.

## Infarct

Acute stroke is more commonly ischemic (87%) than hemorrhagic. Advanced age has been identified as the strongest independent risk factor for cerebrovascular disease.[23] Acute ischemic stroke (AIS) is more common in the elderly, with a mean age for the first AIS of 73.3 years, and 30% of strokes developing in patients older than 80 years.[24,25] Additionally, older adults tend to have worse outcomes after stroke, with more stroke-related death, disability, and subsequent increased rates of dementia compared with younger stroke patients.[23,26] Aging also influences the specific subtype of stroke, with lacunar and atherothrombotic strokes peaking among patients 70 to 74 years old and 75 to 80 years old, respectively; while cardioembolic infarcts increase with age and are the most common subtype in patients older than 80 years.[27]

AIS in the geriatric population may present with typical focal neurological deficits or have a more atypical presentation, including headache, seizure, reduced mobility, altered mental status, falls, and urinary incontinence. The presentation may be further complicated by the presence of baseline disability or neurological deficits.[24,26] Hence, a low threshold should be maintained for imaging suspected strokes in older adults to facilitate timely management.[26] Intravenous recombinant tissue plasminogen activator (IV rt-PA) is approved for treatment of AIS within 3 hours of symptom onset, even in patients older than 80 years, and within 4.5 hours in patients under 80 years of age. The evidence for IV rt-PA in patients over 80 years between 3 and 4.5 hours from symptom onset is not as clear. The risk of symptomatic ICH after IV rt-PA is higher in patients older than 80 years (10%–13% compared with 5%–8% for younger patients).[24,26] Endovascular thrombectomy (EVT) of large-vessel occlusive AIS has been shown to improve the outcomes compared with IV rt-PA alone, even in the elderly.[24,26,28] Timely imaging is crucial for the management of AIS, with recommended door-to-imaging time of less than 20 minutes and door-to-imaging interpretation time of less than 45 minutes.[29,30] NCCT is the initial imaging step to exclude the presence of hemorrhage (which constitutes contraindication for IV rt-PA) or stroke mimics, and to establish the presence and extent of parenchymal ischemic changes manifesting as loss of grey-white matter differentiation giving rise to the "lentiform obscuration" and the "insular ribbon" signs when involving the lentiform nucleus and insular cortex, respectively. This finding can be subtle, especially early after the onset of symptoms, and is best assessed using a dedicated narrow "stroke" window-level setting (Fig. 2.10).[29,31] Frank cortical/subcortical hypodensity and sulcal effacement are usually seen with established infarction. The extent of these changes can be quantified using the Alberta Stroke Program Early CT Score (ASPECTS) by dividing the MCA territory into 10 regions: caudate, lentiform, insula, internal capsule, as well as six cortical

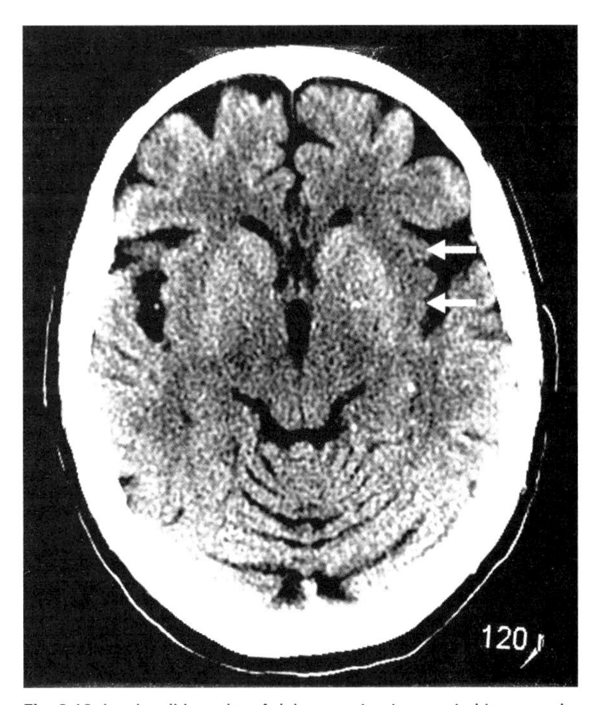


**Fig. 2.10** Insular ribbon sign. Axial noncontrast computed tomography image showing loss of grey-white matter differentiation in the left insula (white arrows) in keeping with the "insular ribbon sign." Please note the use of narrow "stroke" window-level setting.

regions (M1 to M3) at basal ganglia level and (M4 to M6) at supraganglionic level. One point is subtracted for each region showing evidence of ischemia. The hyperdense MCA is an NCCT sign for intraluminal thrombus within the M1 segment of the MCA, with low sensitivity (52%), but when present is a predictor of poor response to IV rt-PA alone.[29]

CTA of the cervical and intracranial arteries is the next imaging step. CTA can identify intracranial large vessel (internal carotid artery and MCA M1 segment) occlusion (LVO) with almost 100% sensitivity (Fig. 2.11). Once LVO is identified, consultation regarding EVT should be initiated, given low recanalization rates with IV rt-PA alone.[29] CTA also allows assessment of the cervical arteries for occlusion, dissection, free floating thrombus (Fig. 2.12), and degree of atherosclerotic stenosis, and to provide a road map for EVT planning.[31]

Multiphasic CTA (mCTA) with additional late arterial and early venous acquisitions allows better assessment of the collaterals status by comparing the density of pial vessels on the affected and healthy sides (Fig. 2.13),

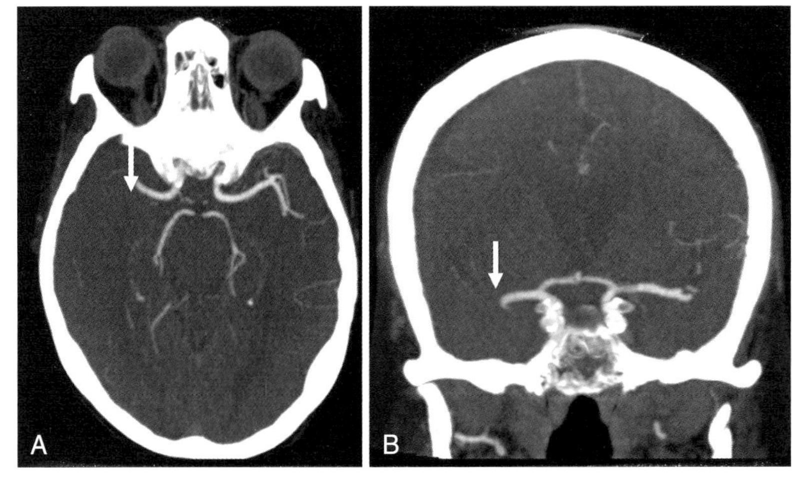


**Fig. 2.11** Axial (A) and coronal (B) computed tomography angiography maximum intensity projection images showing abrupt cutoff of the right middle cerebral arteries (arrows).

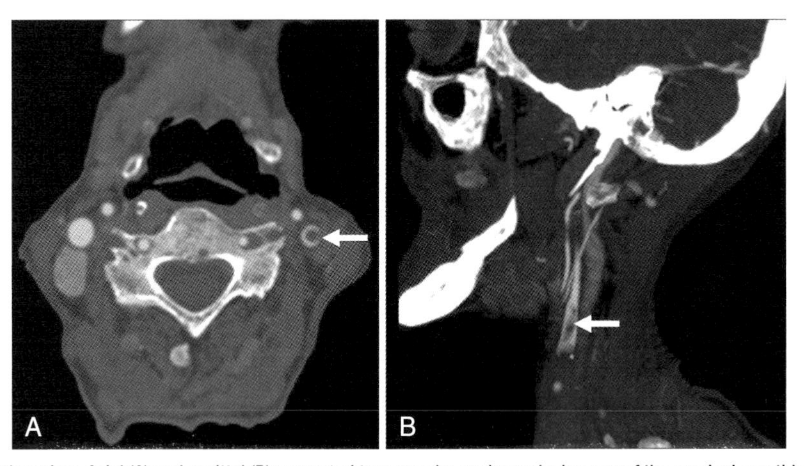


**Fig. 2.12** Free-floating thrombus. Axial (A) and sagittal (B) computed tomography angiography images of the cervical carotid arteries showing intraluminal finger-like filling defect in the proximal left internal carotid artery (arrows in A and B), in keeping with free-floating thrombus.

which predicts the outcome post-EVT, with worse outcome in patients with poor collaterals.[31] The "delayed vessel sign" on mCTA improves detection of distal small occlusions (e.g., MCA M2 or M3 segments). It refers to an artery distal to an occlusion that is better opacified and denser on delayed compared with initial mCTA phases and compared with contralateral equivalent artery (Fig. 2.13).[31,32] CT perfusion allows the identification of the ischemic penumbra, which is potentially salvageable severely ischemic tissue surrounding the infarct core that would benefit from EVT. The identification of cerebral blood flow/volume and mean transit time/time to peak mismatch confirms the presence of penumbra (Fig. 2.14).[31]

MRI with diffusion weighted imaging (DWI) is the gold standard for identification of the extent of core infarct, with diffusion restriction appearing as high signal on diffusion trace images and low signal on the apparent diffusion coefficient maps. Changes can be seen on DWI and on FLAIR within 30 minutes and 6 hours after onset of symptoms, respectively. Susceptibility-sensitive sequences can also identify infarct-related hemorrhage. However, the limited access, especially on emergency after-hour basis, the time needed for patient screening, the presence of contraindications, and patients' claustrophobia limit the role of MRI in the emergency assessment of AIS.[29]

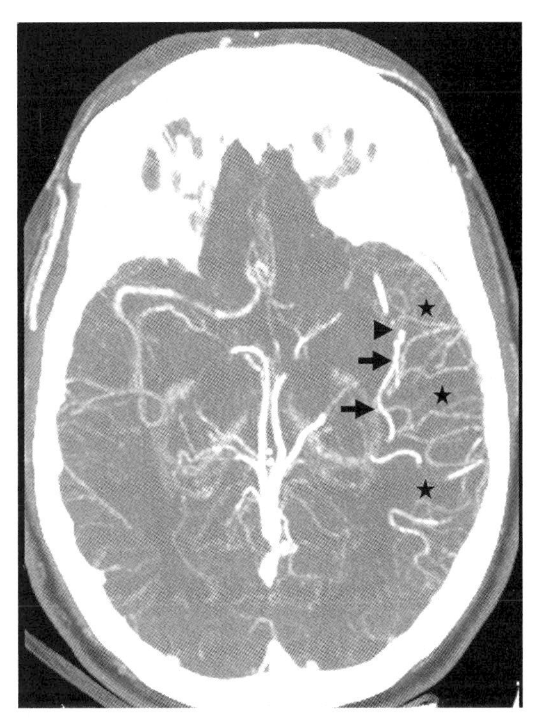

**Fig. 2.13** Delayed vessel sign. Axial maximum intensity projection late angiographic image from multiphasic computed tomography angiography showing delayed vessel sign (arrows) distal to a left middle cerebral artery M2 branch focal occlusion (arrowhead). Please note good collaterals (stars), as evidenced by increased density of pial vessels compared to the right.

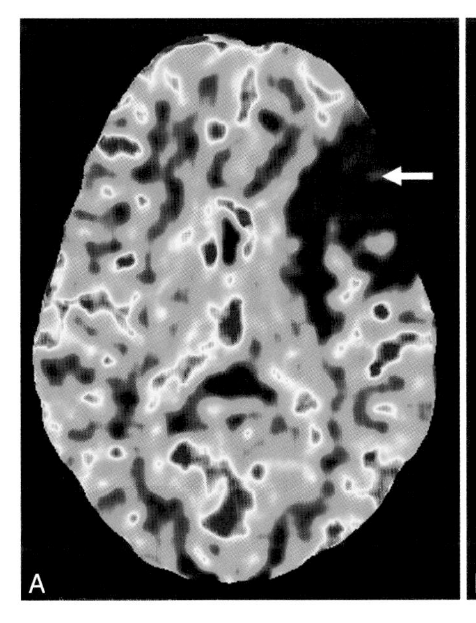


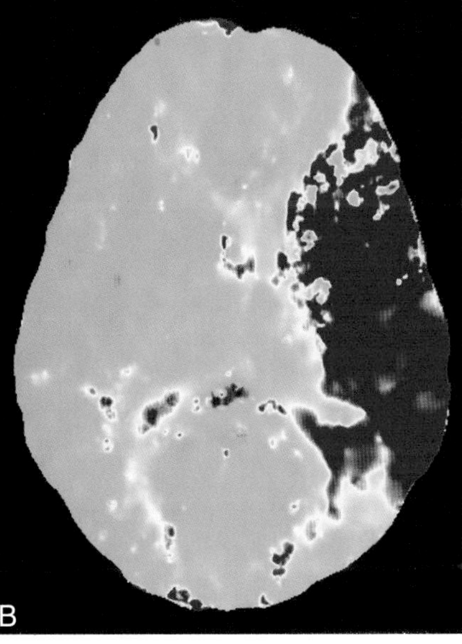


**Fig. 2.14** Infarct on computed tomography perfusion (CTP). Cerebral blood volume (CBV) (A) and time to peak (TTP) (B) CTP maps showing left frontal small area of reduced CBV (white arrow) in keeping with infarct core and a larger area of prolonged TTP involving the right middle cerebral artery territory, in keeping with mismatch and large ischemic penumbra.

## Central Nervous System Infections

### BRAIN

Diagnosis of central nervous system infection in elderly patients is usually delayed due to subtle and nonspecific symptoms including altered mental status, frequent falls, anorexia, or generalized weakness.[24,33] Fever is absent in 20% to 30% of cases,[24] and some geriatric patients may present with normal temperature or even be hypothermic. In addition, age-related dementia, polypharmacy, and concomitant infections make the clinical assessment difficult and limit a reliable clinical history.[3,33]

#### Meningitis

*Streptococcus pneumoniae* is the leading cause of meningitis in older patients with a mortality of about 20%. Other causes of meningitis include *Listeria monocytogenes*, group B streptococcus, and gram-negative bacteria. Otitis, sinusitis, and pneumonia are predisposing conditions and can complicate up to one-third of the cases.[33] Enteroviruses, herpes simplex, arbovirus, cytomegalovirus, and adenovirus are the most frequent causes of viral meningitis.

Imaging findings in bacterial and viral meningitis include thin linear gyriform enhancement along the surface of the brain (Fig. 2.15). Viral meningitis can also cause cranial nerve enhancement (Fig. 2.16).[34] FLAIR images show high signal in the subarachnoid spaces of the sulci and cisterns due to increased protein content.[34]

#### Encephalitis

Herpes simplex encephalitis (HSE) due to herpes virus type 1 accounts for 10% to 15% of cases of encephalitis in older patients. Hypoattenuation in the temporal lobe and insula on head CT are findings suspicious of herpes simplex virus encephalitis. On brain MRI, high signal on FLAIR and T2 sequences (Fig. 2.17), restricted diffusion, and

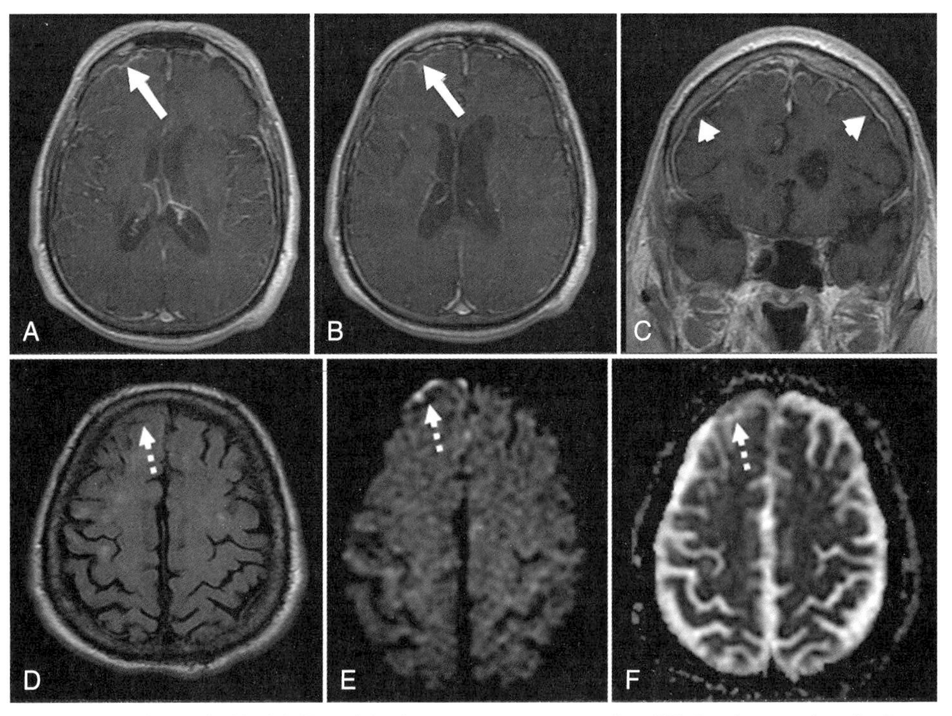


**Fig. 2.15** A 76-year-old male with meningitis. Axial T1-weighted sequences postcontrast (A and B) show leptomeningeal enhancement along the right frontal sulci (arrows). Coronal T1-weighted sequence postcontrast (C) shows bilateral frontal pachymeningeal enhancement (arrowheads). Axial fluid attenuation inversion recovery sequence (D) demonstrates a high-signal extraaxial fluid collection in the right frontal region (dotted arrow) with restricted diffusion (dotted arrows in E and F), consistent with empyema.

patchy parenchymal or gyriform enhancement, typically in the inferior temporal lobe and insula, are findings highly suggestive of HSE.[35]

Adults older than 60 years are 8 to 10 times more likely to present varicella-zoster virus reactivation.[36] Ataxia and seizures are the most common symptoms. CT will demonstrate hypoattenuation in nonspecific areas. Brain MRI shows areas of ischemia in the cortex, grey matter–white matter junction, and deep grey matter. Vasculopathy can be seen with multiple focal areas of stenosis in the intracranial arteries.[35]

West Nile virus encephalitis in older patients is usually acquired through organ transplantation or blood transfusion. Some 1% of cases will develop meningitis, encephalitis, or acute flaccid paralysis.[36] Imaging findings include bilateral high T2-FLAIR areas in the thalami and caudate and lentiform nuclei. Cerebellar and brainstem involvement is also described.[35]

### Intracranial Abscess

Brain abscess is more common in males than females, with a ratio of 2:1 to 3:1.[37] The mechanisms of infection include direct spread from contiguous infection, hematogenous dissemination from a distant source, trauma, and neurosurgical complication. Otitis, mastoiditis, sinusitis, and meningitis are predisposing conditions, while diabetes, alcoholism, and immunosuppression are additional risk factors.[37,38] NCCT shows a round or ovoid lesion with surrounding edema. A ring-enhancing

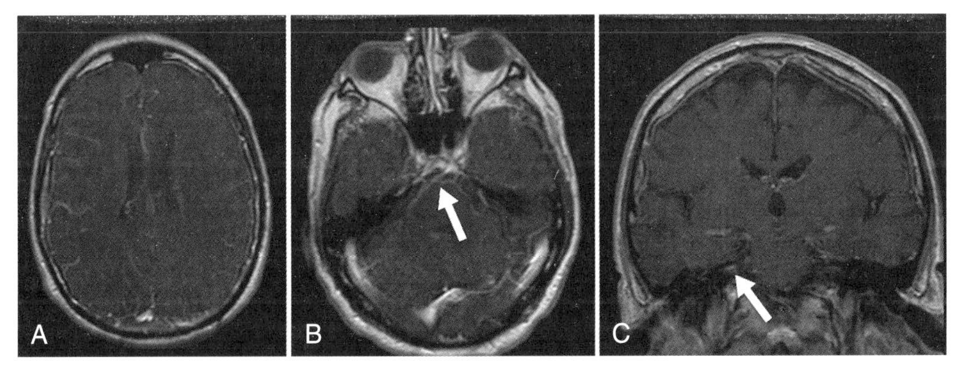


**Fig. 2.16** An 80-year-old male with *Herpes zoster* meningitis. Axial T1-weighted sequences postcontrast (A and B) demonstrate diffuse leptomeningeal enhancement over bilateral cerebral convexities and along the anterior surface of the pons (arrow in B). Coronal T1-weighted sequence postcontrast (C) shows leptomeningeal enhancement involving the VII and VIII cranial nerves on the right side (arrow).

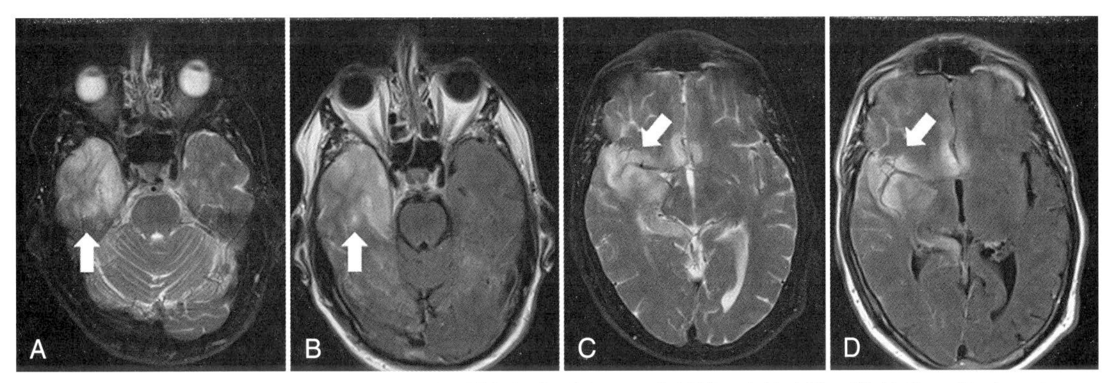


**Fig. 2.17** Herpes simplex encephalitis in a 63-year-old male with behavioral changes. Axial T2-weighted (A) and fluid attenuation inversion recovery (B) sequences show high signal in the right temporal lobe (arrows in A and B), right insula (arrows in C and D), and medial inferior frontal lobes.

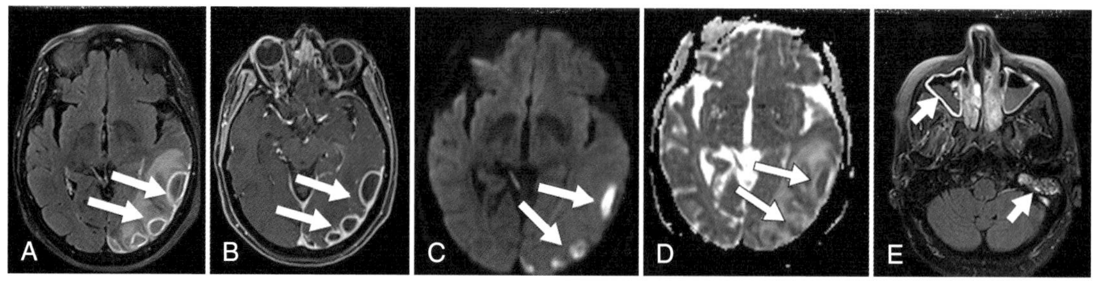


**Fig. 2.18** Brain abscesses in a 72-year-old female with mastoiditis and sinusitis. Axial fluid attenuation inversion recovery (FLAIR) postcontrast (A) and axial T1-weighted postcontrast (B) images show multiple ring-enhancing lesions in the left temporal lobe (arrows). Axial diffusion-weighted imaging and apparent diffusion coefficient (C and D) demonstrate central restricted diffusion within the lesions (arrows). Note the bilateral maxillary sinusitis and left mastoiditis on FLAIR (short arrows on E).

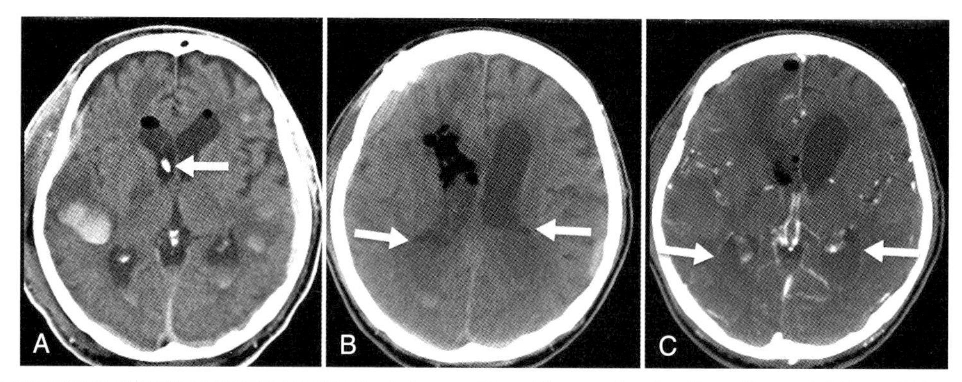


**Fig. 2.19** Postoperative ventriculitis and meningitis after shunt placement in an 82-year-old male with posttraumatic intracranial hemorrhage. Axial computed tomography (CT) image (A) following shunt placement shows the tip of the catheter in the right lateral ventricle (arrow). Axial CT image 1 week after shunt insertion (B) shows a fluid level with high attenuation in the lateral ventricles indicating debris (arrows). Axial CT image with contrast (C) shows ependymal enhancement along the lateral ventricles (arrows) consistent with ventriculitis.

collection with central restricted diffusion is a typical imaging finding on brain MRI (Fig. 2.18).[38,39]

### Device-Related Infection

Cerebrospinal fluid shunts are commonly placed for the treatment of hydrocephalus and to relieve high intracranial pressure in cases of tumors, subarachnoid hemorrhage, intraventricular hemorrhage, and head injuries, which are common conditions in older patients. Introduction of infection at the time of surgery, hematogenous spread from distant site, and contiguous spread are the three routes of shunt-related infections, with secondary development of ventriculomeningitis (Fig. 2.19).[40,41]

## SPINE

Spinal infections in the elderly generally result in longer hospital stays, higher likelihood of failed medical treatment, and higher fatality rate compared with younger patients.[42] Similar to intracranial infections, the diagnosis of spondylodiscitis in the elderly is often delayed, as the signs and symptoms have low specificity.[42] Additionally, low back pain in the elderly is nearly ubiquitous, often from degenerative disease or osteoporotic fractures, which may further confound the diagnosis of infection.

MRI of the spine with and without contrast is the initial imaging modality of choice for patients with suspected spinal infection, and has high sensitivity

(96%), specificity (94%), and accuracy (92%).[43,44] MRI is useful in suggesting the diagnosis of spine infection, evaluating the extent of disease, assessing for cord compression, and helping determine management. Intravenous contrast is beneficial for cases of suspected infection, as it increases lesion conspicuity and helps define the extent of abnormality.[43] CT has great delineation of osseous structures and can evaluate for bony erosions in osteomyelitis; however, the sensitivity for spondylodiscitis (79%) is lower than that of MRI.[43] Radiographs of the spine have low specificity for the evaluation of spondylodiscitis (57%)[45]; hence, MRI is preferred.

### Pyogenic Spondylodiscitis

Bacteria are the most common cause of spinal infection. Among the bacteria, *Staphylococcus aureus* is the most frequent, accounting for 20% to 84% of all cases,[45] with a higher rate of methicillin-resistant *S. aureus* among the elderly population.[46] Pyogenic spondylodiscitis affects mostly the lumbar spine, followed by the thoracic and cervical spine. In general, pyogenic osteomyelitis on imaging is characterized by high signal on T2/short tau inversion recovery (STIR), typically involving the vertebral endplates and disc space, with associated enhancement. Loss of vertebral body height can be noted in more advanced disease. Edema in the adjacent paraspinal soft tissues further supports the diagnosis. Diffuse enhancement of the soft tissues suggests paraspinal phlegmon, while abscess is characterized by a focal fluid collection with rim enhancement. Abscesses can also form in the epidural space and result in cord or cauda equina compression (Fig. 2.20).

### Tuberculous Spondylodiscitis

Tuberculous spinal infections are mostly seen in developing nations but remain a problem worldwide. Tuberculous spondylitis, also known as Pott disease, is more common in the midthoracic or thoracolumbar spine. Chronic disease can cause significant destruction of one or more vertebral bodies, resulting in focal kyphosis of the spine, termed "gibbus deformity." The imaging appearance of osteomyelitis secondary to tuberculosis can be similar to that of

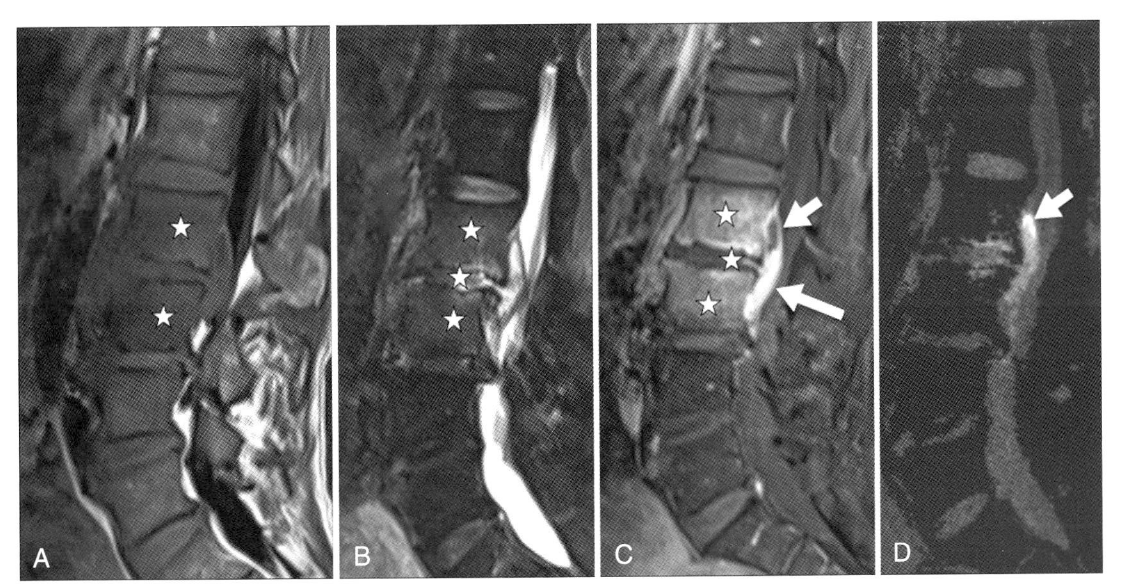


**Fig. 2.20** A 73-year-old male with pyelonephritis and pyogenic discitis and osteomyelitis. Sagittal T1-weighted imaging (A) and short tau inversion recovery (B) sequences show edema in the L2 and L3 vertebral bodies and disc space (stars). Sagittal T1-weighted imaging postcontrast (C) shows diffuse enhancement of the L2 and L3 vertebral bodies and posterior disc (stars), as well as ventral epidural phlegmon (long arrow) and abscess (short arrow). Diffusion-weighted imaging (D) shows restricted diffusion in the ventral epidural space superiorly (short arrow) confirming abscess.

pyogenic osteomyelitis, although focal erosions, vertebral geodes, and intraosseous abscesses have been described. Relative preservation of the disc and calcification of paraspinal abscesses strongly suggest tuberculous etiology (Fig. 2.21).[43]

## Seizures

Contrary to popular belief that epilepsy is more common in young patients, epilepsy is more likely to develop in the elderly.[1] This is secondary to increased risk factors for epilepsy in older adults, such as prior trauma, infarcts, and brain tumors. Epidemiologic studies suggest that aging itself is a risk factor for epilepsy and seizures.[47] The annual incidence of seizures in people over 60 years in the United States is 100 per 100, 000[48]; but at-risk populations, such as nursing home residents, have prevalence rates of epilepsy as high as 9% to 12%.[1]

Seizures are the third most common neurological condition in the elderly population, after stroke and dementia. Acute asymptomatic seizures can be the result of cerebrovascular disease (40%–50%), metabolic disturbance (10%–15%), head trauma (5%–10%), brain infection, neoplasms, or toxins/alcohol.[1] Stroke, in particular, can result in a 20-fold higher risk

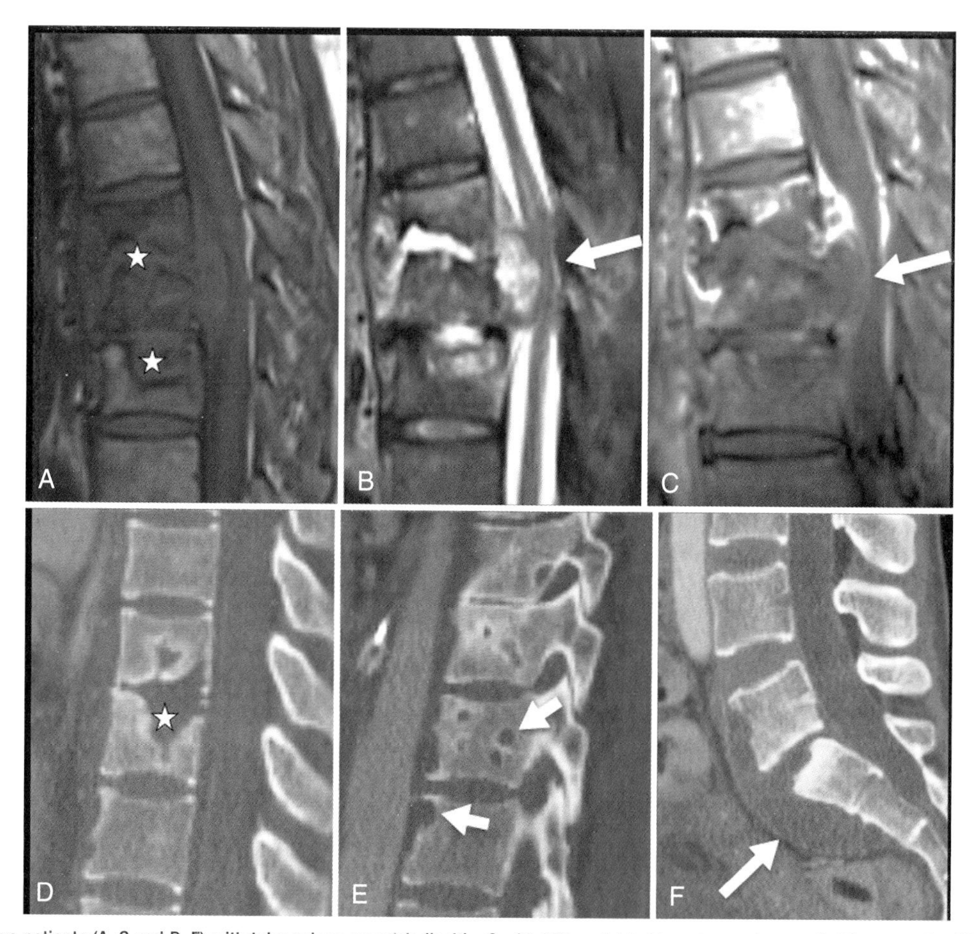


**Fig. 2.21** Two patients (A–C and D–F) with tuberculous spondylodiscitis. Sagittal T1-weighted imaging and computed tomography (CT) images (A and D) show prominent bony erosion of vertebral bodies (stars). Short tau inversion recovery (B) and postcontrast T1-weighted imaging (C) sequences show abscess in the ventral epidural space (arrows) compressing the cord. Multiple erosions and geodes are noted on the sagittal CT (E) (short arrows). Large prevertebral abscess (arrow) is depicted in the lumbosacral spine (F).

of developing epilepsy,[1] while neurodegenerative disorders, such as Alzheimer dementia, can increase the risk of developing seizures by 10 times.[49,50]

Unfortunately, in up to 50% of the elder population with epilepsy, the diagnosis remains unknown,[1] and the rate of correct diagnosis in elderly patients at the time of initial evaluation can be as low as 37%.[51] The lack of accuracy of the clinical examination, particularly in older patients, highlights the value of neuroimaging.

Head CT and MRI are the most common imaging modalities in patients with seizures. NCCT is usually the first imaging tool in these patients, especially in the emergency setting, as it can quickly rule out acute hemorrhage, large-mass lesions, and infarcts. A head CT is indicated when patients present with first time seizures to the ED and may change acute management in 9% to 17% of cases.[52] The presence of abnormalities in CT scans for these patients varies widely, ranging from 3% to 40%.[53] Nevertheless, given the increased risk of strokes and malignancies in the elder population that can result in seizures, a head CT in the emergency setting is required.[53]

MRI is also helpful in the evaluation of seizures, given the more comprehensive assessment of the brain. It identifies and characterizes focal causative lesions, has higher sensitivity for infarct, tumors, gliosis, and parenchymal microhemorrhages, and assesses progression of pathology. In patients with known seizure disorder but with a change in seizure semiology, new neurologic deficit, or no return to previous neurologic baseline, both NCCT head and MRI head are usually appropriate as the initial imaging of patients. MRI head (preferably without and with contrast) is appropriate for the imaging of patients with history of tumor.[54]

Common neuroimaging findings in elderly patients with seizures include cerebral atrophy, white matter changes, ICH, infarcts, gliosis, and granulomas (Fig. 2.22).[55] Less commonly, tumors such as meningioma (Fig. 2.23), glioma, and metastasis are present on imaging. The imaging characteristics of the tumor depend on the type and grade of the tumor; but in general, multiple, well-circumscribed, rounded masses tend to favor metastatic lesions (Fig. 2.24). Hippocampal sclerosis, which is one of the most common causes of temporal lobe epilepsy in childhood and young adults, typically does not present *de novo* in elderly patients.[56]

Periictal changes can also be detected on MRI. Imaging abnormalities in the periictal state include cortical hyperintensity on T2/FLAIR sequences with associate restricted diffusion on DWI, hippocampal swelling, abnormal signal on the ipsilateral thalamus, and increased flow in the ipsilateral brain (Fig. 2.25). Patchy cortical enhancement can also be seen due to breakage of the blood-brain barrier. While these findings can be easily mistaken for tumors or infarctions, they should not follow a vascular territory and usually resolve over hours or days.[57]

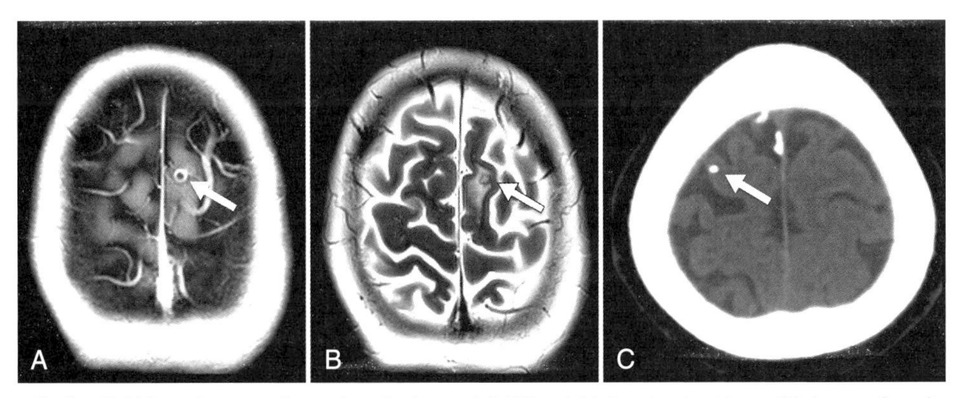


**Fig. 2.22** Two patients with history of neurocysticercosis and seizures. Axial T1-weighted postcontrast image (A) shows a rim-enhancing lesion in the left superior frontal gyrus (arrow), consistent with neurocysticercosis in the colloidal phase. Axial T2-weighted imaging (B) shows surrounding vasogenic edema. Axial computed tomography of the head from a different patient (C) shows a nodular calcified lesion in the right superior frontal gyrus (arrow) without edema, consistent with a calcified granuloma.

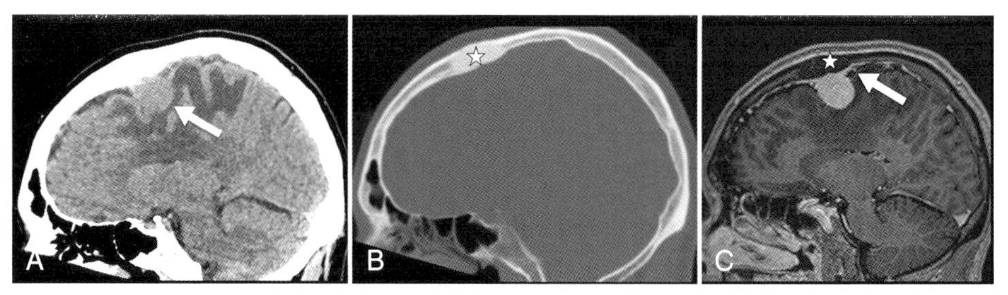


**Fig. 2.23** A 65-year-old-male with meningioma presented with seizures. Sagittal computed tomography (CT) soft tissue window (A) shows an iso- to hyperdense extraaxial mass in the left frontal convexity (arrow), consistent with a meningioma. There is surrounding hypodensity compatible with vasogenic edema. Sagittal CT bone window (B) shows hyperostosis and sclerosis of the adjacent bone (star). Sagittal T1-weighted magnetic resonance imaging (MRI) with contrast (C) shows enhancing meningioma with a dural tail (arrow). Note also bony hyperostosis on MRI (star).

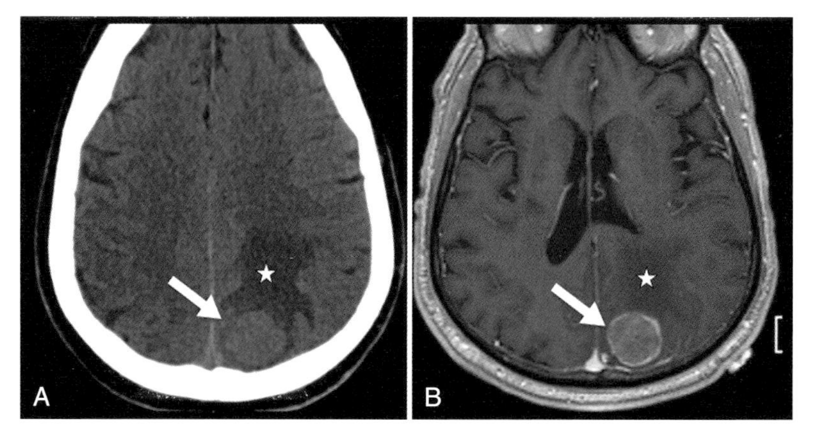


**Fig. 2.24** A 70-year-old-male with lung cancer presented to the emergency department with seizures. Axial computed tomography of the head (A) and axial T1-weighted magnetic resonance imaging with contrast (B) show a rounded, well-defined, enhancing intraaxial mass in the left parietal lobe, consistent with metastasis (arrows). There is surrounding vasogenic edema (stars).

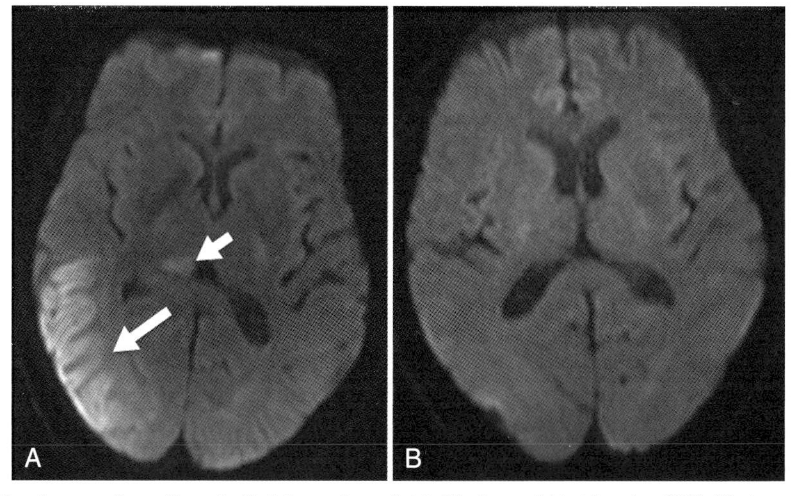


**Fig. 2.25** A 67-year-old-male presenting with acute, first-time seizure. Axial diffusion-weighted imaging (DWI) (A) shows abnormal signal in the right temporal cortex (long arrow) and in the medial ipsilateral thalamus (short arrow). Short-term follow-up DWI (B) shows resolution of signal abnormality, consistent with resolved periictal changes.

## Altered Mental Status

Altered mental status (AMS) is a common presenting complaint among the elderly population in the emergency department.[58] AMS can be broadly thought of in two categories: first is the acute, often-reversible alteration in awareness and cognitive function seen in delirium, and the second is the chronic, irreversible cognitive decline of dementia. These two entities can be difficult to differentiate, as delirium often occurs on a background of long-standing dementia. However, separating these two causes of AMS in the elderly is critical, as each serves as an independent risk factor for mortality, with a distinct differential diagnosis for underlying pathology.[59–61]

Delirium is considered a medical emergency, as it may herald a life-threatening underlying disease process. A patient over 65 years old presenting to the ED with a primary complaint of AMS is highly suggestive of delirium.[62] In the ED, 8% to 17% of all elderly people are delirious on presentation, which increases to 40% in nursing home patients.[63] Patients with delirium have increased length of stay, higher overall hospital costs, and high in-hospital mortality.[64,65]

Delirium is a symptom of illness rather than a distinct pathology, and the differential diagnosis of underlying disease is broad and often multifactorial. For example, delirium may be brought on by infection, acute coronary syndrome, cerebrovascular disease, endocrine and metabolic derangements, drug intoxication, sedative medications, and the postoperative setting.[66,67] In cases of acute or progressively worsening mental status change, a NCCT of the head is an appropriate study, with follow-up MRI of the brain in cases of identified pathology or suspected occult pathology, or to confirm a suspected clinical diagnosis.[68] In one case series of 528 patients with acute-onset delirium, positive findings were found on 11% of CTs and 33% of MRIs, most commonly with hemorrhage, stroke, or metastatic disease as the underlying cause (Fig. 2.26).[69]

Dementia is the fifth leading cause of death in Americans over the age of 65 years, currently affecting over 5 million people, a number expected to increase to 14 million by 2050.[70] All common forms of dementia, including Alzheimer disease (AD), vascular dementia (VaD), frontotemporal dementia (FTD),

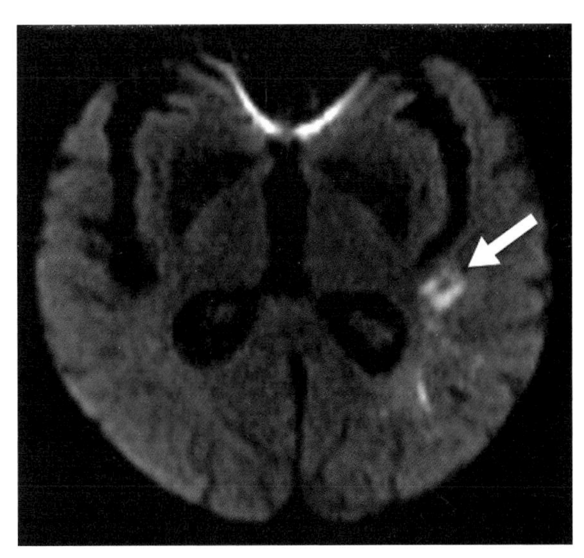

**Fig. 2.26** A 90-year-old woman with "altered mental status," confusing Russian and Polish languages when speaking. Diffusion-weighted images demonstrate an acute infarct in the left temporo-parietal lobes involving Wernicke's area (arrow).

and dementia with Lewy bodies, are clinical diagnoses where imaging aids in the differentiation of dementia subtypes and helps rule out other pathology.[71,72] The American College of Radiologists states that NCCT and MRI of the head are usually appropriate studies for initial workup.[68]

Patients with AD tend to exhibit preferential atrophy of the precuneus and medial temporal lobe/hippocampus (Fig. 2.27), while FTD affects the frontal and temporal lobes primarily (Fig. 2.28). VaD will show evidence of remote strokes, as well as FLAIR white matter hyperintensity seen with chronic microvascular disease. In nonemergent settings, volumetric MRI and advanced imaging modalities such as positron emission tomography are helpful in distinguishing particular subtypes of dementia.[73,74]

## Dizziness and Vertigo

Dizziness is among the most common clinical complaints encountered by clinicians in both the outpatient setting and ED, accounting for up to 4% of all ED visits.[75] Elderly populations are preferentially affected, with up to 30% of people over the age of

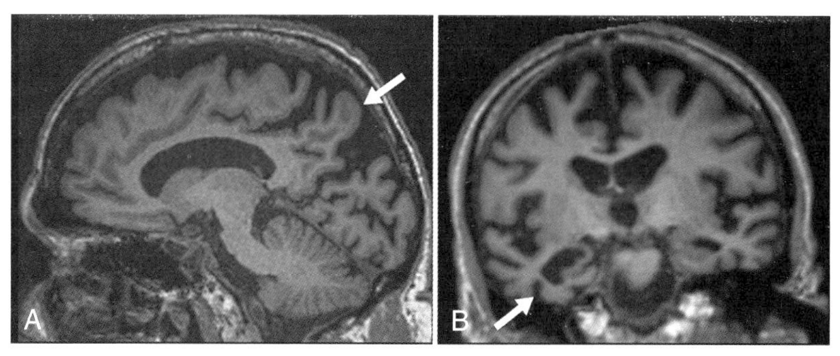


**Fig. 2.27** An 87-year-old man with previously diagnosed Alzheimer disease. T1-weighted sagittal (A) and coronal (B) images demonstrate preferential atrophy of the precuneus and medial temporal lobe, respectively (arrows).

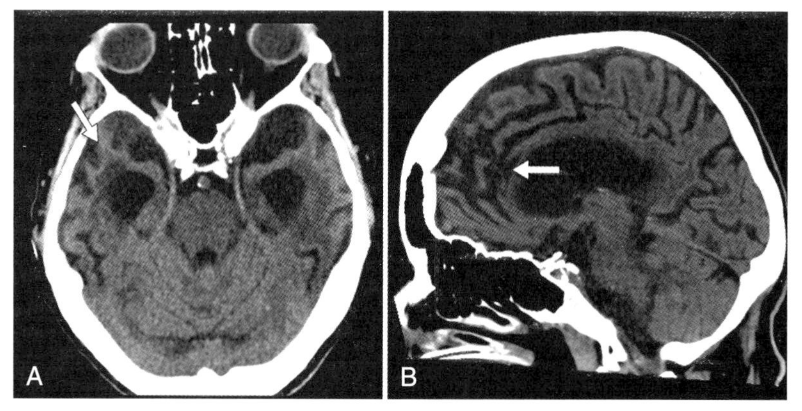


**Fig. 2.28** An 89-year-old woman with frontotemporal dementia and acute mental status change. Axial (A) and sagittal (B) noncontrast computed tomography of the head demonstrates parenchymal volume loss preferentially involving the temporal and frontal lobes, respectively (arrows), suggestive of frontotemporal dementia.

65 years and up to 50% in patients over the age of 85 years experiencing some level of impairment from dizziness.[76,77] While dizziness is a term that may refer to a number of nonspecific symptoms such as lightheadedness, presyncope, and disequilibrium, it can also refer to vertigo. Vertigo, the illusory sense of motion, is closely tied to dysfunction of the vestibular system. An estimated 3% to 4% of patients who present with acute-onset vertigo are experiencing a posterior circulation infarct, many of whom go undiagnosed in the emergency setting, leading to significant morbidity.[78–80] Patients over the age of 40 years who exhibit vestibular dysfunction have a 12-fold increased risk of falling, which is associated with high rates of long-term morbidity and mortality in the elderly.[81,82]

### Nonvestibular Dizziness

For the evaluation of nonvestibular dizziness, the initial workup is dependent on the suspicion of the treating clinician for a neurologic source, as there is a broad differential for this presentation.[80] It should be noted, however, that it is not always possible to delineate forms of dizziness in the elderly, as older patients tend to report less vertigo and more nonspecific dizziness than younger patients with the same condition.[83] As such, there should be a low threshold to obtain either CT or MRI of the brain in these patients.

### Vertigo

Vertigo is classically separated into two categories: peripheral vertigo, which comprises abnormalities relating to the vestibular nerve and inner ear, and

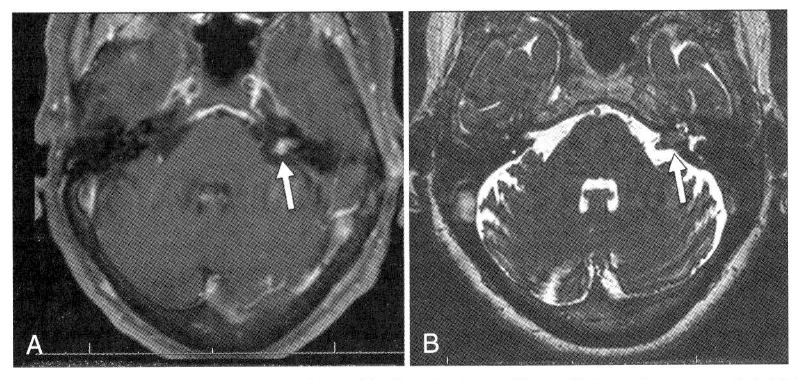


**Fig. 2.29** A 78-year-old woman who presents with vertigo and left-sided hearing loss with vestibular schwannoma. Axial fluid attenuation inversion recovery (A) and high-resolution T2 constructive interference in steady state sequence (CISS), (B) centered in the posterior fossa demonstrate a cone-shaped, homogenously enhancing mass widening the left internal auditory canal (arrows in A and B), highly suggestive of vestibular schwannoma.

central vertigo, which primarily relates to the cerebellum and brainstem nuclei.

In all patients with suspected central vertigo, imaging is a necessity, as the patient should be assumed to have an AIS until proven otherwise. Routine NCCT of the head is often the first imaging study obtained for dizziness, as it is relatively inexpensive and rapidly acquired. However, the diagnostic yield of positive findings in patients with dizziness as a primary complaint is as low as 2.2% on standard CT of the head.[84] In the acute setting, MRI of the brain with special attention to the internal auditory canals (IACs) should be the diagnostic tool of choice.[85] Intravenous contrast allows for better assessment for posterior fossa tumors, such as vestibular schwannomas (Fig. 2.29).

Patients with suspected peripheral vertigo may not require imaging as part of the initial diagnostic workup, as the primary two differential diagnoses of benign positional paroxysmal vertigo and Meniere disease are both clinical diagnoses treated in the outpatient setting. In cases where symptoms persist despite treatment or new neurologic symptoms develop (e.g., headache, visual disturbance, hearing loss), MRI of the brain with special attention to the IACs is the study of choice[85] (Fig. 2.30). CT of the temporal bone is also an acceptable initial imaging tool in the evaluation of peripheral vertigo, as it is superior to MRI in detecting bony abnormalities. It is indicated for suspicion of temporal bone fracture or in posttraumatic vertigo.[86] It is also useful to evaluate for dehiscence of the superior semicircular canal (Fig. 2.31), particularly if there is associated hearing loss or if the vertigo is brought on by loud noises,[87] and to assess for bony erosion, such as in the setting of infection or suspected middle ear tumor.[85]

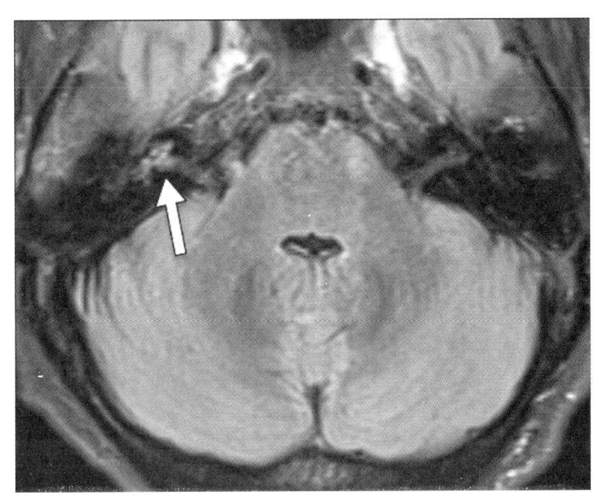

**Fig. 2.30** A 54-year-old woman with acute right-sided hearing loss secondary to labyrinthitis. Magnetic resonance imaging of the brain demonstrates lack of fluid suppression in the right vestibular system on axial fluid attenuation inversion recovery image (arrow), suggesting labyrinthitis.

## Syncope

Syncope, which is transient brief loss of consciousness with inability to maintain postural tone,[88] is responsible for approximately 1.3% of visits to the ED and up to 6% of hospital admissions.[88] The incidence of syncope increases with age, with the prevalence of syncope

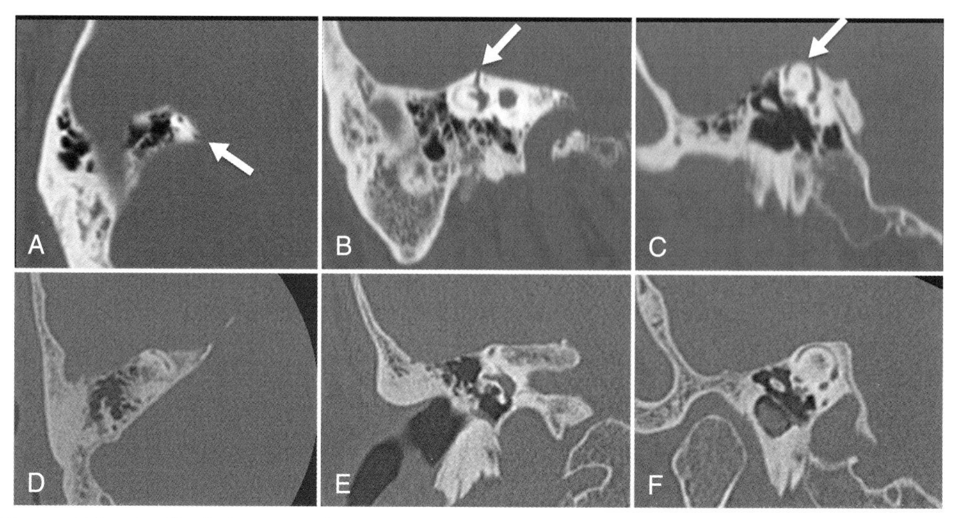


**Fig. 2.31** A 78-year-old female with dizziness secondary to dehiscence of the superior semicircular canal. Axial (A), coronal (B), and Poschl (C) views of a computed tomography scan of the temporal bones show lack of bony covering along the superior semicircular canal (arrows), consistent with dehiscence of the superior semicircular canal. Axial (D), coronal (E,) and Poschl (F) views of a normal inner ear are provided for comparison.

exceeding 20% in patients older than 75 years and an annual incidence of almost 2% in patients older than 80 years.[89] This higher incidence and prevalence in the elderly are due to many factors, including multiple comorbidities, polypharmacy, and age-related changes in cardiovascular function.[89]

Most causes of syncope are unknown (36%), followed by vasovagal/orthostatic (30.4%), cardiac (9%), and neurologic (4%) etiologies. Elderly patients have greater risk of hospitalization and death related to syncope,[90] and patients with neurologic syncope are associated with a threefold risk of stroke.[91]

Patients with syncope secondary to vasovagal reaction, carotid sinus hypersensitivity, and orthostasis tend to have lower long-term mortality, and, if young, typically do not require admission to the hospital. Elderly patients, however, may still require admission to exclude other more serious mechanisms.[92] Cardiac causes of syncope (e.g., dysrhythmias, cardiomyopathy, or cardiac ischemia) or neurologic causes of syncope (e.g., cerebrovascular accident or subarachnoid hemorrhage) need to be carefully evaluated for and excluded before discharge.

The overall consensus among multidisciplinary task forces states that brain CT or MRI are not recommended routinely in cases of uncomplicated syncope, i.e., in the absence of head trauma or neurologic injury.[90] However, some authors suggest that adults older than 60 years presenting with syncope, even if uncomplicated, can benefit from a head CT.[93] Level A recommendations from the American College of Emergency Physicians for the workup of syncope in a patient presenting to the ED include a detailed history, physical examination, and 12-lead electrocardiogram. Any suspicion for neurological injury based on the history and physical examination should prompt neuroimaging.[88] If there is clinical evidence of head injury or the presence of a focal neurologic deficit concerning for infarct or hemorrhage, then head CT or MRI should be obtained. Head CT is usually the first imaging modality for evaluation of intracranial pathology in the ED, although a follow-up MRI of the brain may be beneficial in cases of identified lesions or suspected occult pathology. Intravenous contrast is usually added if neoplasm is suspected. Even though most neuroimaging is negative in cases of syncope, acute abnormal findings can be found in up to 6.4%.[93] These positive cases include most commonly hemorrhage, followed by infarct and intracranial mass.[93]

## Conclusion

Neurological emergencies are common in the elderly population, with increased morbidity and mortality. The physiological changes of aging, coexistence of multiple comorbidities, and atypical presentation of diseases make the diagnosis and management of these patients difficult. Proper clinical, radiological, and specialized assessment is important in order to improve clinical outcome and life quality for these patients.

## REFERENCES


1. Elder CJ, Mendiratta A. Seizures and epilepsy in the elderly: diagnostic and treatment considerations. *Curr Geriatrics Rep*. 2020;9(1):10–17. https://doi.org/10.1007/s13670-020-00310-0.
2. Kahn JH, Magauran BG, Olshaker JS, Shankar KN. Current trends in geriatric emergency medicine. *Emerg Med Clin North Am*. 2016;34(3):435–452. https://doi.org/10.1016/j.emc.2016.04.014.
3. Kulchycki LK, Edlow JA. Geriatric neurologic emergencies. *Emerg Med Clin North Am*. 2006;24(2):273–298. https://doi.org/10.1016/j.emc.2006.01.013.
4. Jolink WMT, Klijn CJM, Brouwers PJAM, Kappelle LJ, Vaartjes I. Time trends in incidence, case fatality, and mortality of intracerebral hemorrhage. *Neurology*. 2015;85(15):1318–1324. https://doi.org/10.1212/WNL.0000000000002015.
5. Lioutas VA, Beiser AS, Aparicio HJ, et al. Assessment of incidence and risk factors of intracerebral hemorrhage among participants in the framingham heart study between 1948 and 2016. *JAMA Neurol*. 2020;77(10):1252–1260. https://doi.org/10.1001/jamaneurol.2020.1512.
6. Angelozzi A, Renda G, Mercuri M. The risk of intracranial hemorrhage with anticoagulation in the elderly: estimates of prevalence and therapeutic strategies. *Am Coll Cardiology*. 2015. Webpage: https://www.acc.org/latest-in-cardiology/articles/2015/12/21/12/59/the-risk-of-intracranial-hemorrhage-with-anticoagulation-in-the-elderly. Accessed April 2021. Updated on 2015.
7. National Trauma Data Bank. National Trauma Data Bank 2010 Annual Report. Trauma. 2010. Webpage: https://www.facs.org/~/media/files/quality%20programs/trauma/ntdb/ntdbannualreport2010.ashx. Accessed April 2021. Updated on 2010
8. Macellari F, Paciaroni M, Agnelli G, Caso V. Neuroimaging in intracerebral hemorrhage. *Stroke*. 2014;45(3):903–908. https://doi.org/10.1161/STROKEAHA.113.003701.
9. Meldon S, Delaney-Rowland S. Subdural hematomas in the elderly: the great neurological imitator. Webpage: https://www.reliasmedia.com 2000;2021. Accessed May 2021, Updated on 2000.
10. Gean AD, Fischbein NJ, Purcell DD, Aiken AH, Manley GT, Stiver SI. Benign anterior temporal epidural hematoma: Indolent lesion with a characteristic CT imaging appearance after blunt head trauma. *Radiology*. 2010;257(1):212–218. https://doi.org/10.1148/radiol.10092075.
11. Mirvis SE, Shanmuganathan K. Trauma radiology: part IV. imaging of acute craniocerebral trauma. *J Intensive Care Med*. 1994;9(6):305–315. https://doi.org/10.1177/088506669400900605.
12. da Rocha AJ, da Silva CJ, Pinto Gama HP, et al. Comparison of magnetic resonance imaging sequences with computed tomography to detect low-grade subarachnoid hemorrhage: Role of fluid-attenuated inversion recovery sequence. *J Comput Assist Tomography*. 2006;30(2):295–303. https://doi.org/10.1097/00004728-200603000-00025.
13. Petridis AK, Kamp MA, Cornelius JF, et al. Aneurysmal subarachnoid hemorrhage-diagnosis and treatment. *Dtsch Arzteblatt Int*. 2017;114(13):226–236. https://doi.org/10.3238/arztebl.2017.0226.
14. Kim JJ, Gean AD. Imaging for the diagnosis and management of traumatic brain injury. *Neurotherapeutics*. 2011;8(1):39–53. https://doi.org/10.1007/s13311-010-0003-3.
15. Aguilar MI, Brott TG. Update in intracerebral hemorrhage. *Neurohospitalist*. 2011;1(3):148–159. https://doi.org/10.1177/1941875211409050.
16. Inzitari D, Giordano GP, Ancona AL, Pracucci G, Mascalchi M, Amaducci L. Leukoaraiosis, intracerebral hemorrhage, and arterial hypertension. *Stroke*. 1990;21(10):1419–1423. https://doi.org/10.1161/01.STR.21.10.1419.
17. Kuhn J, Sharman T. Cerebral Amyloid Angiopathy. StatPearls [Internet]. 2020. Webpage: https://www.ncbi.nlm.nih.gov/books/NBK556105/ Accessed April 2021. Updated on 2020
18. Ohtani R, Kazui S, Tomimoto H, Minematsu K, Naritomi H. Clinical and radiographic features of lobar cerebral hemorrhage: Hypertensive versus non-hypertensive cases. *Intern Med*. 2003;42(7):576–580. https://doi.org/10.2169/internalmedicine.42.576.
19. Al-Mufti F, Amuluru K, Sahni R, et al. Cerebral venous thrombosis in COVID-19: a new york metropolitan cohort study. *AJNR Am J Neuroradiology*. 2021;42(7):1196–1200. https://doi.org/10.3174/ajnr.a7134.
20. Zuurbier SM, Hiltunen S, Lindgren E, et al. Cerebral venous thrombosis in older patients. *Stroke*. 2018;49(1):197–200. https://doi.org/10.1161/STROKEAHA.117.019483.
21. Hottinger AF, DeAngelis LM. Etiology of tumor-related intracranial hemorrhage. *Intracerebral Hemorrhage*. 2009:31. Webpage: https://doi.org/10.1017/CBO9780511691836.004 Accessed April 2021. Updated on May 2010.
22. Mandybur TI. Intracranial hemorrhage caused by metastatic tumors. *Neurology*. 1977;27(7):650–655. https://doi.org/10.1212/wnl.27.7.650.
23. Gupta A, Nair S, Schweitzer AD, et al. Neuroimaging of cerebrovascular disease in the aging brain. *Aging Dis*. 2012;3(5):414–425.
24. Nentwich LM, Grimmnitz B. Neurologic emergencies in the elderly. *Emerg Med Clin North Am*. 2016;34(3):575–599. https://doi.org/10.1016/j.emc.2016.04.009.
25. Kolominsky-Rabas PL, Weber M, Gefeller O, Neundoerfer B, Heuschmann PU. Epidemiology of ischemic stroke subtypes according to TOAST criteria: Incidence, recurrence, and long-term survival in ischemic stroke subtypes: A population-based study. *Stroke*. 2001;32(12):2735–2740. https://doi.org/10.1161/hs1201.100209.
26. Khoujah D, Cobb MJ. Neurologic Emergencies at the extremes of age. *Emerg Med Clin North Am*. 2021;39(1):47–65. https://doi.org/10.1016/j.emc.2020.09.003.
27. Kato Y, Hayashi T, Tanahashi N, Kobayashi S. Cardioembolic stroke is the most serious problem in the aging society: Japan standard stroke registry study. *J Stroke Cerebrovasc Dis*. 2015;24(4):811–814. https://doi.org/10.1016/j.jstrokecerebrovasdis.2014.11.019.
28. Chen CJ, Ding D, Starke RM, et al. Endovascular vs medical management of acute ischemic stroke. *Neurology*. 2015;85(22):1980–1990. https://doi.org/10.1212/WNL.0000000000002176.
29. Rudkin S, Cerejo R, Tayal A, Goldberg MF. Imaging of acute ischemic stroke. *Emerg Radiology*. 2018;25(6):659–672. https://doi.org/10.1007/s10140-018-1623-x.
30. Powers WJ, Rabinstein AA, Ackerson T, et al. Guidelines for the Early Management of Patients With Acute Ischemic Stroke: A Guideline for Healthcare Professionals From the American Heart Association/American Stroke Association. *Stroke*. 2018;49(3):e46–e110. https://doi.org/10.1161/STR.0000000000000158.
31. Byrne D, Walsh JP, Sugrue G, Nicolaou S, Rohr A. CT imaging of acute ischemic stroke. *Can Assoc Radiologists J*. 2020;71(3):266–280. https://doi.org/10.1177/0846537120902068.
32. Byrne D, Sugrue G, Stanley E, et al. Improved detection of anterior circulation occlusions: The delayed vessel sign on multiphase CT angiography. *Am J Neuroradiol*. 2017;38(10):1911–1916. https://doi.org/10.3174/ajnr.A5317.
33. Liang SY. Sepsis and Other Infectious Disease Emergencies in the Elderly. *Emerg Med Clin North Am*. 2016;34(3):501–522. https://doi.org/10.1016/j.emc.2016.04.005.

34. Mohan S, Jain KK, Arabi M, Shah GV. Imaging of meningitis and ventriculitis. *Neuroimaging Clin N Am*. 2012;22(4):557–583. https://doi.org/10.1016/j.nic.2012.04.003.
35. Koeller KK, Shih RY. Viral and prion infections of the central nervous system: Radiologic-pathologic correlation. *Radiographics*. 2017;37(1):199–233. https://doi.org/10.1148/rg.2017160149.
36. Noska A, Tunkel AR. Central nervous system infections in the elderly. *Curr Geriatrics Rep*. 2015;4(1):96–104. https://doi.org/10.1007/s13670-014-0110-9.
37. Chow F. Brain and spinal epidural abscess. *CONTLifelong Learn Neurol*. 2018;24(5):1327–1348. https://doi.org/10.1212/CON.0000000000000649.
38. Rath TJ, Hughes M, Arabi M, Shah GV. Imaging of Cerebritis, Encephalitis, and Brain Abscess. *Neuroimaging Clin N Am*. 2012;22(4):585–607. https://doi.org/10.1016/j.nic.2012.04.002.
39. Swinburne NC, Bansal AG, Aggarwal A, Doshi AH. Neuroimaging in central nervous system infections. *Curr Neurol Neurosci Rep*. 2017;17(6):1–14. https://doi.org/10.1007/s11910-017-0756-8.
40. Seidelman J, Lewis SS. Neurosurgical device-related infections. *Infect Dis Clin North Am*. 2018;32(4):861–876. https://doi.org/10.1016/j.idc.2018.06.006.
41. Stenehjem E, Armstrong WS. Central nervous system device infections. *Infect Dis Clin North Am*. 2012;26(1):89–110. https://doi.org/10.1016/j.idc.2011.09.006.
42. Amadoru S, Lim K, Tacey M, Aboltins C. Spinal infections in older people: an analysis of demographics, presenting features, microbiology and outcomes. *Intern Med J*. 2017;47(2):182–188. https://doi.org/10.1111/imj.13300.
43. Ortiz, A.O, Levitt A, Shah L.M, et al. American College of Radiology ACR Appropriateness Criteria® Suspected Spine Infection. *J Am Coll Radiol: JACR*,18(11s), S488- S501. Webpage: https://AcsearchAcrOrg/Docs/3148734/Narrative 2021;2021. Accessed April 2021. Updated on 2021.
44. Arbelaez A, Restrepo F, Castillo M. Spinal infections: clinical and imaging features. *Top Magnetic Reson Imaging*. 2014;23(5):303–314. https://doi.org/10.1097/RMR.0000000000000032.
45. Mavrogenis AF, Megaloikonomos PD, Igoumenou VG, et al. Spondylodiscitis revisited. *EFORT Open Rev*. 2017;2(11):447–461. https://doi.org/10.1302/2058-5241.2.160062.
46. Nagashima H, Nanjo Y, Tanida A, Dokai T, Teshima R. Clinical features of spinal infection in individuals older than eighty years. *Int Orthop*. 2012;36(6):1129–1234. https://doi.org/10.1007/s00264-011-1440-2.
47. Hauser WA. Seizure Disorders: the changes with age. *Epilepsia*. 1992;33(Suppl 4):S6–S14. https://doi.org/10.1111/j.1528-1157.1992.tb06222.x.
48. Faught E. Epidemiology and drug treatment of epilepsy in elderly people. *Drugs and Aging*. 1999;15(4):255–269. https://doi.org/10.2165/00002512-199915040-00002.
49. Beagle AJ, Darwish SM, Ranasinghe KG, La AL, Karageorgiou E, Vossel KA. Relative incidence of seizures and myoclonus in Alzheimer's disease, dementia with lewy bodies, and fronto-temporal dementia. *J Alzheimer's Dis*. 2017;60(1):211–223. https://doi.org/10.3233/JAD-170031.
50. Thomas RJ. Seizures and epilepsy in the elderly. *Arch Intern Med*. 1997;157(6):605–617.
51. Kellinghaus C, Loddenkemper T, Dinner DS, Lachhwani D, Lüders HO. Seizure semiology in the elderly: a video analysis. *Epilepsia*. 2004;45(3):263–267. https://doi.org/10.1111/j.0013-9580.2004.29003.x.
52. Harden CL, Huff JS, Schwartz TH, et al. Reassessment: neuroimaging in the emergency patient presenting with seizure (an evidence-based review): Report of the Therapeutics and Technology Assessment Subcommittee of the American. *Neurology*. 2007;69(18):1772–1780. https://doi.org/10.1212/01.wnl.0000285083.25882.0e.
53. Jagoda A, Gupta K. The emergency department evaluation of the adult patient who presents with a first-time seizure. *Emerg Med Clin North Am*. 2011;29(1):41–49. https://doi.org/10.1016/j.emc.2010.08.004.
54. Lee RK, Burns J, Ajam AA, et al. ACR appropriateness criteria® seizures and epilepsy. *J Am Coll Radiol*. 2020;17(5S):S293–S304. Webpage: https://acsearch.acr.org/docs/69479/Narrative/, accessed May 2021, updated on 2019.
55. Elangovan S, Thangaraj M, Balamurali K, Arun Kumar M. Neuroimaging in elderly with new-onset unprovoked seizures: a pictorial review. *Int J Contemporary Med Res*. 2017;9:1844–1848.
56. Lozsadi DA, Chadwick DW, Larner AJ. Late-onset temporal lobe epilepsy with unilateral mesial temporal sclerosis and cognitive decline: A diagnostic dilemma. *Seizure*. 2008;17(5):473–476. https://doi.org/10.1016/j.seizure.2007.12.001.
57. Cole AJ. Status epilepticus and periictal imaging. *Epilepsia*. 2004;45(Suppl4):72–77. https://doi.org/10.1111/j.0013-9580.2004.04014.x.
58. Hustey FM, Meldon SW, Smith MD, Lex CK. The effect of mental status screening on the care of elderly emergency department patients. *Ann Emerg Med*. 2003;41(5):678–684. https://doi.org/10.1067/mem.2003.152.
59. Han JH, Shintani A, Eden S, et al. Delirium in the emergency department: An independent predictor of death within 6 months. *Ann Emerg Med*. 2010;56(3):244–252. https://doi.org/10.1016/j.annemergmed.2010.03.003.
60. Golüke NMS, van de Vorst IE, Vaartjes IH, et al. Risk factors for in-hospital mortality in patients with dementia. *Maturitas*. 2019;129:57–61. https://doi.org/10.1016/j.maturitas.2019.08.007.
61. Todd S, Barr S, Roberts M, Passmore AP. Survival in dementia and predictors of mortality: a review. *Int J Geriatr Psychiatry*. 2013;28(11):1109–1124. https://doi.org/10.1002/gps.3946.
62. Han JH, Schnelle JF, Ely EW. The relationship between a chief complaint of "altered mental status" and delirium in older emergency department patients. *Academic Emerg Med*. 2014;21(8):937–940. https://doi.org/10.1111/acem.12436.
63. Inouye SK, Westendorp RGJ, Saczynski JS. Delirium in elderly people. *The Lancet*. 2014;383(9920):911–922. https://doi.org/10.1016/S0140-6736(13)60688-1.
64. Schubert M, Schürch R, Boettger S, et al. A hospital-wide evaluation of delirium prevalence and outcomes in acute care patients: a cohort study. *BMC Health Serv Res*. 2018;18(1):550. https://doi.org/10.1186/s12913-018-3345-x.
65. Leslie DL, Marcantonio ER, Zhang Y, Leo-Summers L, Inouye SK. One-year health care costs associated with delirium in the elderly population. *Arch Intern Med*. 2008;168(1):27–32. https://doi.org/10.1001/archinternmed.2007.4.
66. Kanich W, Brady WJ, Huff JS, et al. Altered mental status: evaluation and etiology in the ED. *Am J Emerg Med*. 2002;20(7):613–617. https://doi.org/10.1053/ajem.2002.35464.
67. Deiner S, Silverstein JH. Postoperative delirium and cognitive dysfunction. *Br J Anaesth*. 2009;103(suppl 1):i41–i46. https://doi.org/10.1093/bja/aep291.
68. Luttrull MD, Boulter DJ, Kirsch CFE, Aulino JM, Broder JS, Chakraborty S, et al. ACR Appropriateness Criteria® acute

mental status change, delirium, and new onset psychosis. *J Am Coll Radiology*. 2019;16(5S):S26–S37.

69. Hijazi Z, Lange P, Watson R, Maier AB. The use of cerebral imaging for investigating delirium aetiology. *Eur J Intern Med*. 2018;52:35–39. https://doi.org/10.1016/j.ejim.2018.01.024.
70. Gaugler J, James B, Johnson T, Scholz K, Weuve J. 2016 Alzheimer's disease facts and figures. *Alzheimer's and Dementia*. 2016;12(4):459–509. https://doi.org/10.1016/j.jalz.2016.03.001.
71. Knopman DS, DeKosky ST, Cummings JL, et al. Practice parameter: diagnosis of dementia (an evidence-based review): report of the quality standards subcommittee of the american academy of neurology. *Neurology*. 2001;56(9):1143–1153. https://doi.org/10.1212/WNL.56.9.1143.
72. Moonis G, Subramaniam RM, Trofimova A, et al. ACR appropriateness criteria® dementia. *J Am Coll Radiology*. 2020;17(5S):S100–S112.
73. Zhang Y, Tartaglia MC, Schuff N, et al. MRI signatures of brain macrostructural atrophy and microstructural degradation in frontotemporal lobar degeneration subtypes. *J Alzheimer's Dis*. 2013;33(2):431–444. https://doi.org/10.3233/JAD-2012-121156.
74. O'Donovan J, Watson R, Colloby SJ, Blamire AM, O'Brien JT. Assessment of regional MR diffusion changes in dementia with Lewy bodies and Alzheimer's disease. *Int Psychogeriatr*. 2014;26(4):627–635. https://doi.org/10.1017/S1041610213002317.
75. Newman-Toker DE, Cannon LM, Stofferahn ME, Rothman RE, Hsieh YH, Zee DS. Imprecision in patient reports of dizziness symptom quality: A cross-sectional study conducted in an acute care setting. *Mayo Clin Proc*. 2007;82(11):1329–1340. https://doi.org/10.4065/82.11.1329.
76. Jönsson R, Sixt E, Landahl S, Rosenhall U. Prevalence of dizziness and vertigo in an urban elderly population. *J Vestib Research: Equilib Orientat*. 2004;14(1):47–52.
77. Colledge NR, Wilson JA, Macintyre CCA, Maclennan WJ. The prevalence and characteristics of dizziness in an elderly community. *Age and Ageing*. 1994;23(2):117–120. https://doi.org/10.1093/ageing/23.2.117.
78. Kerber KA, Brown DL, Lisabeth LD, Smith MA, Morgenstern LB. Stroke among patients with dizziness, vertigo, and imbalance in the emergency department: a population-based study. *Stroke*. 2006;37(10):2484–2487.
79. Arch AE, Weisman DC, Coca S, Nystrom KV, Wira CR, Schindler JL. Missed ischemic stroke diagnosis in the emergency department by emergency medicine and neurology services. *Stroke*. 2016;47(3):668–673. https://doi.org/10.1161/STROKEAHA.115.010613.
80. Newman-Toker DE, Hsieh YH, Camargo CA, Pelletier AJ, Butchy GT, Edlow JA. Spectrum of dizziness visits to US emergency departments: cross-sectional analysis from a nationally representative sample. *Mayo Clin Proc*. 2008;83(7):765–775. https://doi.org/10.4065/83.7.765.
81. Agrawal Y, Carey JP, della Santina CC, Schubert MC, Minor LB. Disorders of balance and vestibular function in US adults: data from the national health and nutrition examination survey, 2001-2004. *Arch Intern Med*. 2009;169(10):938–944. https://doi.org/10.1001/archinternmed.2009.66.
82. Kannus P, Parkkari J, Koskinen S, et al. Fall-induced injuries and deaths among older adults. *J Am Med Assoc*. 1999;281(20):1895–1899. https://doi.org/10.1001/jama.281.20.1895.
83. Fernández L, Breinbauer HA, Delano PH. Vertigo and dizziness in the elderly. *Front Neurol*. 2015;6:144. https://doi.org/10.3389/fneur.2015.00144.
84. Lawhn-Heath C, Buckle C, Christoforidis G, Straus C. Utility of head CT in the evaluation of vertigo/dizziness in the emergency department. *Emerg Radiology*. 2013;20(1):45–49.
85. Sharma A, Kirsch CFE, Aulino JM, et al. ACR Appropriateness Criteria® hearing loss and/or vertigo. *J Am Coll Radiology*. 2018;15(11S):S321–331.
86. Fife TD, Giza C. Posttraumatic vertigo and dizziness. *Semin Neurol*. 2013;33(3):238–243. https://doi.org/10.1055/s-0033-1354599.
87. Minor LB. Superior canal dehiscence syndrome. *Otology & Neurotology*. 2000;21(1):9–19.
88. Kessler C, Tristano JM, de Lorenzo R. The emergency department approach to syncope: evidence-based guidelines and prediction rules. *Emerg Med Clin North Am*. 2010;28(3):487–500. https://doi.org/10.1016/j.emc.2010.03.014.
89. Goyal P, Maurer MS. Syncope in older adults. *J Geriatric Cardiology*. 2016;13(5):380–386. https://doi.org/10.11909/j.issn.1671-5411.2016.05.002.
90. Shen WK, Sheldon RS, Benditt DG, et al. 2017 ACC/AHA/HRS guideline for the evaluation and management of patients with syncope: A report of the American College of Cardiology/American Heart Association task force on clinical practice guidelines and the Heart Rhythm Society. *Circulation*. 2017;136(5):e60–e122. https://doi.org/10.1161/CIR.0000000000000499.
91. Soteriades ES, Evans JC, Larson MG, et al. Incidence and prognosis of syncope. *N Engl J Med*. 2002;347(12):878–885. https://doi.org/10.1056/nejmoa012407.
92. Ouyang H, Quinn J. Diagnosis and evaluation of syncope in the emergency department. *Emerg Med Clin North Am*. 2010;28(3):471–485. https://doi.org/10.1016/j.emc.2010.03.007.
93. Mitsunaga MM, Yoon H-C. Journal club: head CT scans in the emergency department for syncope and dizziness. *Am J Roentgenology*. 2015;204(1):24–28. https://doi.org/10.2214/AJR.14.12993.

Chapter 3

# Neurological Emergencies in Cancer and Immunocompromised Patients

Carlos Zamora, Mauricio Castillo, Paulo Puac-Polanco, and Carlos Torres

## Outline



## Key Points

- Opportunistic central nervous system infections are most commonly seen in patients with human immunodeficiency virus and are usually associated with profound immunosuppression.
- Hematologic disorders are frequent in cancer patients and may lead to neurological complications caused by thrombocytopenia, leukostasis, and prothrombotic states.
- Treatment-induced toxicity is a major cause of morbidity in cancer patients and depends on several factors including dose, route of administration, drug interactions, and patient vulnerability.
- Spinal metastases can lead to cord compression due to intradural masses, pathologic fractures, or epidural extension of disease.

## Introduction

Cancer and immunocompromised patients represent a vulnerable group that can be affected by various neurological emergencies. Patients with malignancies may present with complications that are directly tumor-related (e.g., hemorrhage or hydrocephalus), secondary to systemic effects (e.g., leukostasis, thrombocytopenia, or metabolic derangements), or iatrogenic. Immunosuppression is common in cancer patients and may result from various mechanisms, including neutropenia, impaired cellular or humoral immunity, and immunosuppressive therapies.[1] Additionally, the immunocompromised population includes patients with several primary immune deficiencies and a wide number of secondary causes that include advanced age, metabolic conditions, infection (e.g., human immunodeficiency virus [HIV]), malnutrition, and chronic disorders such as diabetes and systemic lupus erythematosus.[2] In this chapter, we review the relevant imaging characteristics of neurological emergencies that may occur in patients with cancer and immunocompromised conditions.

### IMAGING APPROACH

Computed tomography (CT) remains the preferred imaging modality for acute neurological deterioration, as it allows for rapid detection of acute hemorrhage, mass effect, hydrocephalus, and herniation with high sensitivity.[3] It can also depict focal or diffuse cerebral edema, although the sensitivity for subtle changes and acute ischemia is relatively low compared with magnetic resonance imaging (MRI).[4] In the acute setting, head CT is generally performed without intravenous contrast to detect hemorrhage and to allow visualization of the cerebrospinal fluid (CSF)-filled subarachnoid spaces, which is imperative if a lumbar puncture is being considered.

MRI is the preferred modality to characterize brain pathology due to its high contrast-to-noise ratio. Intravenous contrast is administered when there is suspected infection, malignancy, or an inflammatory or a demyelinating process. In addition to fluid-attenuated inversion recovery (FLAIR), T1- and T2-weighted sequences, diffusion-weighted imaging (DWI), and hemosiderin-sensitive sequences such as susceptibility-weighted imaging should also be routinely obtained. DWI is highly sensitive for the detection of acute infarction and may be able to demonstrate a leading edge of demyelination in progressive multifocal leukoencephalopathy (PML) or other demyelinating processes. DWI is also helpful to detect infection, such as pus in abscesses, meningeal exudates, and ventriculitis, as well as thrombi in certain stages. Advanced MRI techniques such as magnetic resonance spectroscopy (MRS) may be useful in certain situations but are not performed routinely. MRI is susceptible to patient motion artifacts due to longer acquisition times than CT, and therefore may be challenging to perform in critically ill patients.

## TUMOR-RELATED COMPLICATIONS

### Tumoral Hemorrhage

Intracranial hemorrhage occurs in up to 15% of patients with brain tumors and in 57% of such patients presenting with acute neurological syndromes.[5] In cancer patients, hemorrhage most commonly arises from solid tumors and coagulopathies, which are seen in hematologic malignancies and chemotherapy.[6] Mechanisms of tumoral hemorrhage include abnormally friable blood vessels, tumor necrosis, and vascular invasion.[7] Hemorrhage is most commonly intraparenchymal, followed by subarachnoid, intraventricular, subdural, or a combination of all.[6] Melanoma, lung, and breast cancers are the most common primary malignancies to present with hemorrhagic metastases, and long-term anticoagulation confers an increased risk.[6] On CT, hemorrhages at the grey-white matter interfaces and with greater than expected vasogenic edema raise concern for underlying metastases over nontumoral causes such as hypertension or amyloid angiopathy. On MRI, areas of contrast enhancement, mixed signal intensities, and delayed evolution of blood products on serial studies are suspicious for underlying tumor (Fig. 3.1).

### Hydrocephalus

Hydrocephalus can lead to increased intracranial pressure and is an important cause of morbidity in patients with intracranial malignancies. Mechanisms include direct mass effect and increased production (e.g., choroid plexus tumors) or decreased resorption of CSF (e.g., elevated CSF protein, hemorrhage, leptomeningeal disease, and possibly radiation-induced fibrosis of arachnoid granulations).[8] Ventricular obstruction is the most common cause of hydrocephalus and is

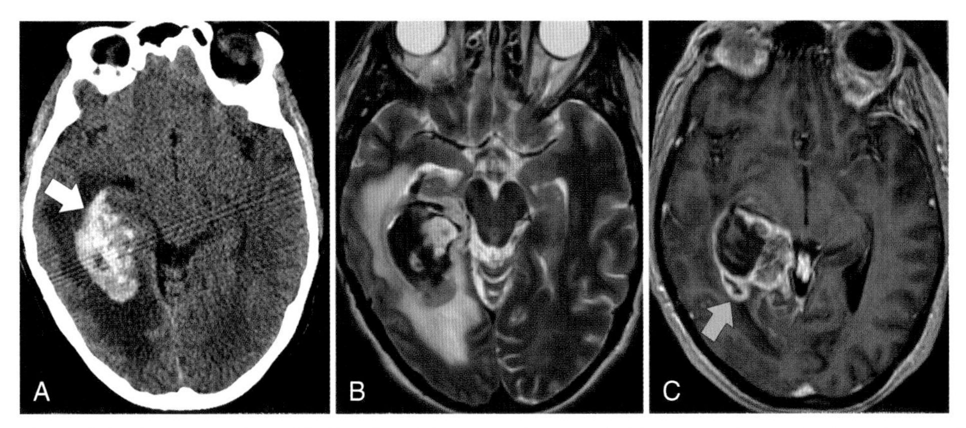


**Fig. 3.1** Hemorrhagic glioblastoma in a patient with altered mental status and seizures. Axial noncontrast computed tomography (A) shows a large hemorrhage in the right temporal lobe (white arrow) with surrounding vasogenic edema. Axial T2-weighted image (B) demonstrates mixed signal intensities. On postcontrast T1-weighted image (C) there are regions of tumoral enhancement (orange arrow).

most frequently seen in tumors involving the posterior fossa, brainstem, and pineal region (Fig. 3.2).[9] Hydrocephalus may develop rapidly in tumors with aggressive growth or in those complicated by hemorrhage.

## COMPLICATIONS RELATED TO IMMUNOSUPPRESSION

### Infections

Immunocompromised patients are susceptible to opportunistic infections from a wide range of microorganisms. In patients with HIV, opportunistic central nervous system (CNS) infections establish a diagnosis of acquired immunodeficiency syndrome (AIDS) and are associated with very low CD4 cell counts (typically below 100/mm$^3$) and increased mortality.[10]

Toxoplasmosis. Toxoplasmosis is caused by *Toxoplasma gondii* and results from reactivation of a latent infection. *T. gondii* is a unicellular protozoan that can infect the CNS in severely immunocompromised patients, usually those with HIV and a CD4 count lower than 100/mm$^3$. Although toxoplasmosis remains the most prevalent opportunistic infection in HIV, its incidence has decreased due to the widespread adoption of combined antiretroviral therapy (ART) and routine prophylaxis against *Pneumocystis jirovecii*.[11,12] Toxoplasmosis leads to necrotic ring-enhancing lesions that are usually multiple and located in the basal ganglia or at grey-white matter junctions. Focal neurologic syndromes are common, and movement disorders are frequently seen when the basal ganglia are involved.[13] Ring-enhancing lesions characteristically present with a peripheral nodule (the "eccentric target" sign) formed by inflamed vessels invaginating into a sulcus.[14] Another distinctive feature is the presence of hypo- and hyperintense concentric rings on T2/FLAIR sequences due to alternating areas of hemorrhage and necrosis (Fig. 3.3).[15] Toxoplasmosis less commonly presents with a diffuse encephalitis.[12]

Fungal infections. Fungal organisms are usually nonpathogenic or lead to limited disease in immunocompetent individuals but are an important cause of morbidity and mortality in immunocompromised hosts. Although invasive fungal infections are commonly seen in AIDS patients and stem cell transplant recipients, they also occur in patients with chronic steroid administration, malignancy, diabetes, indwelling catheters, and intravenous drug use.[16–18] Cryptococcal meningoencephalitis is the most common CNS fungal infection in immunocompromised hosts, with the majority occurring in AIDS patients with low CD4 counts ($<100$/mm$^3$). Cryptococcus is an encapsulated yeast found in decaying wood and soil frequented by birds and contaminated by their droppings.[19] Infection is acquired via inhalation and is disseminated hematogenously to the CNS. The yeast demonstrates a high tropism for the meninges and preferentially spreads along the perivascular spaces of the lenticulostriate and thalamo-perforating arteries.[20] Lesions are typically located in the basal ganglia, thalami, and medial

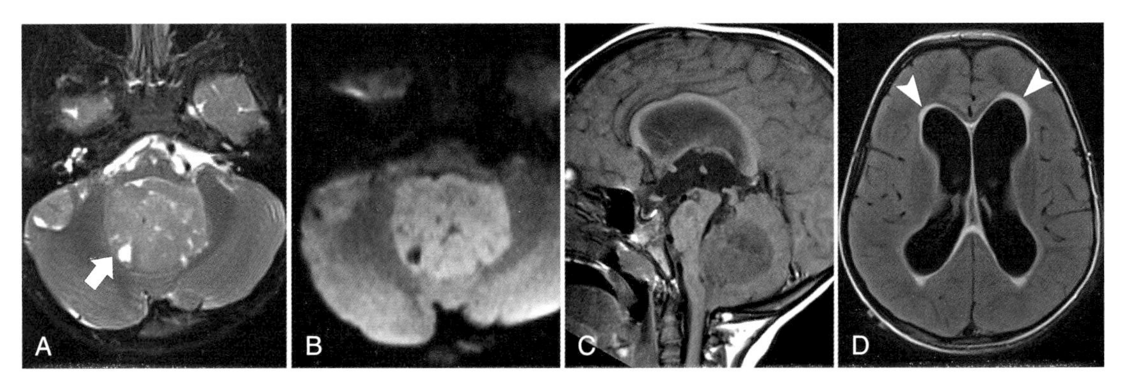


**Fig. 3.2** A 3-year-old male with medulloblastoma. Axial T2 (A) shows a large isointense mass centered in the inferior aspect of the fourth ventricle (white arrow). Note an additional mass along the lateral aspect of the right cerebellum. Diffusion-weighted imaging (B) shows increased signal due to restricted diffusion. Sagittal T1 (C) demonstrates mass effect on the brainstem with crowding of posterior fossa and enlargement of the ventricular system. Axial fluid-attenuated inversion recovery (D) shows hydrocephalus with periventricular interstitial edema (white arrowheads).

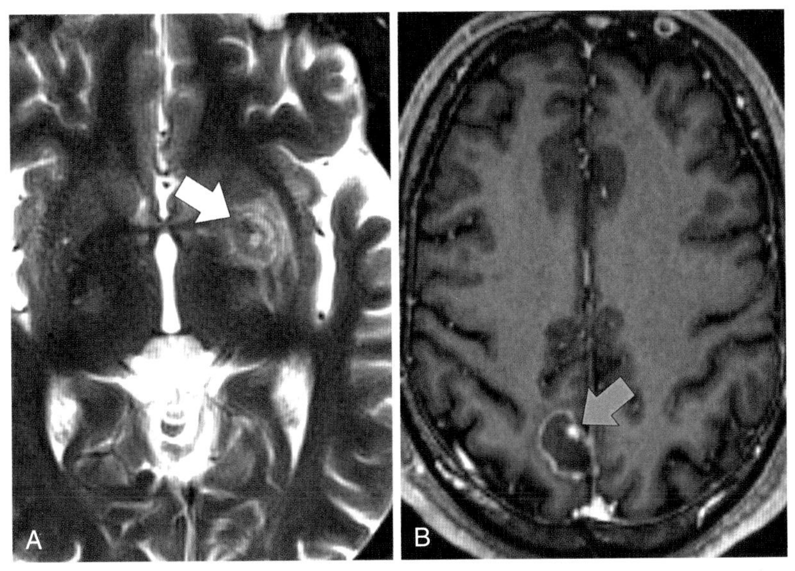


**Fig. 3.3** Toxoplasmosis in a 45-year-old male with human immunodeficiency virus/acquired immunodeficiency syndrome. Axial T2 (A) shows a lesion with concentric hyper- and hypointense signal intensities in the left basal ganglia (white arrow). Axial postcontrast T1 (B) shows an additional lesion in the right parietal lobe with a peripheral nodule resulting in an "eccentric target sign" (orange arrow).

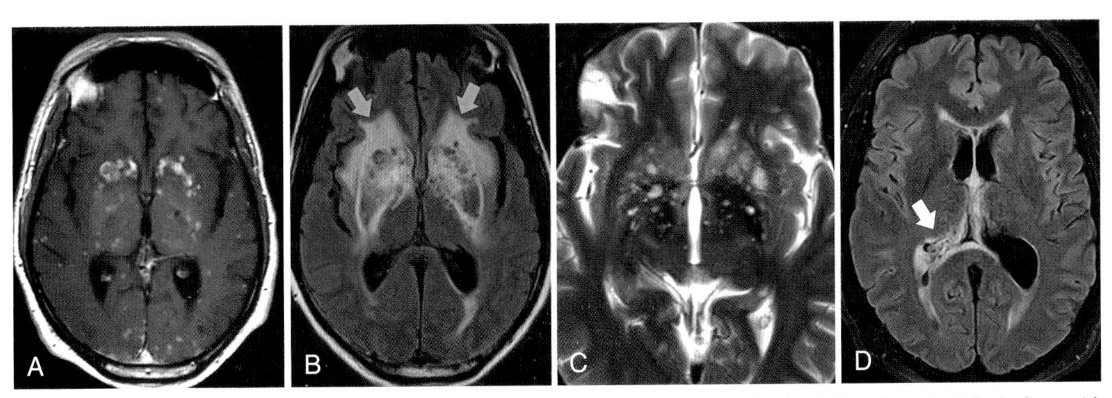


**Fig. 3.4** Cryptococcal meningoencephalitis. Axial postcontrast T1 (A) demonstrates numerous enhancing lesions throughout the brain, most in the basal ganglia. There is extensive associated edema on fluid-attenuated inversion recovery (FLAIR) (orange arrows in B). Axial T2 in a different patient (C) shows multiple cystic appearing lesions in the basal ganglia and anterior thalami consistent with gelatinous pseudocysts. Axial FLAIR in a different patient (D) demonstrates enlargement of the right choroid plexus due to choroid plexitis (white arrow). There is mild associated ventriculomegaly.

cerebellum but can occur anywhere in the brain. On MRI, there may be enhancing granulomatous masses (cryptococcomas) with variable restricted diffusion. Leptomeningeal enhancement is not a prominent feature, and its presence depends on the host's capacity to mount an immune response. Other findings include gelatinous pseudocysts, choroid plexitis, and hydrocephalus (Fig. 3.4).[21,22] Between 50% and 70% of patients have increased intracranial pressure and require therapeutic CSF drainage.[23] A normal brain imaging study does not exclude the possibility of cryptococcal infection.

*Candida* species enter the host via inhalation or by direct inoculation from trauma, surgery, or indwelling catheters. Infection may disseminate hematogenously in immunosuppressed patients, resulting in candidemia. Meningoencephalitis and microabscesses are the most common CNS manifestations, while macroabscesses, mycotic aneurysms, vasculitis, and infarction are rare.[24,25] Imaging findings of meningitis are nonspecific and may appear as leptomeningeal enhancement and/or sulcal FLAIR hyperintensity; however, MRI can be normal. *Candida* abscesses may be indistinguishable from pyogenic ones with ring enhancement and central restricted diffusion, although the degree of enhancement varies depending on the host's immune response.[18,26] Also, compared with pyogenic abscesses, fungal abscesses have a variable appearance, with intermixed areas of facilitated (rather than restricted) diffusion as well as intracavitary projections (Fig. 3.5).[27]

Invasive fungal species can cause aggressive infections in neutropenic patients with hematologic malignancies, and in those with stem cell transplants mortality reaches 50% to 80%.[28] Angioinvasive fungal infections are associated with high mortality and are most commonly caused by *Aspergillus* and *Mucor* species. Immunocompromised individuals are at risk of invasive fungal rhinosinusitis, which can spread to the orbits or intracranially via direct extension or through the valveless emissary veins.[29] The organism can also enter via inhalation and then spread hematogenously.[18] Isolated cerebral infection without sinusitis is highly correlated with intravenous drug use.[30] In immunocompromised patients with sinusitis, inflammatory changes in the pre- and retromaxillary fat planes raise suspicion for angioinvasive fungal infections, which may present with or without osseous erosions. On MRI, the normally T2-hyperintense sinonasal mucosa may appear hypointense and lack contrast enhancement due to necrosis (the "black turbinate" sign) (Fig. 3.6).[31] Intracranially, angioinvasive hyphal forms such as *Mucor* or *Aspergillus* are likely to result in parenchymal disease (Fig. 3.7).[18] Intracranial infection can lead to encephalitis with varying degrees of enhancement and abscess formation. Areas of T1 hyperintensity and T2 hypointensity may be present, which have been attributed to iron, manganese, hemorrhage, and/or hemosiderin-laden macrophages.[18,32,33]

Viral infections. Herpes simplex encephalitis (HSE) is the most common fatal sporadic encephalitis and is caused by the herpes simplex virus type 1.[34] Although recurrent mucocutaneous viral infections are common in immunocompromised patients, the incidence of HSE is not increased in them, presumably because CNS damage results from both direct viral injury and indirect immune-mediated factors.[35] The imaging hallmark of HSE is profound cortical edema affecting the medial temporal lobes, insula, cingulate

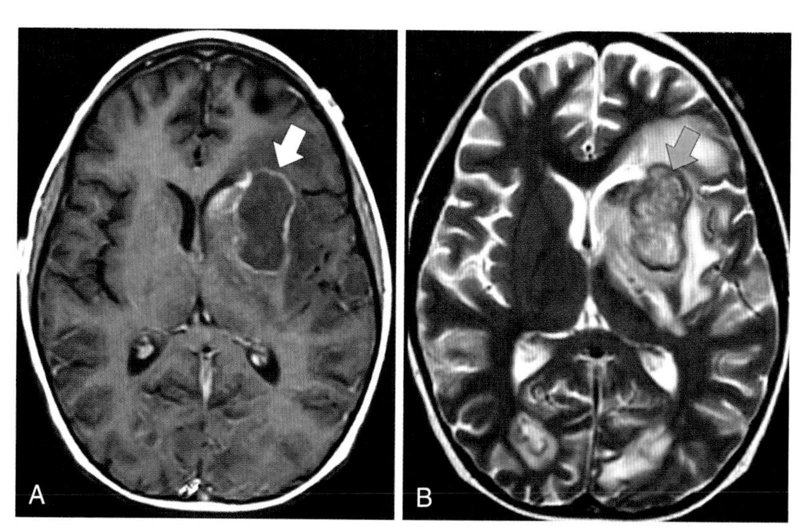


**Fig. 3.5** Fungal abscess. Axial postcontrast T1 (A) shows a ring-enhancing mass centered in the left basal ganglia (white arrow). On axial T2 (B) the lesion has a heterogeneous appearance, with numerous intracavitary projections (orange arrow).

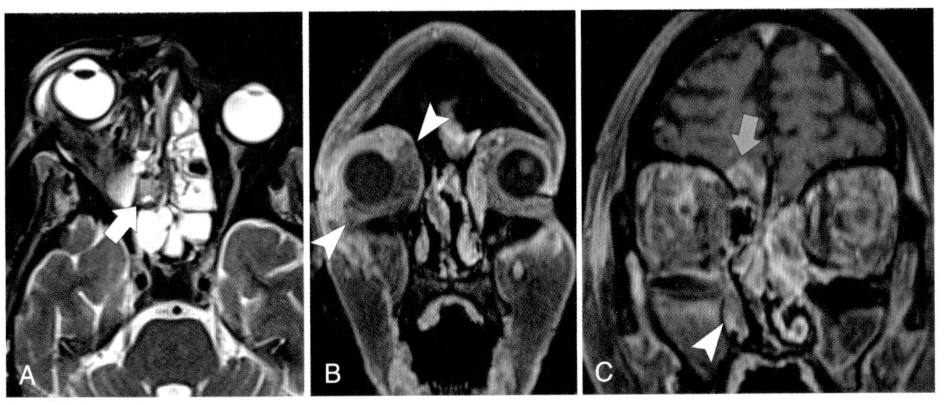


**Fig. 3.6** Invasive fungal sinusitis with orbital and intracranial extension in an 18-year-old female with acute lymphoblastic leukemia. Axial T2 (A) shows a hypointense appearance of the usually bright sinus mucosa (white arrow). There are extensive inflammatory changes in the right orbit with deformity of the proptotic globe. Coronal postcontrast T1 images (B, C) show areas of lack of enhancement in the right orbit and inferior turbinate due to devitalized tissue (white arrowheads). There is intracranial extension through the cribriform plate (orange arrow).

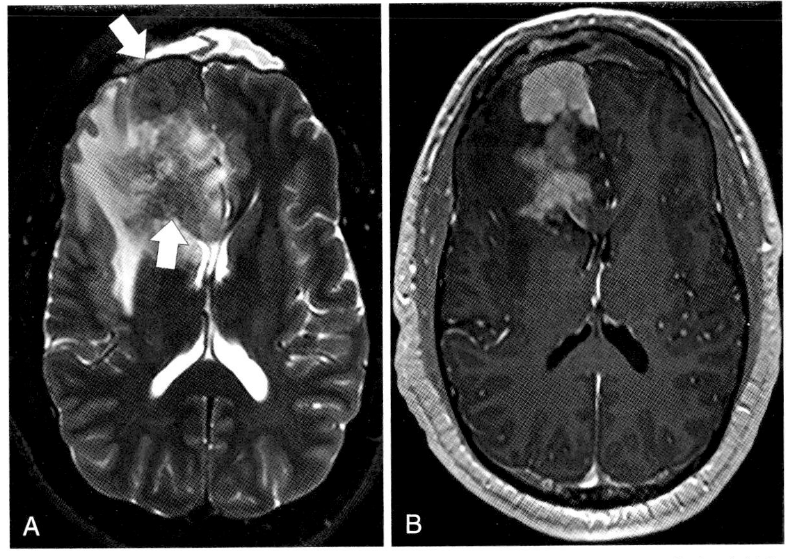


**Fig. 3.7** Invasive fungal sinusitis with intracranial extension. Axial T2 (A) shows extensive vasogenic edema in the right frontal lobe and subinsular white matter. There are areas of T2 hypointensity (white arrows) that demonstrate avid enhancement on postcontrast T1 (B).

gyrus, and inferior frontal lobes. Although the diagnosis may be suspected on CT, MRI with DWI is the imaging study of choice due to its higher sensitivity. In the acute stage, MRI shows restricted diffusion involving the limbic system that may be unilateral or bilateral and asymmetric. Patchy or gyral enhancement is common after several days, and hemorrhage is also frequent (Fig. 3.8).[36] Atypical presentations of HSE have been reported in immunocompromised patients, with widespread cortical, brainstem, or cerebellar involvement.[37]

Varicella-zoster virus is another neurotropic herpesvirus that causes varicella (chickenpox) as a primary infection.[38] The virus remains latent in neural tissues and may become reactivated later in life in the form of a vesicular rash (shingles) or with infection

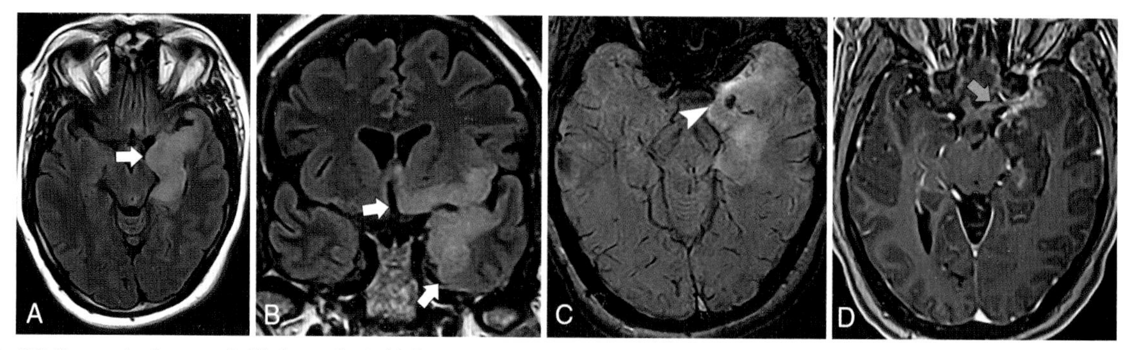


**Fig. 3.8** Herpes simplex encephalitis in a patient with fever, altered mental status, and seizures. Axial (A) and coronal (B) fluid-attenuated inversion recovery show marked cortical/gyral swelling in the left temporal and frontal lobes (white arrows) extending to the fornix. Susceptibility-weighted imaging (C) shows a small focus of hemorrhage (white arrowhead). Note areas of enhancement on postcontrast T1 (orange arrow, D).

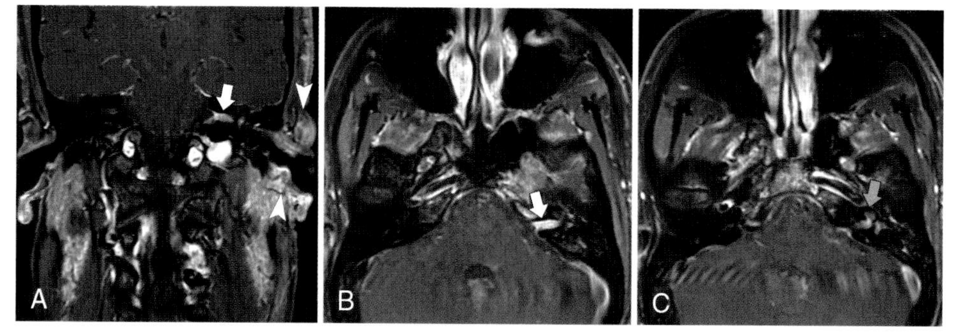


**Fig. 3.9** Ramsay-Hunt syndrome in a patient with human immunodeficiency virus. Coronal (A) and axial (B, C) postcontrast T1 show avid enhancement in the left internal auditory canal (white arrows). Note enhancing inflammatory changes in the left external auditory canal and surrounding tissues (white arrowheads in A). There is also enhancement of the left cochlea and vestibule (orange arrow in C) due to associated labyrinthitis.

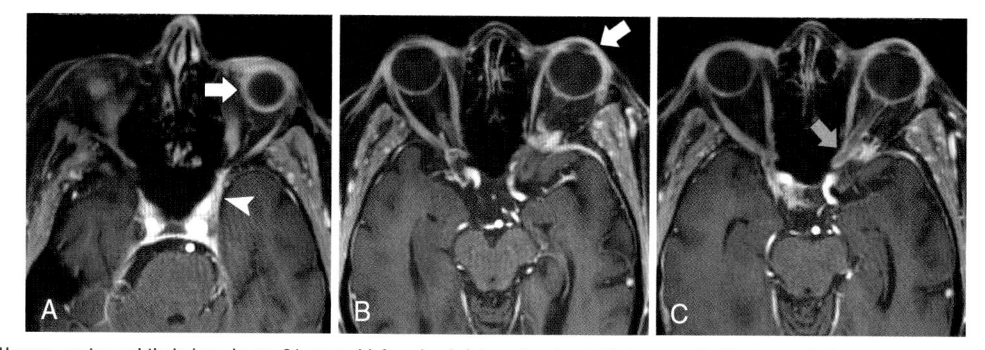


**Fig. 3.10** Herpes zoster ophthalmicus in an 81-year-old female. Axial postcontrast T1 images (A–C) demonstrate asymmetric thickening and enhancement of the left cavernous sinus (arrowhead). There is thickening and enhancement of the left sclera (white arrows) and abnormal enhancement along the left optic nerve sheath (orange arrow).

of the geniculate ganglion (Ramsay Hunt syndrome/ herpes zoster oticus) or ophthalmic division of the trigeminal nerve (herpes zoster ophthalmicus) (Figs. 3.9 and 3.10).[39,40] Such infections are more common and severe in immunocompromised patients. Reactivation rarely results in meningoencephalitis, myelitis, or radiculitis.[41] Patients can also develop a vasculitis involving small and large vessels, which may lead to infarction or hemorrhage (Fig. 3.11).[42] Unifocal large-vessel vasculitis usually affects the middle cerebral artery and appears to be more common in immunocompetent individuals. Vasculitis in immunocompromised patients is more commonly multifocal (Fig. 3.12).[43] MRI is the study of choice for evaluation of intracranial involvement and should include dedicated high-resolution sequences for evaluation of cranial neuropathies and ophthalmic involvement. On MRI, enhancement of the facial nerve and geniculate ganglion in Ramsay Hunt syndrome may be indistinguishable from Bell's palsy, and therefore the presence of otic pain or vesicular eruption are important clues for the diagnosis.[44,45] Compared with Bell's palsy, patients with Ramsay Hunt syndrome are more likely to have more severe and persistent facial paralysis.[44]

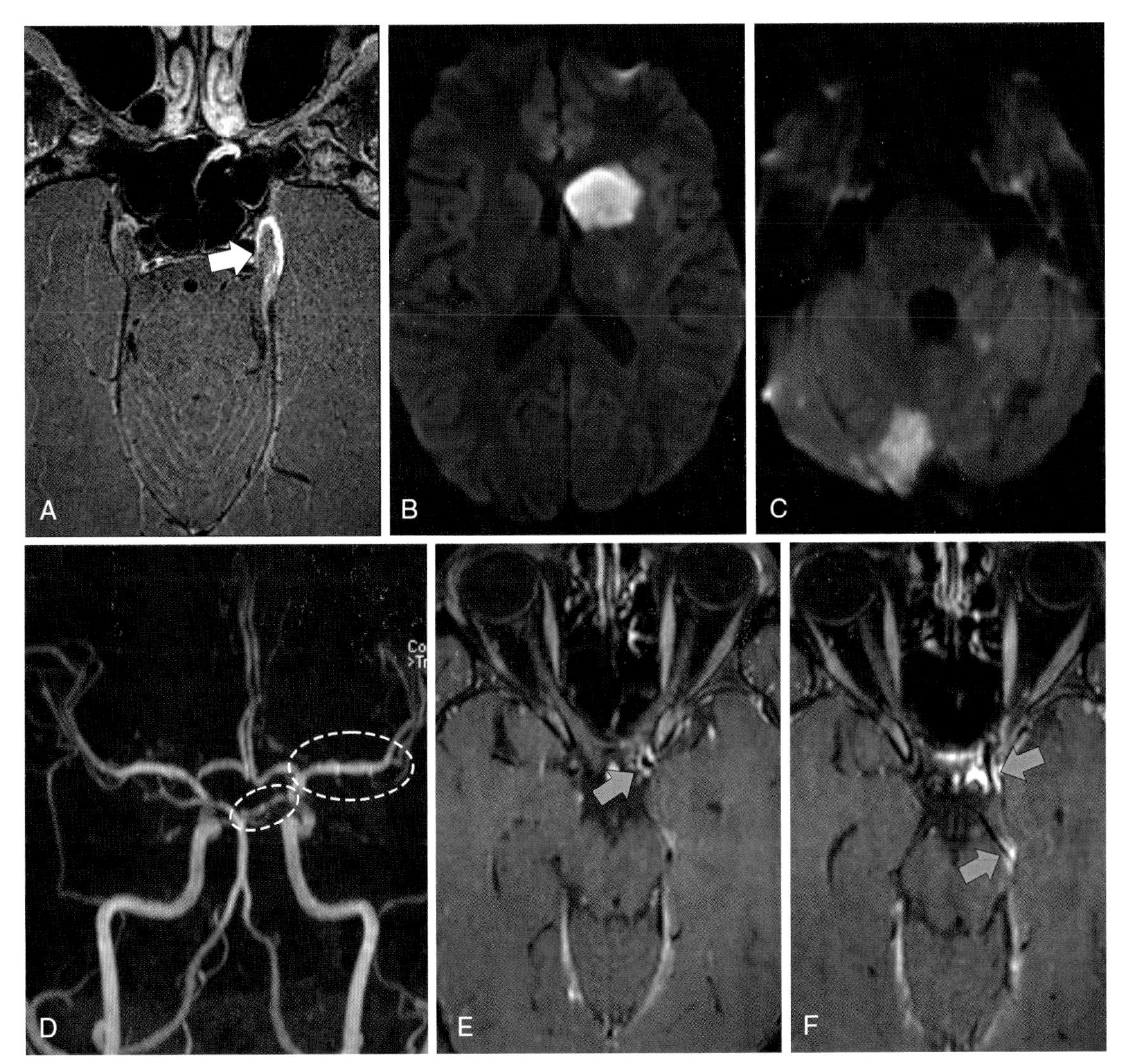


**Fig. 3.11** Reactivation of varicella zoster virus infection in a 24-year-old female with systemic lupus erythematosus on corticosteroids. Axial postcontrast T1 shows enhancement of the left trigeminal nerve cisternal segment and ganglion (white arrow). Axial diffusion-weighted imaging (B, C) shows acute infarcts in the left striatum and bilateral cerebellum. Frontal view time-of-flight three-dimensional magnetic resonance angiography reconstruction (D) demonstrates abnormal "beading" of the left posterior cerebral and middle cerebral arteries (dashed ovals). Axial postcontrast T1 vessel wall imaging (E, F) shows perivascular and vessel wall enhancement of the left internal carotid and left posterior cerebral arteries in keeping with vasculitis (orange arrows).

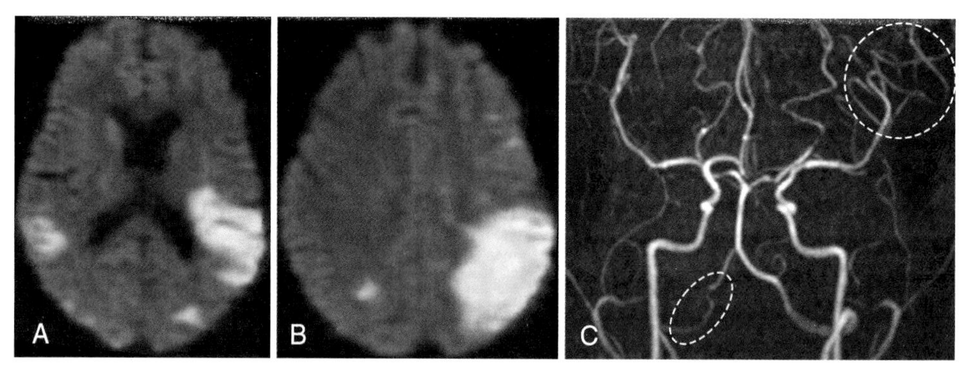


**Fig. 3.12** Varicella zoster virus vasculitis in a patient with acquired immunodeficiency syndrome. Axial diffusion-weighted imaging (A, B) shows multifocal areas of restricted diffusion compatible with acute infarcts. Frontal view time-of-flight three-dimensional magnetic resonance angiography reconstruction (C) shows segments of mild luminal narrowing and irregularity in right vertebral and distal left middle cerebral arteries (dashed circle and oval).

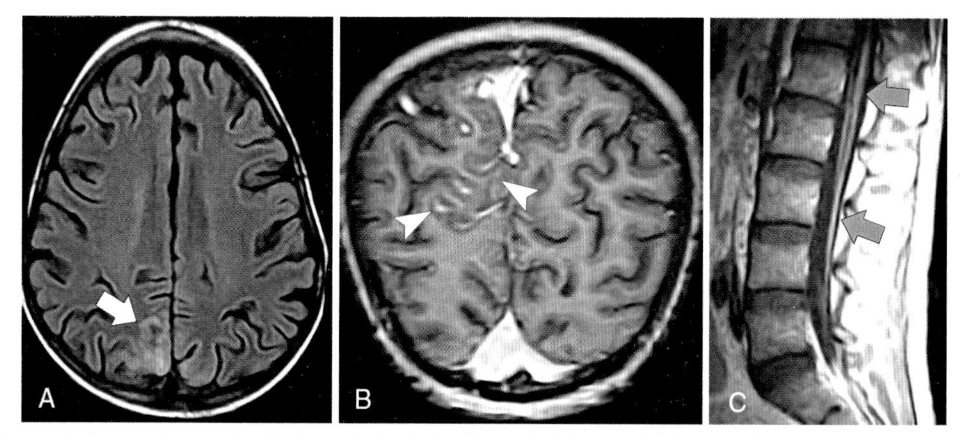


**Fig. 3.13** Cytomegalovirus meningoencephalitis in an adult patient with acquired immunodeficiency syndrome. Axial fluid-attenuated inversion recovery (A) shows edema in the right parietal lobe (white arrow) with associated leptomeningeal enhancement on postcontrast T1 (white arrowheads in B). Sagittal T1 of the lumbar spine (C) shows enhancement along the cauda equina due to radiculitis (orange arrows).

Cytomegalovirus is another member of the herpesvirus family that can result in latent infection. Encephalitis is a rare complication that develops in patients who are severely immunosuppressed, usually in the setting of AIDS. Imaging findings are nonspecific and can present in the form of encephalitis, ventriculitis, myelitis, and/or radiculitis (Fig. 3.13).[46]

The JC virus is a polyoma virus with a high rate of seropositivity among the general population, where it causes an asymptomatic latent infection.[47] Reactivation may lead to PML, a devastating demyelinating disease that occurs almost exclusively in patients with profound cell-mediated immunosuppression. Most affected patients have HIV or hematologic malignancies or are being treated with immunosuppressive or immunomodulatory drugs, most notably natalizumab.[48] PML initially affects the subcortical white matter in an asymmetric fashion and involves the U fibers. Extension to the corpus callosum and involvement of the parietooccipital white matter and middle cerebellar peduncles are common.[49] MRI is the modality of choice, and a normal study argues strongly against the diagnosis.[49] PML lesions have no significant mass effect and no significant contrast enhancement, although faint peripheral enhancement has been reported.[47] On DWI, newer and larger lesions may show an advancing edge of restricted diffusion corresponding to cytotoxic edema (Fig. 3.14).[50]

Immune Reconstitution Inflammatory Syndrome (IRIS). Usually occurring in the setting of HIV, IRIS presents with paradoxical clinical deterioration after a patient is placed on ART and regains the capacity to mount an immune response. Onset after initiation of ART is variable and depends on underlying opportunistic infections, ranging from weeks to months.[51] The inflammatory response may lead to worsening manifestations of a known or unknown infection.[52] A wide number of organisms have been implicated in IRIS, including cytomegalovirus, cryptococcus, JC virus, and *Mycobacterium tuberculosis*.[53] Incidence is inversely associated with CD4 count at the time of ART initiation, with counts typically below 100/mm$^3$.[53] However, IRIS has also been described in non-HIV patients with tuberculosis, where the CD4 count may be higher. Although usually self-limited, IRIS is associated with poor outcomes when there is involvement of the CNS.[54] Its imaging hallmarks are edema, mass effect, and contrast enhancement at the site of previous infection, which are best visualized on MRI (Fig. 3.15).[55,56]

Tuberculosis. Tuberculosis saw a resurgence due to the AIDS pandemic, the emergence of multidrug-

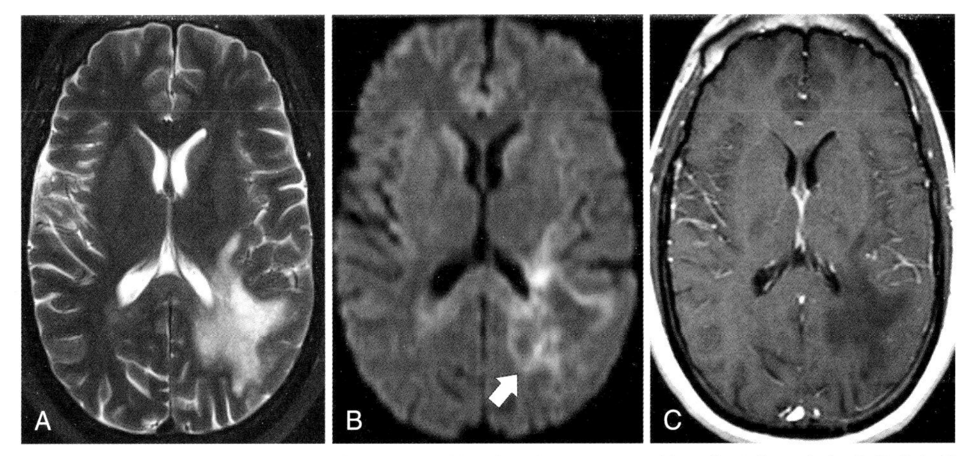


**Fig. 3.14** Progressive multifocal leukoencephalopathy in a 30-year-old male on long-term steroids and natalizumab due to Crohn's disease. Axial T2 (A) shows confluent signal abnormality in the left parietal lobe extending to the corpus callosum and involving the U fibers. On diffusion-weighted imaging (B) there is a leading edge of demyelination with restricted diffusion (white arrow). Postcontrast T1 (C) shows no evidence of enhancement.

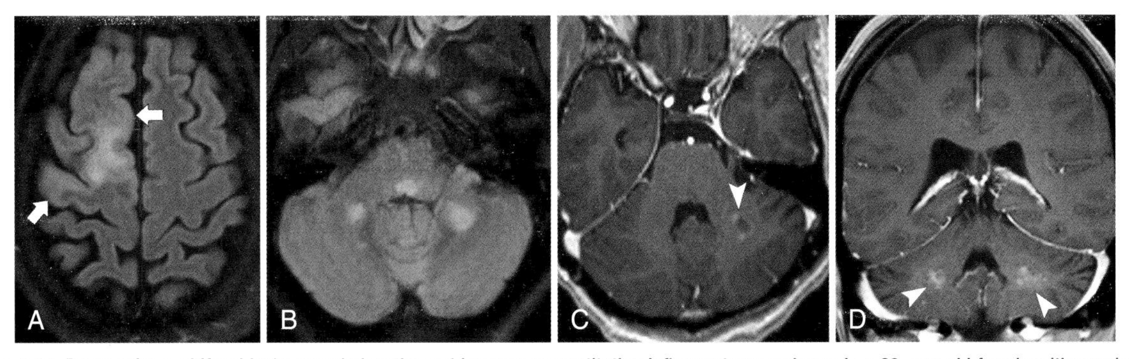


**Fig. 3.15** Progressive multifocal leukoencephalopathy and immune reconstitution inflammatory syndrome in a 29-year-old female with acquired immunodeficiency syndrome. Axial fluid-attenuated inversion recovery (A) shows signal abnormality in the right frontal lobe with mild mass effect and sulcal effacement (white arrows). There are additional lesions in the posterior fossa (B) with corresponding contrast enhancement (arrowheads on C and D).

resistant mycobacteria, and socioeconomic factors. It continues to be one of the leading causes of death caused by a single infectious agent worldwide, and was only surpassed in 2020 as the top infectious cause of mortality by SARS-CoV-2.[57] *M. tuberculosis* primarily infects the lungs and then progresses to other sites depending on the host's immune status.[58] CNS involvement occurs in 10% of non-HIV patients, and its risk is substantially higher in those with HIV, who are more likely to present with a disseminated infection.[59] Most patients are severely immunosuppressed, with CD4 counts below 100/mm$^3$.[60] The main route of dissemination to the CNS is hematogenous, with development of meningeal or parameningeal granulomas that then burst to release infection into the subarachnoid spaces.[61] Tuberculosis may cause meningitis (the dominant form), axial or extra-axial masses/granulomas, or disseminated infection. The classic imaging finding is a thick basal meningeal exudate with avid contrast enhancement, although such an appearance is less common in patients with HIV.[62] This exudate leads to vascular and cranial nerve encasement resulting in vasculitis, infarction, and cranial neuropathies.[63] Noncaseating tuberculomas appear as avidly contrast-enhancing solid masses that are typically hypointense on T2. Some undergo caseation with ring enhancement and others liquefy, resulting in a T2-hyperintense center that may be indistinguishable from a bacterial abscess.[64] A miliary pattern with punctate enhancing lesions may be seen in patients with disseminated disease. Conglomerate ring-enhancing granulomas are a feature that is suggestive of tuberculosis (Fig. 3.16).[65] Hydrocephalus is common.[63]

Nocardia. Nocardiosis is a rare infection caused by a gram-positive bacillus that primarily affects immunocompromised individuals. Infection in hospitalized patients most commonly involves the lungs followed by the CNS, and disseminated disease occurs in one-third of patients.[66,67] Imaging findings are nonspecific, with abscesses being most common, followed by meningitis or a combination of both (Fig. 3.17).[67]

Relevant imaging findings for the diseases discussed above are summarized in Table 3.1.

### CD8 Encephalitis

This is a severe form of immune-mediated acute encephalitis that was recently described in HIV patients receiving ART but with otherwise adequately controlled disease.[68, 69] Pathologically, it is characterized by massive cerebral infiltration with CD8 lymphocytes, astrocytosis, and microglial activation that predominantly occurs along the perivascular spaces.[70] On imaging, there is linear enhancement along the perivascular spaces, with varying degrees of surrounding edema (Fig. 3.18).[70]

## VASCULAR

### Hematologic Disorders

Thrombocytopenia is common in cancer patients and is most frequently caused by chemotherapy. Myeloablative treatments such as those used in leukemia and stem cell transplant patients confer the highest risk.[71] Other causes include tumor replacement of

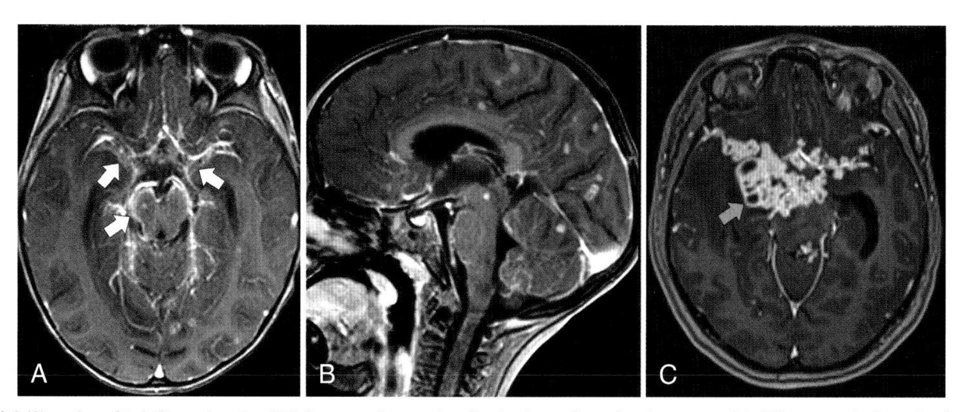


**Fig. 3.16** Axial (A) and sagittal (B) postcontrast T1 images show extensive leptomeningeal enhancement (white arrows) along the basal cisterns, brainstem, and posterior fossa in a 19-month-old male with central nervous system tuberculosis. Note numerous small parenchymal granulomas in keeping with disseminated disease. Axial postcontrast T1 in a different patient (C) shows conglomerate ring-enhancing granulomas in the basal cisterns (orange arrow).

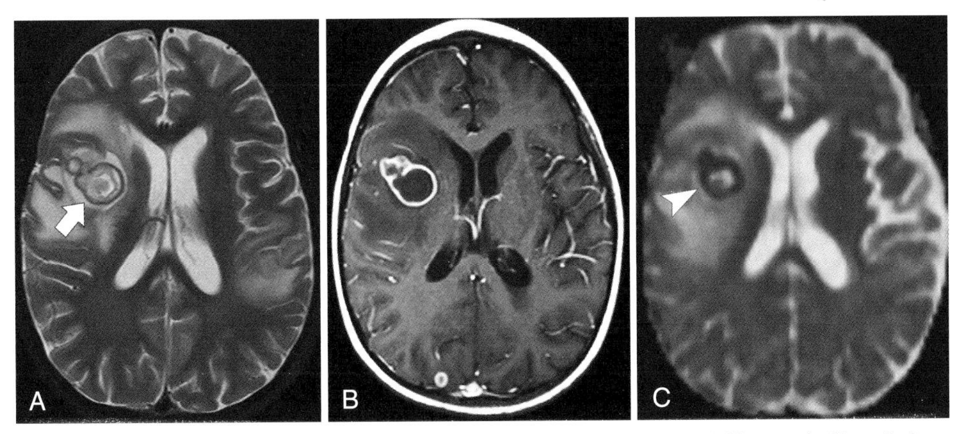


**Fig. 3.17** Nocardial abscesses. Axial T2 (A) shows a well-circumscribed mass in the right frontal lobe (white arrow) with marked surrounding vasogenic edema. There is associated ring enhancement (B) and internal regions of restricted diffusion (arrowhead in C). Note additional small abscess in the right posterior parietal lobe (B).

**TABLE 3.1 Imaging Findings in Opportunistic Infections**

| | |
|---|---|
| Toxoplasmosis | - Lesions in basal ganglia and grey-white matter junction.<br>- T2/FLAIR: concentric hyper- and hypointense rings.<br>- Postcontrast T1: peripheral enhancing nodule (eccentric target sign). |
| Fungus | Cryptococcus:<br>- Basal ganglia, thalamus, and medial cerebellum.<br>- Gelatinous pseudocysts, cryptococcomas.<br>- Variable enhancement.<br>Candida:<br>- Micro- or macroabscesses, mycotic aneurysms, vasculitis.<br>Acute invasive fungal sinusitis:<br>- T2-hypointense and nonenhancing mucosa (black turbinate sign). |
| Viruses | Herpes simplex encephalitis:<br>- Cortical edema in medial temporal lobes, insula, cingulate gyrus, inferior frontal lobes.<br>- Restricted diffusion in the acute setting.<br>- Enhancement and hemorrhage are common.<br>Varicella-zoster virus:<br>- Ramsay Hunt syndrome: enhancement of facial nerve may be indistinguishable from Bell's palsy. Accompanied by otic pain and vesicular eruption.<br>- Herpes zoster ophthalmicus: involvement of cavernous sinus and orbital structures due to infection of the ophthalmic division of trigeminal nerve.<br>Cytomegalovirus:<br>- Nonspecific findings. May appear as meningoencephalitis, ventriculitis, myelitis, and/or radiculitis.<br>Progressive multifocal leukoencephalopathy:<br>- Confluent white matter lesions involving U fibers, usually bilateral but asymmetric.<br>- No enhancement or mass effect, otherwise suspect IRIS.<br>- Newer and larger lesions may have a leading edge of restricted diffusion. |
| Tuberculosis | - Basal meningeal exudates are common.<br>- Granulomas may be solid (noncaseating) and hypointense on T2, caseating, or with a fluid center.<br>- Conglomerate ring-enhancing lesions are typical.<br>- May result in hydrocephalus, cranial neuropathies, or infarction. |
| Nocardia | - Nonspecific findings. May present with abscesses, meningitis, or a combination of both. |

*FLAIR*, fluid-attenuated inversion recovery; *IRIS*, immune reconstitution inflammatory syndrome.

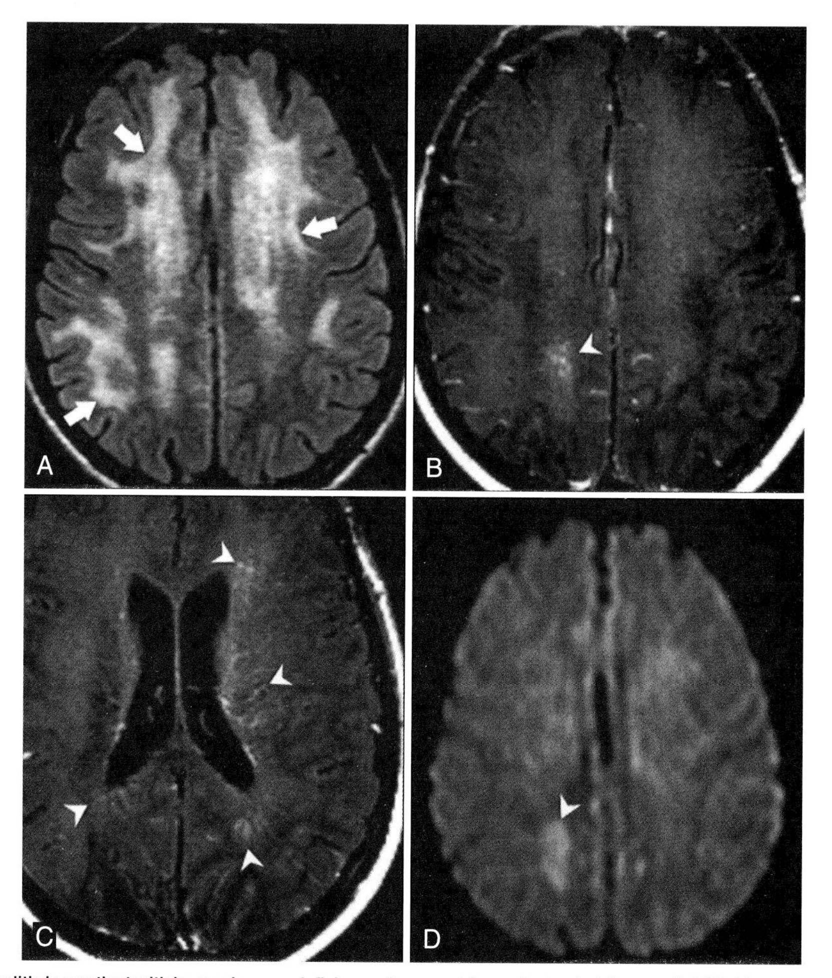


**Fig. 3.18** CD8 encephalitis in a patient with human immunodeficiency virus receiving antiretroviral therapy. Axial fluid-attenuated inversion recovery (A) shows extensive regions of white matter edema bilaterally (white arrows). Axial postcontrast T1 (B, C) demonstrates linear enhancement along perivascular spaces bilaterally (arrowheads). Diffusion-weighted imaging (D) shows areas of increased signal intensity (arrowhead). Used with permission from Lescure FX, Moulignier A, Savatovsky J, et al. CD8 encephalitis in HIV-infected patients receiving cART: a treatable entity. Clin Infect Dis. 2013;57(1):101-108.

the bone marrow or spleen, disseminated intravascular coagulation, thrombotic thrombocytopenic purpura, hemolytic uremic syndrome, and secondary immune thrombocytopenia associated with lymphoproliferative malignancies.[70,72] Patients are at increased risk of life-threatening hemorrhages and frequently require platelet transfusions.[72]

Leukostasis is a complication leading to hyperviscosity in patients with leukemia and is typically seen with white blood cell counts greater than 100,000/$mm^3$.[6] The pathological hallmark is the presence of white blood cell plugs and leukemic nodules in the microvasculature that cause vascular disruption and intracranial hemorrhages as well as small infarctions (Fig. 3.19).[73]

Prothrombotic states are also common in cancer patients and are a leading cause of mortality due to ischemia and venous thrombosis, which may be complicated by hemorrhagic infarction (Fig. 3.20). Multiple mechanisms that lead to hypercoagulable states include production of procoagulant factors, cytokine release, endothelial damage, stasis, and chemotherapy.[74]

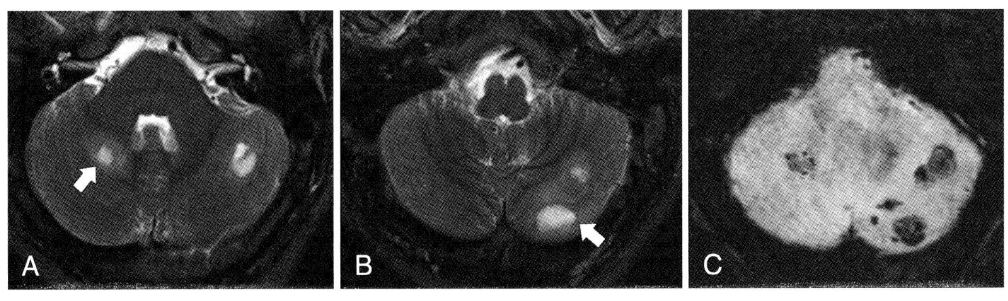


**Fig. 3.19** Leukostasis in a 38-year-old male with leukemia and white blood cell count of 245,000/mm$^3$. Axial T2 (A, B) shows multiple lesions in the cerebellum bilaterally (white arrows) with signal dropout on the susceptibility-weighted imaging sequence compatible with hemorrhages (C).

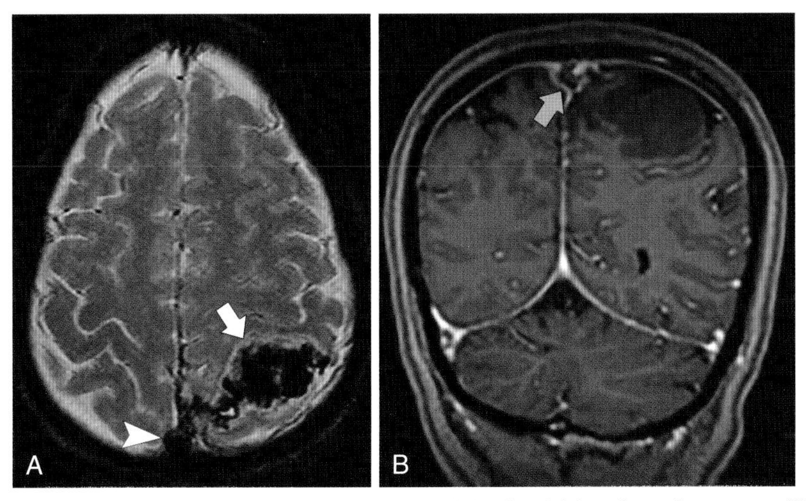


**Fig. 3.20** Thrombosis of the superior sagittal sinus with hemorrhagic venous infarction. Axial gradient echo sequence (A) shows signal dropout in the left parietal lobe due to hemorrhage (white arrow). There is also increased susceptibility artifact in the superior sagittal sinus related to thrombosis (arrowhead). On coronal postcontrast T1 (B) there is a filling defect due to thrombus within the superior sagittal sinus (orange arrow).

## METABOLIC

### Osmotic Demyelination

Osmotic demyelination is associated with rapid correction of hyponatremia but may also be seen in other conditions regardless of shifts in sodium levels, including hyperosmolar states, liver disease, malnutrition, and cancer.[75] Clinical manifestations depend of the extent of the injury and include ataxia, quadriparesis, and ophthalmoplegia, although some patients may be asymptomatic despite the presence of imaging abnormalities.[76,77] As is usually the case with metabolic and toxic insults, lesions tend to be symmetric. The pons is the most commonly affected site, and there is preservation of peripheral and transverse fibers and corticospinal tracts. Other areas that may be affected are the basal ganglia, thalami, extreme and external capsules, grey-white matter junctions, and hippocampi (Fig. 3.21).[78] On MRI, restricted diffusion is common acutely, and some lesions show contrast enhancement.[77,79]

### Wernicke's Encephalopathy

Wernicke's encephalopathy (WE) is caused by thiamine deficiency and is commonly associated with alcoholism. However, nonalcoholic WE is being increasingly recognized in cancer patients and is

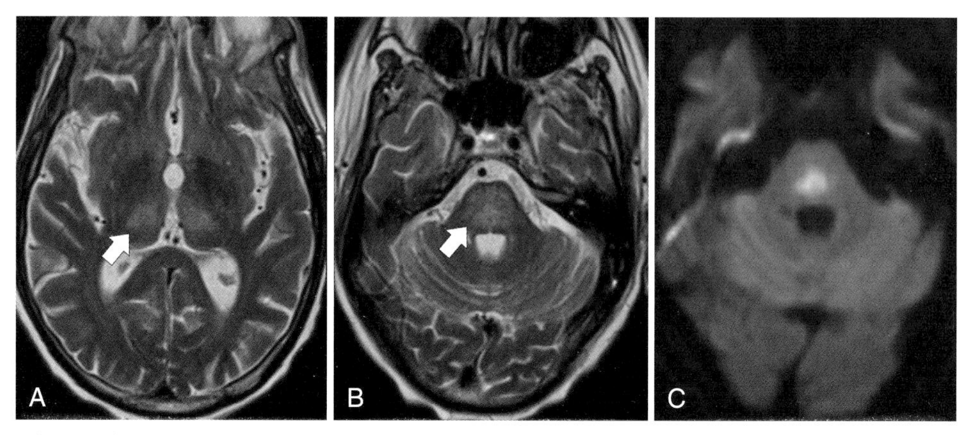


**Fig. 3.21** Osmotic demyelination in a 57-year-old male. Axial T2 (A, B) shows a bilateral and symmetric signal abnormality in the thalami and brainstem (white arrows). Diffusion-weighted imaging (C) shows corresponding central restricted diffusion in the pons.

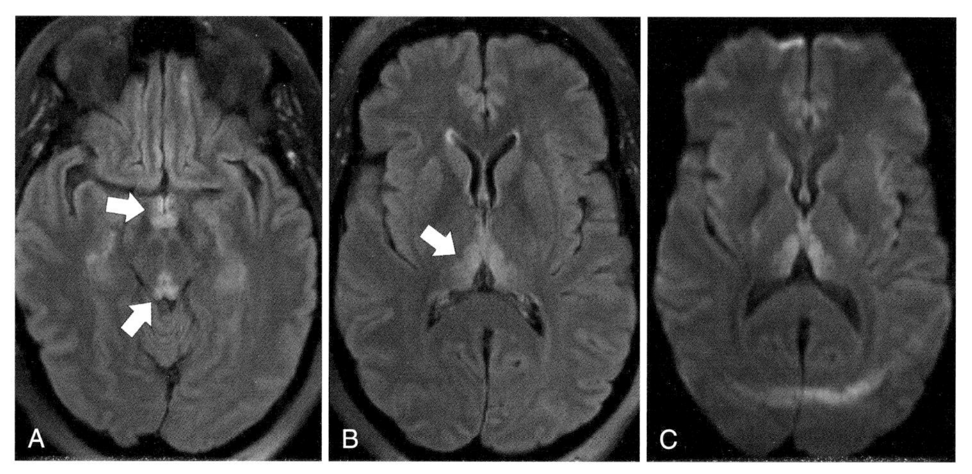


**Fig. 3.22** Wernicke encephalopathy. Axial fluid-attenuated inversion recovery (A, B) shows bilateral and symmetric signal abnormality in the mammillary bodies, hypothalamus, periaqueductal gray, tectal plate, and medial thalami (white arrows). There is increased signal on diffusion-weighted imaging (C) due to restricted diffusion.

due to malabsorption, vomiting, physiologic stress, and high cellular turnover.[80] Findings on MRI are characteristic, with symmetric T2/FLAIR hyperintensity most commonly in the medial thalami, mammillary bodies, hypothalamus, tectum, periaqueductal grey matter, and putamina (Fig. 3.22). Less commonly affected areas include the cerebellum, dorsal medulla, and cortex.[81] Enhancement can be present in the mammillary bodies and thalami and is more common in alcohol abuse, while involvement of the cortex is more common in nonalcoholic WE.[82]

## TREATMENT-RELATED COMPLICATIONS

Treatment-induced CNS toxicity is a major cause of morbidity in patients with cancer. Neurotoxicity depends on a variety of factors that include dose delivered, route of administration, interactions with other agents, and individual patient vulnerability. Herein, we highlight the clinical and imaging features of several well-known CNS adverse events of cancer therapy.

### Drug-Induced

Acute Leukoencephalopathy. Acute methotrexate (MTX) neurotoxicity is a well-known complication most typically seen in children with acute lymphocytic leukemia.[83] Patients present with stroke-like symptoms during the first to second weeks after drug administration.[83,84] On MRI, unilateral or bilateral areas of restricted diffusion are present in the centra semiovale in the acute phase, with subsequent changes on FLAIR and T2-weighted images (Fig. 3.23).[83,84] Symptoms and most imaging findings resolve on follow-up MRI studies. Subsequent MTX administration is generally not associated with recurrence or exacerbation of symptoms and MRI findings.[83]

Posterior Reversible Encephalopathy Syndrome. Posterior reversible encephalopathy syndrome (PRES) is a manifestation of acute leukoencephalopathy in cancer treatment. PRES has been reported with multiple drug therapies, such as antiangiogenic agents (bevacizumab), biological agents (ipilimumab), and commonly with traditional chemotherapy (cyclosporine, cyclophosphamide).[85] Patients present with headaches, confusion, visual changes, and seizures. MRI typically shows abnormal T2/FLAIR signal hyperintensities in the white matter, with predominance in the parietal and occipital lobes (Fig. 3.24).[85] Chemotherapy-induced PRES is

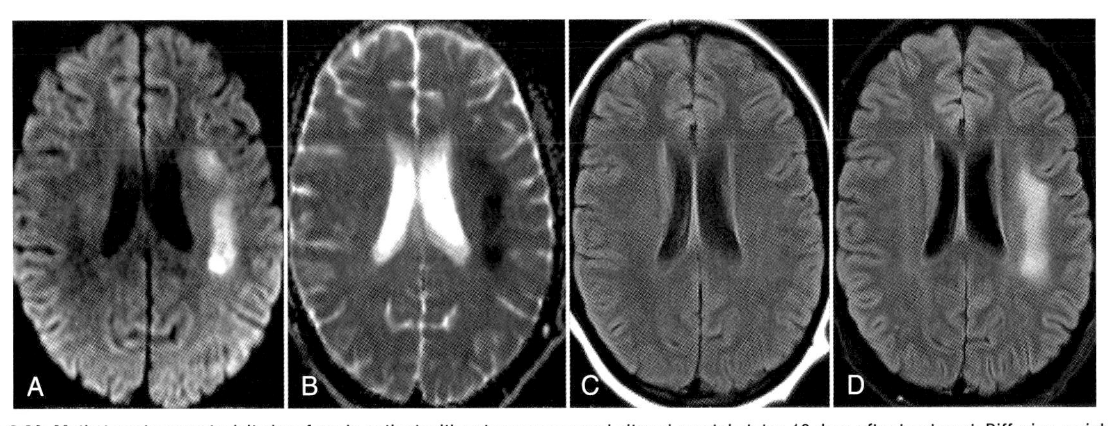


**Fig. 3.23** Methotrexate neurotoxicity in a female patient with osteosarcoma and altered mental status 10 days after treatment. Diffusion-weighted imaging (A) and apparent diffusion coefficient map (B) show an area of restricted diffusion in the left corona radiata without signal abnormality on fluid-attenuated inversion recovery (FLAIR) (C). Follow-up imaging 7 days after symptom onset (D) showed increased signal changes on FLAIR with resolution of the restricted diffusion (not shown).

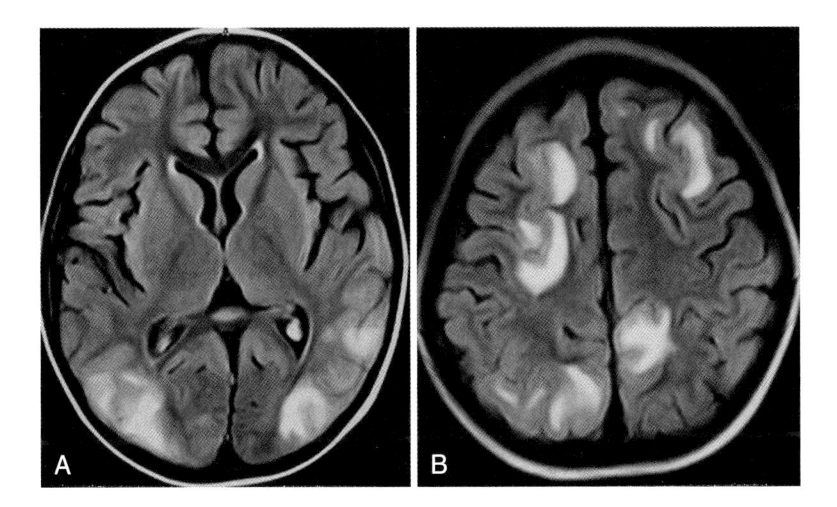


**Fig. 3.24** Patient with diffuse large B-cell lymphoma and 4-week history of increasing confusion after chemotherapy. Axial fluid-attenuated inversion recovery images (A and B) show bilateral symmetric increased signal in the subcortical white matter of the occipital, frontal, and parietal lobes consistent with posterior reversible encephalopathy syndrome.

thought to be secondary to a direct effect of cytotoxic therapy on endothelial function, although high blood pressure and hypoalbuminemia also contribute in some patients.[85] The clinical and imaging features of this syndrome are reversible once the causative agent has been discontinued.

Hypophysitis. Immune checkpoint inhibitors (i.e., ipilimumab) are the preferred treatments for many advanced solid tumors such as melanoma, lung, and renal cancer.[86] While they prolong survival and may lead to disease-free survival, treatment may be jeopardized by the development of numerous adverse effects, including hypophysitis.[86] Ipilimumab-induced hypophysitis typically occurs 8 weeks (6–14 weeks) after treatment.[86] Patients present with headaches, visual field impairments, hypopituitarism, diabetes insipidus, and hyperprolactinemia.[86, 87]

MRI is essential to assess the extent of disease and mass effect and to exclude other space-occupying lesions. Imaging findings typically demonstrate mild to moderate diffuse enlargement of the pituitary gland, loss of normal posterior pituitary signal intensity on precontrast images, and variable enlargement of the infundibulum, and the findings may simulate those of metastasis to the gland (Fig. 3.25).[87] Findings are reversible within 6 weeks, but only approximately 35% to 50% of patients recover pituitary-thyroid axis function.[86]

### Radiation-Induced

Radiation necrosis. Radiation necrosis (RN) is the most serious complication of radiotherapy, occurring in 3% to 24% of patients.[88, 89] The risk of RN is proportional to radiation dose (>50 Gy), fraction size (>2.5 Gy), and associated systemic therapies, such as chemotherapy and targeted therapy.[88, 90] Time elapsed after completion of radiotherapy is an essential factor to consider when making the diagnosis of RN, because 85% of cases occur within 2 years, and most commonly during the first year (60%).[88] The clinical presentation is nonspecific, including headache, focal neurologic symptoms, seizures, and cognitive impairment. RN may be a self-limited condition that resolves with conservative treatment. However, other cases require surgical excision and/or treatment with steroids and antiangiogenesis drugs.

The imaging diagnosis of RN is challenging due to its shared features with tumor recurrence. Both present as solid and/or necrotic contrast-enhancing lesions with variable surrounding vasogenic edema. Analysis of lesion components on conventional imaging in addition to advanced MRI techniques helps discriminate RN from tumor recurrence (Table 3.2). In general, the presence of a "Swiss cheese," "cut green pepper," or "spreading wave front" types of contrast enhancement,[91] restricted diffusion in the nonenhancing necrosis,[92,93] and a "cold" or low relative cerebral

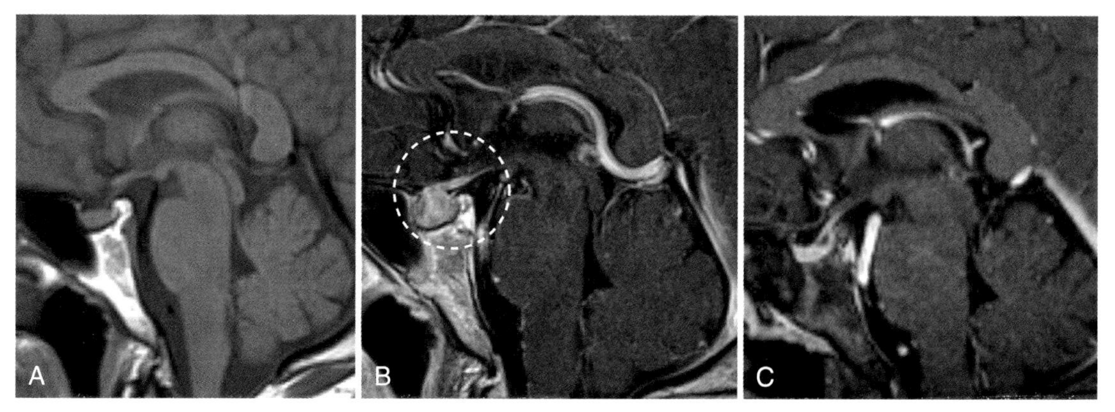


**Fig. 3.25** Female patient with melanoma presenting with fatigue and headaches. Sagittal T1 without contrast (A), before treatment, shows a normal pituitary gland. A sagittal T1-weighted sequence postcontrast (B) shows interval enlargement and diffuse enhancement of the pituitary gland and infundibulum (B, dashed circle) 2 months after ipilimumab administration, consistent with hypophysitis. One month after steroid placement and immunotherapy cessation, a sagittal T1-weighted sequence postcontrast (C) shows resolution of the pituitary/infundibulum enlargement.

**TABLE 3.2 Imaging Findings in Radiation Necrosis Versus Tumor Recurrence**

| Imaging Feature | Radiation Necrosis | Tumor Recurrence |
|---|---|---|
| "Swiss cheese" or "wavefront" patterns of enhancement | +++ | + |
| Lesion quotient[a] | + | +++ |
| Restricted diffusion in central necrosis | +++ | + |
| Restricted diffusion in solid enhancement | + | +++ |
| MRS: elevated Cho/Cr[b] | + | +++ |
| MRS: elevated Cho/NAA[c] | + | +++ |
| MRS: lipid-lactate peak | +++ | ++ |
| Perfusion: rCVB enhancing component | + | +++ |

[a]The lesion quotient is defined as the ratio of T2 hypointensity within the enhancing nodule on contrast-enhanced T1-weighted image (<0.3 indicates radiation necrosis)[9,91]
[b]A choline-creatine ratio threshold >1.11 favors tumor recurrence[18,95]
[c]A choline–N-acetyl aspartate ratio threshold >1.17 favors tumor recurrence[18,95]
*MRS*, Magnetic resonance spectroscopy; *rCVB*, relative cerebral blood volume; *NAA*, N-acetyl aspartate; *Cho*, choline; *Cr*, creatine.

blood volume in the solid enhancing component favor RN (Fig. 3.26).[91] The diagnostic performance of MRI increases when a combined approach of imaging techniques (i.e., perfusion, contrast-enhanced T1-weighted imaging, DWI, and MRS) is used to differentiate tumor recurrence from RN.[94]

Lastly, it is important to note that RN and tumor recurrence are not mutually exclusive, and that both entities can coexist within a single lesion. Therefore, a lesion may be classified as "predominant RN" or "predominant tumor recurrence" based on its predominant imaging features (Table 3.1).[89]

Myelitis. Radiation myelitis (RM) is a rare but increasingly detected complication, given the widespread and growing use of spine radiotherapy.[96] Once thought to represent a devastating disease, RM may be a transitory condition with clinical improvement in some cases.[96] Similar to other complications of radiotherapy, the incidence of RM is strongly dependent on radiation dose/fraction. RM is rare (<1%) when the maximum dose is limited to 13 Gy in a single fraction or 20 Gy in three fractions.[97] Khan et al.[96] reported a diagnostic delay since symptom onset of 6 months in a case series.

Symptoms at presentation are similar to other causes of myelopathy, including paresthesias, pain, motor weakness, and urinary incontinence.[89,96] The most common features on MRI include longitudinally extensive (thoracic > cervical) T2 signal abnormality involving the central or entire cord (Fig. 3.27).[89,96] Other findings include cord expansion (~50%) and contrast enhancement (45%).[96] These imaging features are nonspecific and can be encountered with transverse myelitis and other diseases. There is, however, a key finding that may help in the diagnosis of RM: the presence of T1 hyperintensity of the vertebrae included in the field of radiation due to fatty marrow replacement after radiotherapy (Fig. 3.27).[89,96] The differential diagnosis includes transverse myelitis, recurrent tumor, or metastatic tumor, as well as paraneoplastic myelitis in the context of prior history of malignancy.

Vasculopathy. Radiation therapy can induce a spectrum of slowly evolving lesions involving the vascular system, including radiation-induced arteritis (steno-occlusive and Moyamoya-like vasculopathy), intracranial aneurysms, and cavernous malformations (CM).[89] The first usually manifests with transient ischemic attacks, infarcts, or seizures; while the second and third can present with symptomatic intracranial hemorrhage. These entities share a primary pathogenic mechanism, where endothelial cells are directly damaged after irradiation.[89]

Radiation-induced aneurysms are a rare late complication of radiation therapy that may develop over a median period of 12 years after treatment.[89,98] These aneurysms are usually encountered in the anterior circulation, are saccular in morphology, and may occur in the surgical bed of tumors such as glioblastoma.[98] It has been suggested that, compared with ordinary aneurysms, radiation-induced aneurysms arise directly from the arterial wall rather than from a branching site, are more prone to rupture, and are more complicated to repair due to their fragile nature.[98] More

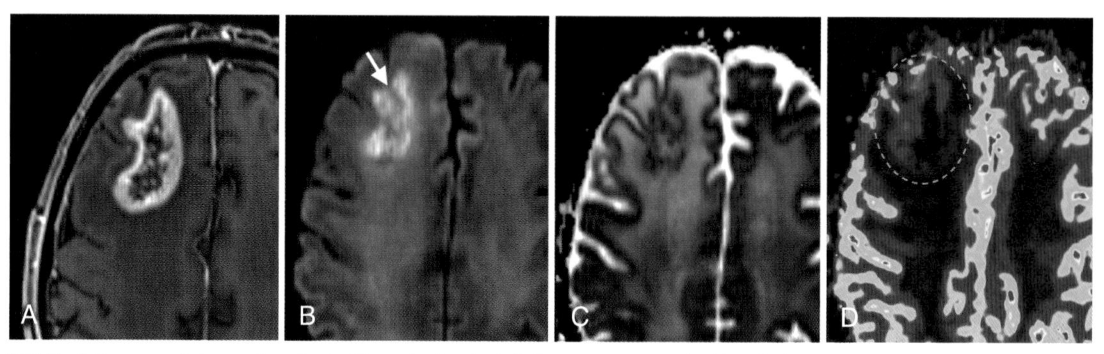


**Fig. 3.26** Radiation necrosis in a male patient with cerebral metastatic lung cancer treated with radiation therapy 14 months prior. There is a centrally necrotic ring-enhancing lesion in the right frontal lobe (A) with internal foci of enhancement giving the appearance of a "cut green pepper." The lesion shows restricted diffusion (B C) in the central non-enhancing portion of the lesion (B, arrow). Dynamic susceptibility contrast magnetic resonance perfusion shows very low relative cerebral blood volume (D, dashed circle), "cold perfusion," in the lesion and adjacent tissues.

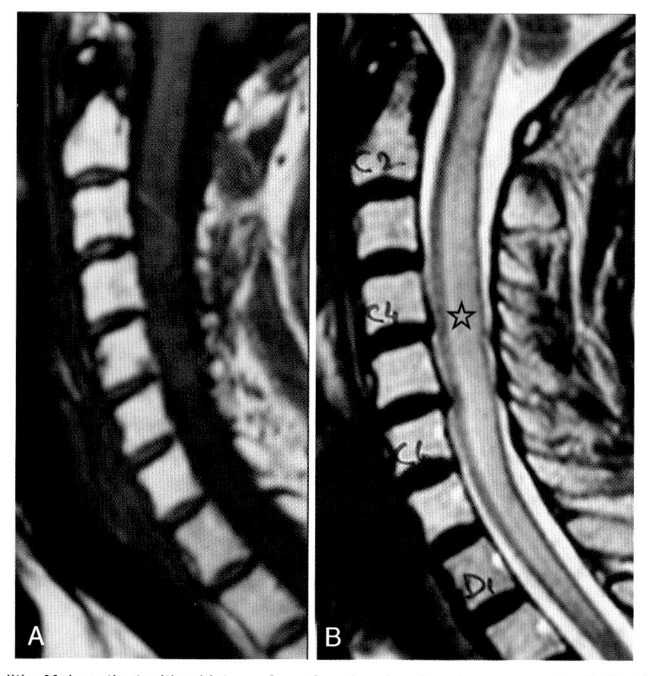


**Fig. 3.27** Radiation-induced myelitis. Male patient with a history of previous head and neck cancer and radiation therapy. Sagittal T1 (A) and T2 (B) images show cervical cord expansion associated with longitudinally extensive high T2 signal of the cord (B, asterisk), from the cervicomedullary junction to the upper thoracic spine. In addition, the marrow signal intensity of the cervical and thoracic vertebrae is diffusely increased in the T1- and T2-weighted images, consistent with fatty marrow replacement secondary to radiation therapy.

than half of the radiation-induced aneurysms present with hemorrhage, and subarachnoid hemorrhage is the most common presentation.[98] The imaging workup and diagnosis are based on CT-angiography, MR-angiography, or catheter cerebral angiogram, and prior history of brain irradiation.

Another type of vascular injury after radiotherapy is the development of CMs. Radiation-induced CMs are age- and radiation dose–dependent: they develop faster and at lower total dosage ($\leq$30 Gy) if radiotherapy is given during the first decade of life.[99] Based on these factors, the median time between radiation therapy and diagnosis ranges from 4.8 to 10.5 years (the higher the dosage, the shorter the latency period).[99,100] MRI usually demonstrates a heterogeneous T2 signal lesion with a dark peripheral rim of hemosiderin and blooming on T2*-weighted images (Fig. 3.28).[89,99,100] Radiation-induced CMs are more likely to be multiple and cause symptomatic hemorrhage compared with nonradiation CMs.[100]

Delayed Emergent Complications of Radiation Therapy. Stroke-like migraine attacks after radiation therapy (SMART) syndrome is a rare complication occurring a few years to decades following cranial irradiation. Most patients reported in the literature have had a total radiation dose of at least 50 Gy or relatively high fractionated doses.[101] Patients present with migraine-like headaches and focal neurological symptoms mimicking stroke, which are usually reversible. Findings on MRI are characteristic, with prominent cortical and/or leptomeningeal enhancement and T2/FLAIR cortical hyperintensity confined to the radiation field.[101] Restricted diffusion is variable.[102] Periictal pseudoprogression (PIPG) has also been rarely described and thought to be on the same spectrum as SMART syndrome. Although MRI findings are similar, patients with PIPG primarily present with epileptic seizures, whereas headaches and stroke-like symptoms are not a common feature (Fig. 3.29).[103] MRI findings normalize within a few months in both conditions but may recur in some patients.[101,103]

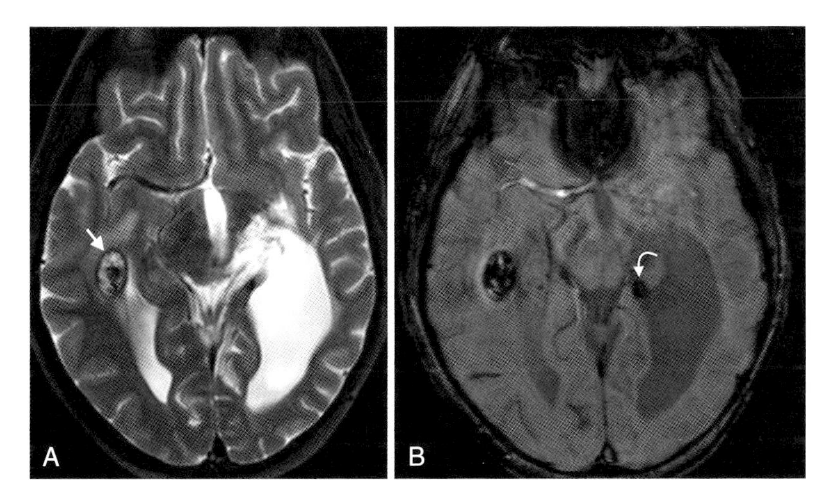


**Fig. 3.28** Radiation-induced cavernomas. Male patient with a history of prior tumor resection and radiotherapy. Axial T2 (A) image shows a focal lesion with a "popcorn" appearance, heterogeneous T2 signal, and a hypointense rim in the right temporal lobe (A, arrow) consistent with a cavernoma. Susceptibility-weighted imaging shows significant susceptibility artifact of this lesion and an additional smaller cavernoma (B, curved arrow) in the tail of the left hippocampus.

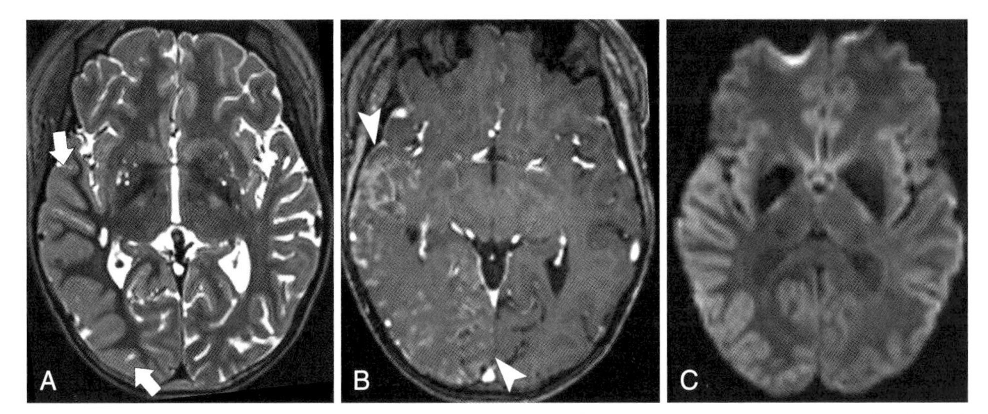


**Fig. 3.29** Periictal pseudoprogression. Axial T2 (A) shows cortical edema with hyperintensity in the right temporal and parietal lobes (white arrows). There is leptomeningeal enhancement on the postcontrast T1 image (arrowheads, B) and increased diffusion-weighted imaging signal intensity in the same territory (C).

## OTHER INTRACRANIAL CONDITIONS

### Seizures and Status Epilepticus

Seizures are a common complication in patients with brain tumors and can also be a manifestation of intracranial infection, PRES, drug toxicities, and RN. Patients with intracranial malignancies may not have a history of seizures, and in some of them the diagnosis of cancer is made only after they present with status epilepticus.[104] In patients with brain metastases, the presence of more than two lesions and location in the temporal or occipital lobes are factors leading to an increased risk of seizures.[105] CT shows emergent findings in 12% of all patients presenting with first-time seizures, with tumors accounting for 4% of underlying lesions.[106] MRI is useful to characterize an epileptogenic lesion and to evaluate for underlying lesions in hemorrhages of unknown etiology. In patients with status epilepticus, one may see T2/FLAIR hyperintensity with or without restricted diffusion in the cerebral cortex, subcortical white matter, hippocampi, medial temporal lobes, and pulvinar nuclei of the thalami (Fig. 3.30).[107] Various imaging modalities may show hyperperfusion during the seizure episode and hypoperfusion in the postictal state.[108]

### Paraneoplastic Encephalitis

Paraneoplastic encephalitis is an autoimmune inflammatory process directed against intracellular neuronal proteins. Several onconeuronal antibodies have been described and vary by tumor type, with the most common being anti-Hu (small cell lung cancer), anti-Ma/Ta (testicular cancer), and anti-CV2 (small cell lung cancer and thymoma). Patients usually present with behavioral and psychiatric manifestations over days to weeks. Seizures are common, and a minority of patients may present with fever.[109] Neurological manifestations often precede the cancer diagnosis. Paraneoplastic encephalitis typically affects the limbic system (hippocampus, medial temporal lobe, hypothalamus, and cingulate gyrus), brainstem, and/or cerebellum, although any part of the CNS may be involved.[109] Most patients have abnormal MRI, with T2/FLAIR hyperintense signal abnormalities and variable patchy contrast enhancement (Fig. 3.31). Restricted diffusion is rare.[110] Bilateral hypertrophic olivary degeneration is rarely seen in patients with paraneoplastic brainstem encephalitis.[111]

## SPINAL COMPLICATIONS

### Metastatic Spinal Cord Compression

Metastatic spinal cord compression is estimated to occur in approximately 15% of patients with advanced cancer, although its true incidence is unknown.[112] Breast, lung, and prostate cancers account for over 60% of cases.[113] Spinal cord compression can occur due to intradural masses and pathologic fractures as bone is weakened and replaced by tumor, or by

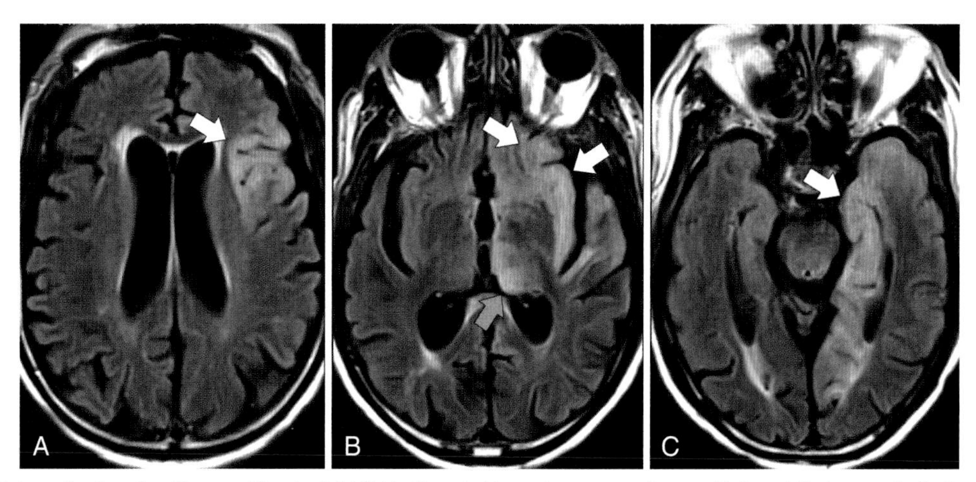


Fig. 3.30 Status epilepticus in a 72-year-old male. Axial fluid-attenuated inversion recovery images (A, B, and C) show cortical edema in the left frontal lobe, insula, and medial temporal lobe including the hippocampus (white arrows). There is also signal abnormality in the pulvinar nucleus of left thalamus (orange arrow in B). Polymerase chain reaction in cerebrospinal fluid was negative for herpes simplex virus.

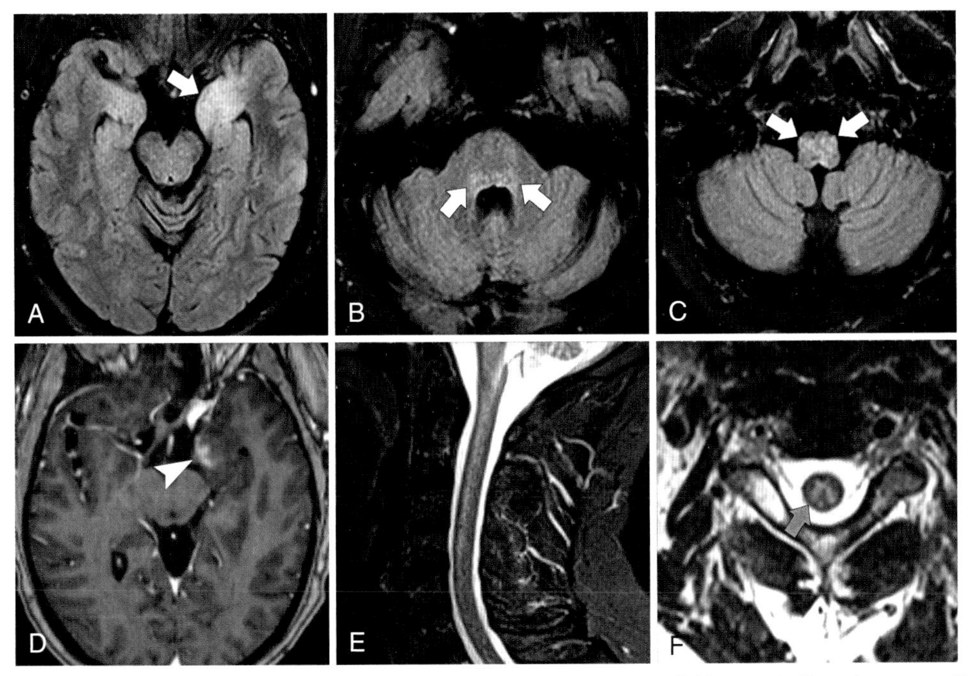


**Fig. 3.31** Paraneoplastic encephalomyelitis in a 42-year-old male with renal cell carcinoma. Axial fluid-attenuated inversion recovery (A, B, C) shows edema of the temporal lobes, left greater than right, and subtle signal abnormalities in the pons and inferior olivary nuclei (white arrows). Postcontrast T1 (D) shows a small region of enhancement in the left temporal lobe (white arrowhead). Sagittal short tau inversion recovery (E) and axial T2 (F) of the cervical spine demonstrate longitudinally extensive signal abnormality due to myelopathy (orange arrow).

epidural extension of disease. The spinal instability neoplastic score is used to identify patients who may benefit from surgical intervention.[114] Lytic lesions, those occurring at junctional spine segments, those involving the posterior elements, those associated with listhesis, and those leading to greater than 50% collapse of the vertebral body are likely unstable and warrant surgical consultation.[115] The extent of spinal involvement by epidural disease is best defined on MRI (Figs. 3.32 and 3.33). This is assessed by the epidural spinal cord compression scale, which helps determine which patients will benefit from radiation therapy as initial treatment (Table 3.2).[116]

### Spinal Infection

Immunocompromised patients are at increased risk of spondylodiscitis from bacterial, fungal, or tuberculous organisms, which usually spread hematogenously from distant sources.[117] Atypical infections are more commonly seen in immunosuppressed conditions.[117,118] Because the intervertebral disc in adults is avascular, the infection starts at the endplate and subsequently spreads to adjacent structures. In children, the disc is vascularized and represents the usual site of initial infection.[119] Tuberculous spondylodiscitis frequently spares the disc and has a predilection for subligamentous spread, presumably due to *M. tuberulosis*'s lack of proteolytic enzymes.[120] Epidural phlegmon or abscess can result in spinal cord compression, and these phenomena are seen in a small number of cancer patients who present for spinal irradiation (Fig. 3.34).[121] CT is useful to depict erosive changes in bone. The extent of bone marrow edema and spinal canal involvement, as well as differentiation between abscess and phlegmon, are best demonstrated with MRI. Severe infections can disseminate to the CNS with leptomeningeal involvement and radiculomyelitis. In addition, some opportunistic infections can directly involve the CNS. This is most commonly seen in tuberculous meningitis, which is associated with radiculomyelitis in 39% of patients.[122]

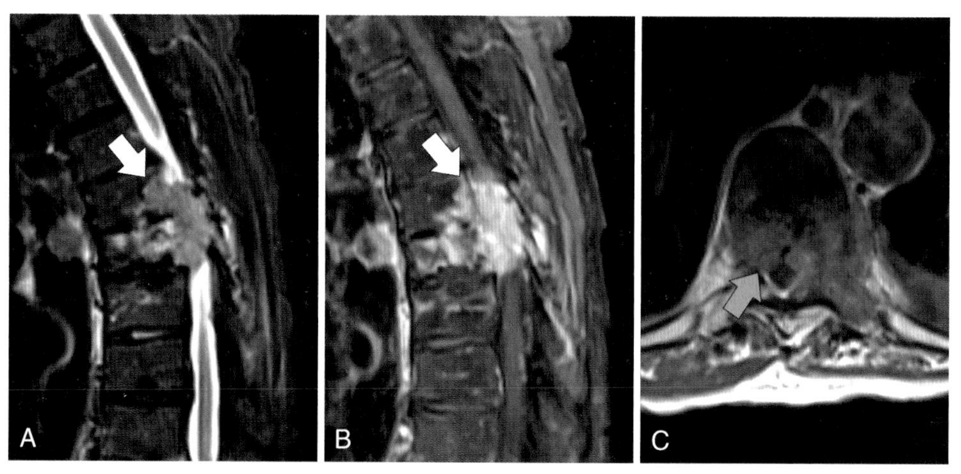


**Fig. 3.32** Vertebral metastases with spinal invasion in a 79-year-old female with breast cancer. Sagittal short tau inversion recovery (A) and postcontrast T1 (B) show avidly contrast-enhancing vertebral metastases in the midthoracic spine encroaching on the spinal canal (white arrows). Axial postcontrast T1 (C) shows epidural extension of disease with the typical "curtain sign" in the ventral epidural space (orange arrow).

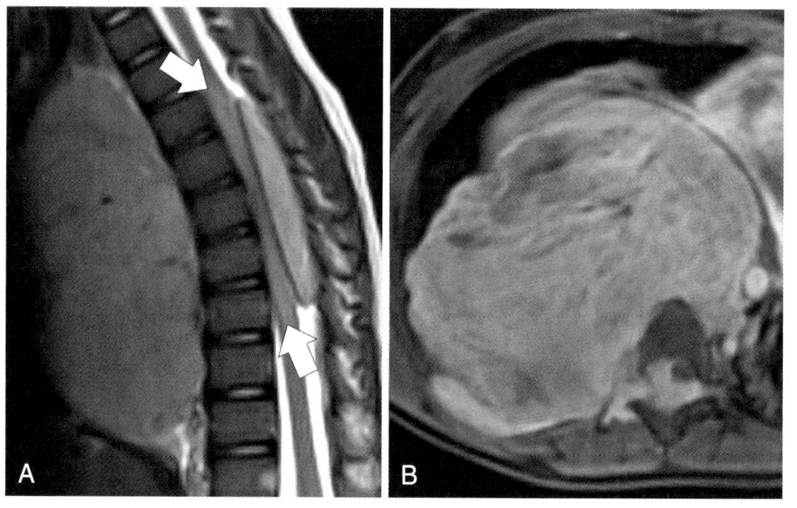


**Fig. 3.33** Neuroblastoma with invasion of the spinal canal in a 22-month-old male. Sagittal T2 (A) shows a large thoracic mass compressing the spinal cord due to epidural extension. Note increased spinal cord signal due to myelopathy (white arrows). The mass shows avid enhancement on postcontrast T1 (B).

## Paraneoplastic Myelitis and Radiculoneuritis

Paraneoplastic myelitis is rare and can occur in isolation or concurrent with encephalitis. Similar to paraneoplastic encephalitis, neurologic manifestations commonly precede the diagnosis of cancer.[123] Patients can present with acute or subacute myelopathic symptoms or a more insidious course.[111] The most commonly implicated onconeuronal antibodies are anti-Hu, anti-CV2, and, rarely, anti-amphiphysin.[123,124] The most common imaging finding is longitudinally extensive myelopathy with T2 hyperintensity and variable contrast enhancement on MRI (Fig. 3.31).[111] Signal abnormalities and contrast enhancement restricted to the lateral columns

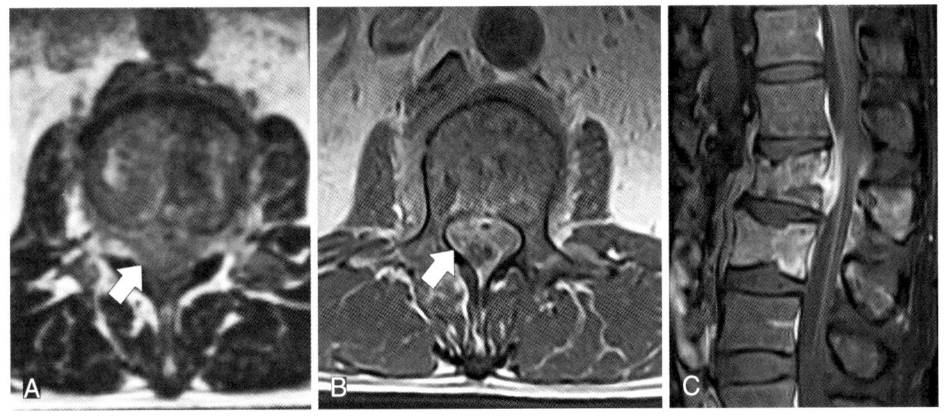


**Fig. 3.34** Vertebral osteomyelitis with epidural phlegmon. Axial T2 (A) and postcontrast T1 (B) show abnormal tissue resulting in near-complete effacement of the spinal canal (white arrows). Sagittal fat-saturated T1 (C) demonstrates diffuse enhancement of the epidural tissue consistent with phlegmon. There are prevertebral inflammatory changes.

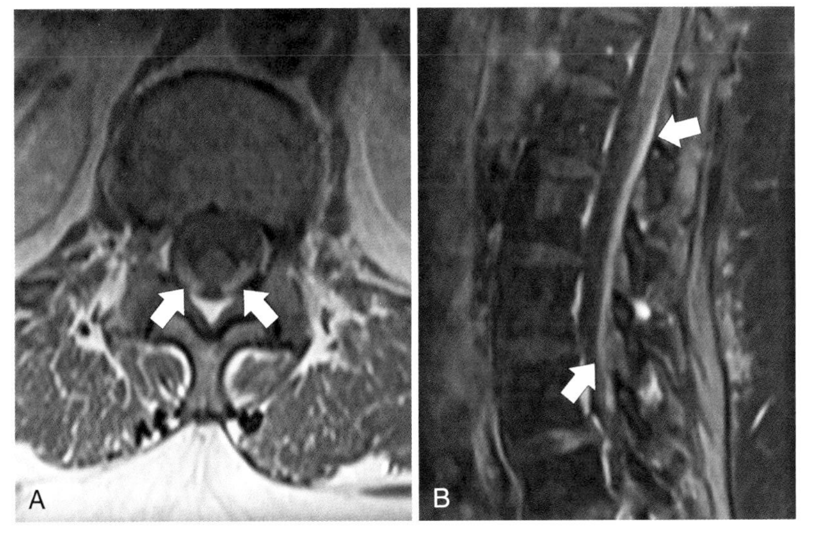


**Fig. 3.35** Paraneoplastic radiculitis in a 67-year-old female patient with carcinosarcoma. Axial (A) and sagittal (B) postcontrast T1 show diffuse enhancement of the dorsal nerve roots of the cauda equina (white arrows).

of the spinal cord have been described in a subset of patients.[123] Radiculoneuritis is rare, with a few reports related to anti-Hu and anti-CV2 antibodies. The most common presentation is sensory neuropathy; however, patients may develop ascending weakness mimicking Guillain-Barré syndrome (Fig. 3.35). Imaging findings are nonspecific and not well characterized due to a paucity of large patient series. On MRI, there is variable enhancement of spinal nerve roots that may show preferential ventral or dorsal distribution.[111]

## Conclusion

Neurological complications in cancer and immunocompromised patients are associated with increased morbidity and mortality. Mechanisms are varied and include direct tumoral effects, increased susceptibility to infections, systemic disturbances, autoimmune processes, and iatrogenic complications. Knowledge of characteristic imaging findings, clinical presentation, and treatment history are essential to provide an accurate diagnosis.

## REFERENCES


1. Thirumala R, Ramaswamy M, Chawla S. Diagnosis and management of infectious complications in critically ill patients with cancer. *Crit Care Clin*. 2010;26(1):59–91.
2. Raje N, Dinakar C. Overview of immunodeficiency disorders. *Immunology Allergy Clin North Am*. 2015;35(4):599–623.
3. ACR Appropriateness Criteria®—Acute mental status change, delirium, and new onset psychosis. American College of Radiology. https://acsearch.acr.org/docs/3102409/Narrative/.
4. Chalela JA, Kidwell CS, Nentwich LM, et al. Magnetic resonance imaging and computed tomography in emergency assessment of patients with suspected acute stroke: a prospective comparison. *Lancet*. 2007;369(9558):293–298.
5. Kondziolka D, Bernstein M, Resch L, et al. Significance of hemorrhage into brain tumors: clinicopathological study. *J Neurosurg*. 1987;67(6):852–857.
6. Navi BB, Reichman JS, Berlin D, et al. Intracerebral and subarachnoid hemorrhage in patients with cancer. *Neurology*. 2010;74(6):494–501.
7. Lieu AS, Hwang SL, Howng SL, Chai CY. Brain tumors with hemorrhage. *J Formos Med Assoc*. 1999;98(5):365–367.
8. Hong B, Polemikos M, Heissler HE, Hartmann C, Nakamura M, Krauss JK. Challenges in cerebrospinal fluid shunting in patients with glioblastoma. *Fluids Barriers CNS*. 2018;15(1):16.
9. Wong TT, Liang ML, Chen HH, Chang FC. Hydrocephalus with brain tumors in children. *Child's Nerv system: ChNS: Off J Int Soc Pediatric Neurosurg*. 2011;27(10):1723–1734.
10. Vivithanaporn P, Heo G, Gamble J, et al. Neurologic disease burden in treated HIV/AIDS predicts survival: a population-based study. *Neurology*. 2010;75(13):1150–1158.
11. Stansell JD, Osmond DH, Charlebois E, et al. Predictors of pneumocystis carinii pneumonia in HIV-infected persons. Pulmonary Complications of HIV Infection Study Group. *Am J Respiratory Crit Care Med*. 1997;155(1):60–66.
12. Bowen LN, Smith B, Reich D, Quezado M, Nath A. HIV-associated opportunistic CNS infections: pathophysiology, diagnosis and treatment. *Nat Rev Neurol*. 2016;12(11):662–674.
13. Tse W, Cersosimo MG, Gracies JM, Morgello S, Olanow CW, Koller W. Movement disorders and AIDS: a review. *Parkinsonism & Relat Disord*. 2004;10(6):323–334.
14. Kumar GG, Mahadevan A, Guruprasad AS, et al. Eccentric target sign in cerebral toxoplasmosis: neuropathological correlate to the imaging feature. *JMRI*. 2010;31(6):1469–1472.
15. Mahadevan A, Ramalingaiah AH, Parthasarathy S, Nath A, Ranga U, Krishna SS. Neuropathological correlate of the "concentric target sign" in MRI of HIV-associated cerebral toxoplasmosis. *JMRI*. 2013;38(2):488–495.
16. Rees JR, Pinner RW, Hajjeh RA, Brandt ME, Reingold AL. The epidemiological features of invasive mycotic infections in the San Francisco Bay area, 1992-1993: results of population-based laboratory active surveillance. *Clin Infect Dis*. 1998;27(5):1138–1147.
17. Richardson M, Lass-Florl C. Changing epidemiology of systemic fungal infections. *Clin Microbiology Infect*. 2008;14 (Suppl 4):5–24.
18. Mathur M, Johnson CE, Sze G. Fungal infections of the central nervous system. *Neuroimaging Clin North Am*. 2012;22(4):609–632.
19. Pyrgos V, Seitz AE, Steiner CA, Prevots DR, Williamson PR. Epidemiology of cryptococcal meningitis in the US: 1997-2009. *PLoS ONE*. 2013;8(2):e56269.
20. Liu TB, Perlin DS, Xue C. Molecular mechanisms of cryptococcal meningitis. *Virulence*. 2012;3(2):173–181.
21. Kumari R, Raval M, Dhun A. Cryptococcal choroid plexitis: rare imaging findings of central nervous system cryptococcal infection in an immunocompetent individual. *Br J Radiology*. 2010;83(985):e14–e17.
22. Xia S, Li X, Shi Y, et al. A retrospective cohort study of lesion distribution of HIV-1 infection patients with cryptococcal meningoencephalitis on MRI: correlation with immunity and immune reconstitution. *Medicine*. 2016;95(6):e2654.
23. Chang CC, Perfect JR. Repeated therapeutic lumbar punctures in cryptococcal meningitis - necessity and/or opportunity? *Curr OpInfect Dis*. 2016;29(6):539–545.
24. Goralska K, Blaszkowska J, Dzikowiec M. Neuroinfections caused by fungi. *Infection*. 2018;46(4):443–459.
25. Sanchez-Portocarrero J, Perez-Cecilia E, Corral O, Romero-Vivas J, Picazo JJ. The central nervous system and infection by Candida species. *Diagnostic Microbiology Infect Dis*. 2000;37(3):169–179.
26. Jain KK, Mittal SK, Kumar S, Gupta RK. Imaging features of central nervous system fungal infections. *Neurol India*. 2007;55(3):241–250.
27. Luthra G, Parihar A, Nath K, et al. Comparative evaluation of fungal, tubercular, and pyogenic brain abscesses with conventional and diffusion MR imaging and proton MR spectroscopy. *AJNR*. 2007;28(7):1332–1338.
28. Chen CY, Sheng WH, Cheng A, et al. Invasive fungal sinusitis in patients with hematological malignancy: 15 years experience in a single university hospital in Taiwan. *BMC Infect Dis*. 2011;11:250.
29. Chikley A, Ben-Ami R, Kontoyiannis DP. Mucormycosis of the central nervous system. *J Fungi (Basel)*. 2019;5(3):59.
30. Stave GM, Heimberger T, Kerkering TM. Zygomycosis of the basal ganglia in intravenous drug users. *Am J Med*. 1989; 86(1):115–117.
31. Safder S, Carpenter JS, Roberts TD, Bailey N. The "Black Turbinate" sign: An early MR imaging finding of nasal mucormycosis. *AJNR*. 2010;31(4):771–774.
32. Almutairi BM, Nguyen TB, Jansen GH, Asseri AH. Invasive aspergillosis of the brain: radiologic-pathologic correlation. *Radiographics*. 2009;29(2):375–379.
33. Marzolf G, Sabou M, Lannes B, et al. Magnetic resonance imaging of cerebral aspergillosis: imaging and pathological correlations. *PLoS ONE*. 2016;11(4):e0152475.
34. Kennedy PG. Viral encephalitis: causes, differential diagnosis, and management. *J Neurology, Neurosurgery, Psychiatry*. 2004;75(Suppl 1):i10–i15.
35. Piret J, Boivin G. Innate immune response during herpes simplex virus encephalitis and development of immunomodulatory strategies. *Rev Med Virology*. 2015;25(5):300–319.
36. Hauer L, Pikija S, Schulte EC, Sztriha LK, Nardone R, Sellner J. Cerebrovascular manifestations of herpes simplex virus infection of the central nervous system: a systematic review. *J neuroinflammation*. 2019;16(1):19.
37. Tan IL, McArthur JC, Venkatesan A, Nath A. Atypical manifestations and poor outcome of herpes simplex encephalitis in the immunocompromised. *Neurology*. 2012;79(21):2125–2132.
38. Ahmed AM, Brantley JS, Madkan V, Mendoza N, Tyring SK. Managing herpes zoster in immunocompromised patients. *Herpes*. 2007;14(2):32–36.
39. Gilden D, Cohrs RJ, Mahalingam R, Nagel MA. Neurological disease produced by varicella zoster virus reactivation without rash. *Curr Top Microbiology Immunology*. 2010;342:243–253.
40. Tran KD, Falcone MM, Choi DS, et al. Epidemiology of herpes zoster ophthalmicus: recurrence and chronicity. *Ophthalmology*. 2016;123(7):1469–1475.

41. Nagel MA, Gilden D. Neurological complications of varicella zoster virus reactivation. *Curr OpNeurol*. 2014;27(3):356–360.
42. Nagel MA, Cohrs RJ, Mahalingam R, et al. The varicella zoster virus vasculopathies: clinical, CSF, imaging, and virologic features. *Neurology*. 2008;70(11):853–860.
43. Gilden DH, Lipton HL, Wolf JS, et al. Two patients with unusual forms of varicella-zoster virus vasculopathy. *N Engl J Med*. 2002;347(19):1500–1503.
44. Sweeney CJ, Gilden DH. Ramsay Hunt syndrome. *J Neurology, Neurosurgery, Psychiatry*. 2001;71(2):149–154.
45. Tada Y, Aoyagi M, Tojima H, et al. Gd-DTPA enhanced MRI in Ramsay Hunt syndrome. *Acta Oto-Laryngologica Supplementum*. 1994;511:170–174.
46. Singer EJ, Valdes-Sueiras M, Commins D, Levine A. Neurologic presentations of AIDS. *Neurologic Clin*. 2010;28(1):253–275.
47. Cortese I, Reich DS, Nath A. Progressive multifocal leukoencephalopathy and the spectrum of JC virus-related disease. *Nat Rev Neurol*. 2021;17(1):37–51.
48. Kartau M, Sipila JO, Auvinen E, Palomaki M, Verkkoniemi-Ahola A. Progressive multifocal leukoencephalopathy: current insights. *Degener Neurol Neuromuscul Dis*. 2019;9:109–121.
49. Sahraian MA, Radue EW, Eshaghi A, Besliu S, Minagar A. Progressive multifocal leukoencephalopathy: a review of the neuroimaging features and differential diagnosis. *Eur J Neurology: Off J Eur Federation Neurological Societies*. 2012; 19(8):1060–1069.
50. Bergui M, Bradac GB, Oguz KK, et al. Progressive multifocal leukoencephalopathy: diffusion-weighted imaging and pathological correlations. *Neuroradiology*. 2004;46(1):22–25.
51. Murdoch DM, Venter WD, Van Rie A, Feldman C. Immune reconstitution inflammatory syndrome (IRIS): review of common infectious manifestations and treatment options. *AIDS Res Ther*. 2007;4:9.
52. Armstrong WS. The immune reconstitution inflammatory syndrome: a clinical update. *Curr Infect Dis Rep*. 2013;15(1):39–45.
53. Muller M, Wandel S, Colebunders R, et al. Immune reconstitution inflammatory syndrome in patients starting antiretroviral therapy for HIV infection: a systematic review and meta-analysis. *Lancet Infect Dis*. 2010;10(4):251–261.
54. Bahr N, Boulware DR, Marais S, Scriven J, Wilkinson RJ, Meintjes G. Central nervous system immune reconstitution inflammatory syndrome. *Curr Infect Dis Rep*. 2013;15 (6):583–593.
55. Gheuens S, Ngo L, Wang X, Alsop DC, Lenkinski RE, Koralnik IJ. Metabolic profile of PML lesions in patients with and without IRIS: an observational study. *Neurology*. 2012;79(10):1041–1048.
56. Post MJ, Thurnher MM, Clifford DB, et al. CNS-immune reconstitution inflammatory syndrome in the setting of HIV infection, part 1: overview and discussion of progressive multifocal leukoencephalopathy-immune reconstitution inflammatory syndrome and cryptococcal-immune reconstitution inflammatory syndrome. *AJNR Am J neuroradiology*. 2013;34(7):1297–1307.
57. Chakaya J, Khan M, Ntoumi F, et al. Global Tuberculosis Report 2020 - Reflections on the Global TB burden, treatment and prevention efforts. *Int J Infect Dis*. 2021;113(Suppl 1): S7–S12.
58. Smith I. Mycobacterium tuberculosis pathogenesis and molecular determinants of virulence. *Clin Microbiology Rev*. 2003;16(3):463–496.
59. Bourgi K, Fiske C, Sterling TR. Tuberculosis meningitis. *Curr Infect Dis Rep*. 2017;19(11):39.
60. Leeds IL, Magee MJ, Kurbatova EV, et al. Site of extrapulmonary tuberculosis is associated with HIV infection. *Clin Infect Dis*. 2012;55(1):75–81.
61. Wilkinson RJ, Rohlwink U, Misra UK, et al. Tuberculous meningitis. *Nat Rev Neurol*. 2017;13(10):581–598.
62. Katrak SM, Shembalkar PK, Bijwe SR, Bhandarkar LD. The clinical, radiological and pathological profile of tuberculous meningitis in patients with and without human immunodeficiency virus infection. *J Neurological Sci*. 2000;181(1-2):118–126.
63. Dian S, Hermawan R, van Laarhoven A, et al. Brain MRI findings in relation to clinical characteristics and outcome of tuberculous meningitis. *PLoS ONE*. 2020;15(11):e0241974.
64. Chaudhary V, Bano S, Garga UC. Central nervous system tuberculosis: an imaging perspective. *Can Assoc Radiologists J*. 2017;68(2):161–170.
65. Kim TK, Chang KH, Kim CJ, Goo JM, Kook MC, Han MH. Intracranial tuberculoma: comparison of MR with pathologic findings. *AJNR*. 1995;16(9):1903–1908.
66. Beaman BL, Beaman L. Nocardia species: host-parasite relationships. *Clin Microbiology Rev*. 1994;7(2):213–264.
67. Anagnostou T, Arvanitis M, Kourkoumpetis TK, Desalermos A, Carneiro HA, Mylonakis E. Nocardiosis of the central nervous system: experience from a general hospital and review of 84 cases from the literature. *Medicine*. 2014;93(1):19–32.
68. Miller RF, Isaacson PG, Hall-Craggs M, et al. Cerebral CD8+ lymphocytosis in HIV-1 infected patients with immune restoration induced by HAART. *Acta Neuropathologica*. 2004;108(1):17–23.
69. Lucas SB, Wong KT, Nightingale S, Miller RF. HIV-associated CD8 encephalitis: A UK case series and review of histopathologically confirmed cases. *Front Neurol*. 2021;12:628296.
70. Lescure FX, Moulignier A, Savatovsky J, et al. CD8 encephalitis in HIV-infected patients receiving cART: a treatable entity. *Clin Infect Dis*. 2013;57(1):101–108.
71. Liebman HA. Thrombocytopenia in cancer patients. Thromb Res. *133*. 2014;Suppl 2:S63–S69.
72. Carlson KS, DeSancho MT. Hematological issues in critically ill patients with cancer. *Crit Care Clin*. 2010;26(1):107–132.
73. Koenig MK, Sitton CW, Wang M, Slopis JM. Central nervous system complications of blastic hyperleukocytosis in childhood acute lymphoblastic leukemia: diagnostic and prognostic implications. *J Child Neurol*. 2008;23(11):1347–1352.
74. Caine GJ, Stonelake PS, Lip GY, Kehoe ST. The hypercoagulable state of malignancy: pathogenesis and current debate. *Neoplasia*. 2002;4(6):465–473.
75. Ashrafian H, Davey P. A review of the causes of central pontine myelinosis: yet another apoptotic illness? *Eur J neurology: Off J Eur Federation Neurological Societies*. 2001;8(2):103–109.
76. Brown WD. Osmotic demyelination disorders: central pontine and extrapontine myelinolysis. *Curr OpNeurol*. 2000;13 (6):691–697.
77. Haynes HR, Gallagher PJ, Cordaro A, Likeman M, Love S. A case of chronic asymptomatic central pontine myelinolysis with histological evidence of remyelination. *Forensic Sci Med Pathol*. 2018;14(1):106–108.
78. Alleman AM. Osmotic demyelination syndrome: central pontine myelinolysis and extrapontine myelinolysis. *SemUltrasound, CT, MR*. 2014;35(2):153–159.
79. Graff-Radford J, Fugate JE, Kaufmann TJ, Mandrekar JN, Rabinstein AA. Clinical and radiologic correlations of central pontine myelinolysis syndrome. *Mayo Clin Proc Mayo Clin*. 2011;86(11):1063–1067.
80. Isenberg-Grzeda E, Alici Y, Hatzoglou V, Nelson C, Breitbart W. Nonalcoholic thiamine-related encephalopathy

(Wernicke-Korsakoff syndrome) among inpatients with cancer: A series of 18 cases. *Psychosomatics*. 2016;57(1):71–81.
81. de Oliveira AM, Paulino MV, Vieira APF, et al. Imaging patterns of toxic and metabolic brain disorders. *Radiographics*. 2019;39(6):1672–1695.
82. Zuccoli G, Santa Cruz D, Bertolini M, et al. MR imaging findings in 56 patients with Wernicke encephalopathy: nonalcoholics may differ from alcoholics. *AJNR Am J neuroradiology*. 2009;30(1):171–176.
83. Rollins N, Winick N, Bash R, Booth T. Acute methotrexate neurotoxicity: findings on diffusion-weighted imaging and correlation with clinical outcome. *AJNR*. 2004;25(10):1688–1695.
84. Inaba H, Khan RB, Laningham FH, Crews KR, Pui CH, Daw NC. Clinical and radiological characteristics of methotrexate-induced acute encephalopathy in pediatric patients with cancer. *Ann Oncol*. 2008;19(1):178–184.
85. Stone JB, DeAngelis LM. Cancer-treatment-induced neurotoxicity: focus on newer treatments. *Nat Rev Clin Oncol*. 2016;13(2):92–105.
86. Martins F, Sofiya L, Sykiotis GP, et al. Adverse effects of immune-checkpoint inhibitors: epidemiology, management and surveillance. *Nat Rev Clin Oncol*. 2019;16(9):563–580.
87. Carpenter KJ, Murtagh RD, Lilienfeld H, Weber J, Murtagh FR. Ipilimumab-induced hypophysitis: MR imaging findings. *AJNR*. 2009;30(9):1751–1753.
88. Ruben JD, Dally M, Bailey M, Smith R, McLean CA, Fedele P. Cerebral radiation necrosis: incidence, outcomes, and risk factors with emphasis on radiation parameters and chemotherapy. *Int J Radiat Oncology, Biology, Phys*. 2006; 65(2):499–508.
89. Katsura M, Sato J, Akahane M, Furuta T, Mori H, Abe O. Recognizing radiation-induced changes in the central nervous system: where to look and what to look for. *Radiographics*. 2021;41(1):224–248.
90. Colaco RJ, Martin P, Kluger HM, Yu JB, Chiang VL. Does immunotherapy increase the rate of radiation necrosis after radiosurgical treatment of brain metastases? *J Neurosurg*. 2016;125(1):17–23.
91. Shah R, Vattoth S, Jacob R, et al. Radiation necrosis in the brain: imaging features and differentiation from tumor recurrence. *Radiographics*. 2012;32(5):1343–1359.
92. Zakhari N, Taccone MS, Torres C, et al. Diagnostic accuracy of centrally restricted diffusion in the differentiation of treatment-related necrosis from tumor recurrence in high-grade gliomas. *AJNR*. 2018;39(2):260–264.
93. Alcaide-Leon P, Cluceru J, Lupo JM, et al. Centrally reduced diffusion sign for differentiation between treatment-related lesions and glioma progression: a validation study. *AJNR*. 2020;41(11):2049–2054.
94. Kim HS, Goh MJ, Kim N, et al. Which combination of MR imaging modalities is best for predicting recurrent glioblastoma? Study of diagnostic accuracy and reproducibility. *Radiology*. 2014;273(3):831–843.
95. Khan M, Ambady P, Kimbrough D, et al. Radiation-induced myelitis: initial and follow-up MRI and clinical features in patients at a single tertiary care institution during 20 years. *AJNR*. 2018;39(8):1576–1581.
96. Kirkpatrick JP, van der Kogel AJ, Schultheiss TE. Radiation dose-volume effects in the spinal cord. *Int J Radiat Oncology, Biology, Phys*. 2010;76(3 Suppl):S42–S49.
97. Nanney 3rd AD, El Tecle NE, El Ahmadieh TY, et al. Intracranial aneurysms in previously irradiated fields: literature review and case report. *World Neurosurg*. 2014;81(3-4):511–519.
98. Heckl S, Aschoff A, Kunze S. Radiation-induced cavernous hemangiomas of the brain: a late effect predominantly in children. *Cancer*. 2002;94(12):3285–3291.
99. Cutsforth-Gregory JK, Lanzino G, Link MJ, Brown Jr. RD, Flemming KD. Characterization of radiation-induced cavernous malformations and comparison with a nonradiation cavernous malformation cohort. *J Neurosurg*. 2015;122(5):1214–1222.
100. Kerklaan JP, Lycklama a Nijeholt GJ, Wiggenraad RG, Berghuis B, Postma TJ, Taphoorn MJ. SMART syndrome: a late reversible complication after radiation therapy for brain tumours. *J Neurol*. 2011;258(6):1098–1104.
101. Singh TD, Hajeb M, Rabinstein AA, et al. SMART syndrome: retrospective review of a rare delayed complication of radiation. *Eur J neurology: Off J Eur Federation Neurological Societies*. 2021;28(4):1316–1323.
102. Rheims S, Ricard D, van den Bent M, et al. Peri-ictal pseudoprogression in patients with brain tumor. *Neuro-oncology*. 2011;13(7):775–782.
103. Fox J, Ajinkya S, Greenblatt A, et al. Clinical characteristics, EEG findings and implications of status epilepticus in patients with brain metastases. *J Neurological Sci*. 2019;407:116538.
104. Wu A, Weingart JD, Gallia GL, et al. Risk factors for preoperative seizures and loss of seizure control in patients undergoing surgery for metastatic brain tumors. *World Neurosurg*. 2017;104:120–128.
105. Kotisaari K, Virtanen P, Forss N, Strbian D, Scheperjans F. Emergency computed tomography in patients with first seizure. *Seizure*. 2017;48:89–93.
106. Williams JA, Bede P, Doherty CP. An exploration of the spectrum of peri-ictal MRI change; a comprehensive literature review. *Seizure*. 2017;50:19–32.
107. Gaxiola-Valdez I, Singh S, Perera T, Sandy S, Li E, Federico P. Seizure onset zone localization using postictal hypoperfusion detected by arterial spin labelling MRI. *Brain: a J Neurol*. 2017;140(11):2895–2911.
108. Oyanguren B, Sanchez V, Gonzalez FJ, et al. Limbic encephalitis: a clinical-radiological comparison between herpetic and autoimmune etiologies. *Eur J Neurology: Off J Eur Federation Neurological Societies*. 2013;20(12):1566–1570.
109. Forster A, Griebe M, Gass A, Kern R, Hennerici MG, Szabo K. Diffusion-weighted imaging for the differential diagnosis of disorders affecting the hippocampus. *Cerebrovasc Dis*. 2012;33(2):104–115.
110. Madhavan AA, Carr CM, Morris PP, et al. Imaging review of paraneoplastic neurologic syndromes. *AJNR*. 2020;41 (12):2176–2187.
111. Loblaw DA, Laperriere NJ, Mackillop WJ. A population-based study of malignant spinal cord compression in Ontario. *Clin Oncol*. 2003;15(4):211–217.
112. Boussios S, Cooke D, Hayward C, et al. Metastatic spinal cord compression: unraveling the diagnostic and therapeutic challenges. *Anticancer Res*. 2018;38(9):4987–4997.
113. Fisher CG, Schouten R, Versteeg AL, et al. Reliability of the Spinal Instability Neoplastic Score (SINS) among radiation oncologists: an assessment of instability secondary to spinal metastases. *Radiat Oncol (London, Engl)*. 2014;9:69.
114. Huisman M, van der Velden JM, van Vulpen M, et al. Spinal instability as defined by the spinal instability neoplastic score is associated with radiotherapy failure in metastatic spinal disease. *spine J: Off journal North Am Spine Soc*. 2014;14(12):2835–2840.
115. Bilsky MH, Laufer I, Fourney DR, et al. Reliability analysis of the epidural spinal cord compression scale. *J Neurosurg Spine*. 2010;13(3):324–328.

116. Nickerson EK, Sinha R. Vertebral osteomyelitis in adults: an update. *Br Med Bull*. 2016;117(1):121–138.
117. Tsantes AG, Papadopoulos DV, Vrioni G, et al. Spinal infections: an update. *Microorganisms*. 2020;8(4):476.
118. Urban JP, Smith S, Fairbank JC. Nutrition of the intervertebral disc. *Spine (Phila Pa 1976)*. 2004;29(23):2700–2709.
119. Hong SH, Choi JY, Lee JW, Kim NR, Choi JA, Kang HS. MR imaging assessment of the spine: infection or an imitation? *Radiographics*. 2009;29(2):599–612.
120. Rades D, Bremer M, Goehde S, Joergensen M, Karstens JH. Spondylodiscitis in patients with spinal cord compression: a possible pitfall in radiation oncology. *Radiotherapy Oncol*. 2001;59(3):307–309.
121. Garg RK, Malhotra HS, Gupta R. Spinal cord involvement in tuberculous meningitis. *Spinal Cord*. 2015;53(9):649–657.
122. Flanagan EP, McKeon A, Lennon VA, et al. Paraneoplastic isolated myelopathy: clinical course and neuroimaging clues. *Neurology*. 2011;76(24):2089–2095.
123. Graber JJ, Nolan CP. Myelopathies in patients with cancer. *Arch Neurol*. 2010;67(3):298–304.
124. Plotkin M, Eisenacher J, Bruhn H, et al. 123I-IMT SPECT and 1H MR-spectroscopy at 3.0 T in the differential diagnosis of recurrent or residual gliomas: a comparative study. *J Neuro-Oncology*. 2004;70(1):49–58.

Chapter 4

# Chest Emergencies in Pregnant Patients

Joseph Mansour, Demetrios A. Raptis, and Sanjeev Bhalla

## Outline



## Key Points

- In pregnant patients presenting with signs of acute myocardial infarction with no known history of coronary artery disease, spontaneous coronary artery dissection should be suspected.
- Patients with preexisting vascular conditions, such as aortopathies and hereditary hemorrhagic telangiectasia, should be closely followed throughout pregnancy, as these conditions can exacerbate.
- In a pregnant patient with suspected pulmonary embolism, the fetal radiation dose does not significantly differ between a perfusion scan and computed tomography; however, the radiation dose to the breast is lower with a perfusion scan.
- Whenever possible, imaging that does not utilize ionizing radiation or gadolinium contrast agents should be used to minimize risk to the fetus.

## Introduction

Pregnancy causes changes in the hemodynamics and hormones that can induce stress, unmask underlying preexisting conditions, or increase the risk of certain cardiothoracic conditions. Examples of such entities include cardiomyopathy, coronary artery dissection, and pulmonary embolism, among others. Maternal cardiovascular complications account for more than 25% of all pregnancy-related deaths in the United States.[1] Imaging plays an essential role in both diagnosing these entities and guiding treatment throughout pregnancy and in the postpartum period.

## Imaging Approach

Echocardiography is currently the first-line modality for evaluation of cardiac function, given its availability and lack of ionizing radiation. Echocardiography is able to assess biventricular systolic function, detect hemodynamic derangement and wall motion abnormalities, and identify complications such as thrombus. It may be limited by poor acoustic windows, especially in women in late pregnancy or in the immediate postpartum period.

Cardiac magnetic resonance (CMR) has become the gold standard examination for cardiac volumetric and flow quantification due to high soft tissue contrast resolution, high accuracy, and reproducibility.[2] CMR is particularly useful for identifying masses, especially thrombus. Intravenous gadolinium contrast should not be administered, especially in the first trimester, as repeated doses of gadolinium have been shown to be teratogenic in animal studies.[3,4] Gadolinium is considered safe for women who are breastfeeding. While there is no data to suggest fetal harm from magnetic resonance, there are theoretical concerns such as fetal acoustic damage and teratogenesis. Pregnant patients should undergo magnetic resonance imaging (MRI) in a 1.5-T scanner, as most of the data in the literature are derived from scanners with 1.5 T or less.[5]

Whenever possible, imaging modalities that do not utilize ionizing radiation are preferred. Chest radiography is a quick and useful modality to assess for cardiac enlargement and pulmonary edema in patients presenting with dyspnea. With computed tomography (CT), the risk of radiation to the mother is similar to that of nonpregnant women, with the only exception being the breast tissue. Pregnant females have more sensitive breast tissue due to tissue proliferation.[6] Radiation effects on the fetus depend on both the dose and the age of the fetus. The embryo is most sensitive during the first 2 weeks after conception, which usually results in failure of implantation.[7] Most of the data regarding the effects on radiation on the fetus are extrapolated from exposure after the atomic bomb detonations of Hiroshima and Nagasaki.[8,9] In general, a fetal absorbed dose of less than 50 mGy is considered safe with regards to teratogenic or abortive effects[10]; this dose is rarely exceeded with the advent of lower-dose protocols. Techniques such as decreasing the kilovoltage or tube current and reducing the exposure time, modulating the dose, adjusting the collimation and scan length, and increasing the pitch can be employed to lower radiation dose. For reference, a retrospective coronary CT is estimated to deliver a fetal dose of approximately 3 mGy.[11] While iodinated contrast material can cross the placenta, it has no teratogenic effects.[12]

## Cardiac Complications

### HEART FAILURE

There are two categories of heart failure: heart failure with reduced ejection fraction and heart failure with preserved ejection fraction. Pregnancy can result in exacerbation of maternal cardiovascular conditions, such as hypertension, or lead to the development of new conditions such as cardiomyopathy. These conditions may result in heart failure, which accounts for approximately 9% of hospitalized maternal-related deaths.[13] Even though heart failure accounts for less than 2% of pregnancy-related hospitalization, more than 60% of pregnancy-related heart failure diagnoses occur in postpartum patients.[13] Patients with preexisting comorbidities such as cardiomyopathy, valvular disease, diabetes, and hypertension are more likely to develop heart failure. Heart failure patients are also more likely to develop pregnancy-associated conditions, such as preeclampsia and diabetes.[13]

Heart failure in the pregnant or postpartum patient can be a result of increased vascular resistance, decreased left ventricular function, or valvular dysfunction. Preeclampsia, hypertrophic cardiomyopathy, and pulmonary hypertension can be accentuated during pregnancy and lead to increased vascular resistance resulting in heart failure. Cardiomyopathies including peripartum cardiomyopathy (PPCM), inherited disorders, drug reactions, or ischemia can cause left ventricular dysfunction and heart failure. Valvular disease in the setting of endocarditis or rheumatic heart disease can also lead to heart failure.[14]

#### Clinical Manifestations

Pregnant patients with heart failure usually develop symptoms related to right, left, or biventricular dysfunction. Changes related to pregnancy can have signs and symptoms that overlap with those of heart failure. For example, mildly elevated jugular pressure and lower extremity edema are findings that are not uncommonly encountered in pregnancy and occur due to physiologic changes.[15] Additionally, pregnant women can experience dyspnea as a result of increased, progesterone-induced, respiratory drive.[15,16] It is believed that this overventilation is a physiologic response to increase carbon dioxide excretion to create a higher gradient between the fetal and maternal circulation.[16] Signs and symptoms that should prompt a workup for heart failure include orthopnea, paroxysmal nocturnal dyspnea, palpitations, and syncope. Worrisome findings on physical examination include cyanosis, resting tachycardia, collapsing pulse, hypo- or hypertension, pulsatile and elevated jugular pressures, auscultatory findings of pulmonary edema, and signs of respiratory distress.[14]

### Imaging Manifestations

Chest radiography is the first imaging modality in a pregnant patient presenting with dyspnea or lower extremity edema. In patients with left-sided heart failure, the chest radiograph will show interstitial signs of pulmonary edema and, in more severe forms of edema, perihilar airspace opacification. The cardiac silhouette is usually enlarged, and pleural effusions are usually present. Echocardiography has the same utility as in nonpregnant patients, offering evaluation for ventricular and valvular function. CT is not used in the evaluation of patients with heart failure, unless it is indicated to exclude other causes of dyspnea, such as pulmonary embolism.

CMR is useful for diagnosing the underlying etiology of the patient's heart failure, as it allows for assessment of function, volume, morphology, and tissue characterization. In the postpartum patient, gadolinium should be used. Patterns of myocardial enhancement are particularly useful for characterization of myocardial processes such as subendocardial enhancement in the setting of ischemia or subepicardial and midmyocoardial enhancement in myocarditis. Patients with dilated cardiomyopathy will have a dilated poorly functioning left ventricle with midmyocardial enhancement. Other underlying etiologies may be suggested by function and morphology of the left ventricle alone, such as takotsubo, which manifests with characteristic apical ballooning.

## PERIPARTUM CARDIOMYOPATHY

PPCM refers to left ventricular dysfunction and cardiac failure that occurs in the peripartum period. While relatively uncommon, the incidence is rising, with an incidence in the United States ranging from 1 in 1000 to 4000 live births.[17] The rise in the number of cases may be due to increased awareness, workup, and diagnosis. Risk factors that are becoming more prevalent include age, where more than half of the cases occur in women over the age of 30 years,[18] increased incidence of cardiovascular risk factors (i.e., diabetes, hypertension, and obesity), and increased multifetal pregnancies.[18,19] Additionally, more than 40% of PPCM occurs in Black American women, who are three times more likely than White Americans to develop this condition.[20]

### Clinical Presentation

While most cases occur in the week after delivery, PCCM can also less commonly occur in the second or third trimesters. Current international guidelines define PCCM as symptomatic left ventricular dysfunction, with or without ventricular dilation, with an ejection fraction of less than 45% occurring from the last month of pregnancy to up to 5 months after delivery.[21,22] This definition can help distinguish PCCM from an unmasked preexisting cardiomyopathy due to pregnancy, which usually occurs earlier, in the late second trimester.[23] The exact pathophysiology of the disease remains unknown, with many proposed etiologies, including viral, nutritional, autoimmune, genetic, and hormonal causes, among others.[24] Some postulate that the physiologic stress of pregnancy may expose an underlying genetic susceptibility or cardiovascular disease. Clinically, these patients present with signs of heart failure, including orthopnea and paroxysmal nocturnal dyspnea. During late pregnancy, it may be difficult to distinguish the PCCM from normal physiologic changes. Physical examination signs of PCCM include tachycardia, lower extremity edema, pulmonary rales, and elevated jugular venous pressure. Life-threatening presentation can occur with acute respiratory distress from low cardiac output heart failure, requiring emergent medical and mechanical support.

### Imaging Manifestations

Echocardiography can help distinguish PPCM from other pregnancy-related cardiac diseases. Findings of PPCM include reduced systolic and diastolic left ventricular function (Fig. 4.1); left ventricular dilation is not always necessarily present and therefore not included in the major criteria for diagnosis of this entity.[4] CMR can be utilized for more accurate assessment of left ventricular function and volumes, as well as to evaluate for the potential complication of cardiac thrombus. Thrombus will typically appear as a mass within the ventricle that does not enhance on postcontrast imaging.[25] High inversion times of 450 to 600 ms will show the thrombus to be of homogeneously low signal intensity compared with the surrounding blood pool.[25]

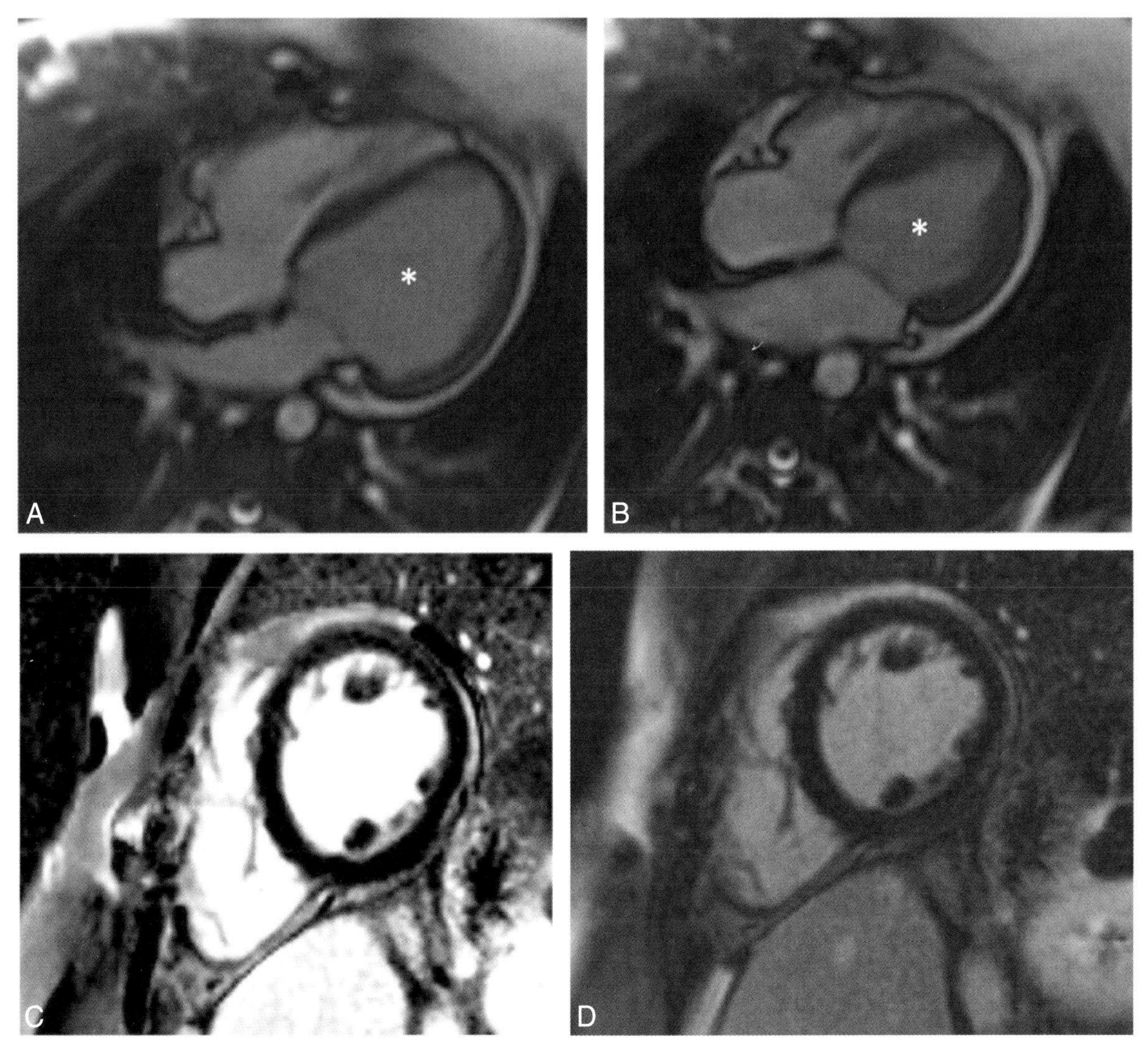


**Fig. 4.1** Peripartum cardiomyopathy. A 21-year-old female with presents with new-onset left ventricular dysfunction shortly after childbirth. Cardiac magnetic resonance was performed. Four-chamber images in end-diastole (A) and end-systole (B) show a dilated left ventricle (*) and reduced systolic function. Postcontrast magnitude inversion recovery (C) and phase-sensitive inversion recovery (D) images in short axis views show no myocardial enhancement to suggest an infiltrative cardiomyopathy or infarct.

## AORTIC DISSECTION AND AORTOPATHIES

While aortic dissection rarely occurs in women of child-bearing age, approximately half of all cases of dissection in women under the age of 40 years occur in pregnant patients.[26] Patients with conditions that increase the risk for developing dissection, such as Marfan syndrome and bicuspid aortic valve, may undergo prophylactic prepartum surgery to mitigate, but are usually followed more closely with imaging. High-risk patients in which the aorta rapidly dilates to greater than 5 cm during pregnancy rarely require surgical repair while pregnant.[27]

### Clinical Manifestations

Aneurysmal aortic dilatation usually does not result in symptoms, unless there is direct compression of adjacent structures or resultant dissection or rupture. Rarely, dilatation of the descending aorta can cause compression of the recurrent laryngeal nerve, which results in hoarseness, or compression of the esophagus resulting in dysphagia.[28] Aortic root dilation can also result in symptoms of heart failure from lack of aortic valve coaptation. Symptoms of dissection include sudden-onset chest pain that may radiate to the back and abdomen. The most critical complication of an aneurysm is rupture, usually presenting with severe chest pain, hypotension, and shock from either hemorrhagic or hemopericardium, resulting in tamponade. Patients with rupture may have diminished or absent lower extremity pulses.[29]

### Imaging

Surveillance imaging is required in high-risk patients. Echocardiography can be used to visualize the aortic root and the ascending aorta. MRI can provide a comprehensive analysis of the aorta, as the aortic arch and descending aorta can be well visualized without ionizing radiation. MRI can also visualize a dissection flap, if present, and establish the extent of the dissection, as the entire thoracic abdominal aorta can be imaged (Fig. 4.2). On black blood spin echo sequences, the false lumen may be hyperintense due to slow flow and turbulence that leads to loss of a normal flow void.[30,31] On bright blood sequences, the hypointense dissection flap can be seen surrounded by increased signal in both the true and false lumen.[31,32] CT is often utilized in the emergency setting, as it offers faster image acquisition and great spatial resolution for vascular structures. Any stranding or hemorrhage in the mediastinum should raise suspicion for rupture. Noncontrast CT is useful for detection of intramural hematoma, which will appear as a hyperattenuating crescent in the aortic wall.[32] Postcontrast images will show the dissection flap when surrounded by contrast in both the false and true lumen (Fig. 4.3).[32]

## ACUTE CORONARY SYNDROME AND MYOCARDIAL INFARCTION

Acute coronary syndrome (ACS) is relatively uncommon during pregnancy but is more common compared with age-matched nonpregnant patients.[33] ACS is more frequent in the third trimester and can occur secondary to atherosclerotic disease and nonatherosclerotic entities, including spontaneous coronary artery dissection (SCAD).[33] It is estimated that 27% to 40% of cases of myocardial infarction in pregnancy are related to atherosclerosis.[34,35]

SCAD accounts for approximately 43% of cases of myocardial infarction.[34] The majority of cases of SCAD occur in women, with around 30% of cases occurring in pregnant or peripartum patients.[36] Multivessel SCAD can also occur. The cause of increased incidence in pregnancy is unknown, but it has been theorized that hemodynamic changes result in increased shear forces, or hormonal changes induce changes within the walls of the vasculature, making the blood vessels prone to dissection.[37]

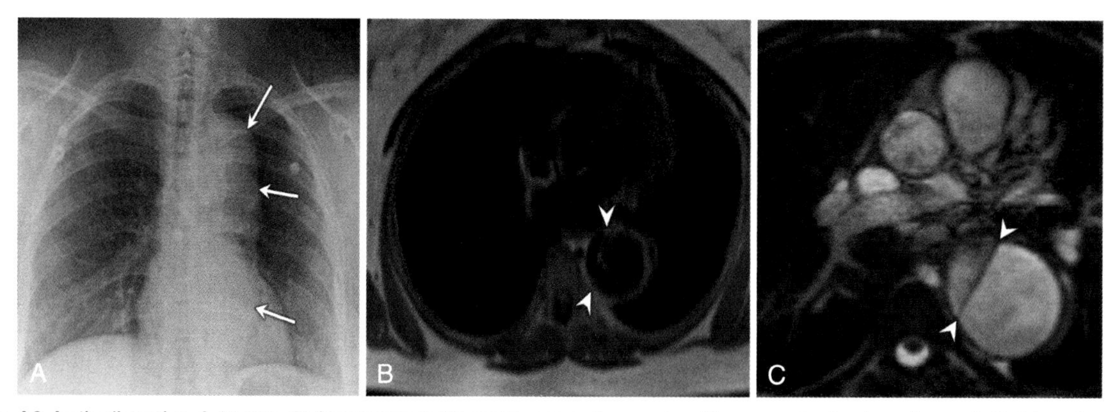


**Fig. 4.2** Aortic dissection. A 27-year-old female who is 10 weeks pregnant presents with severe chest pain and uncontrolled hypertension. Anteroposterior chest radiograph (A) shows a dilated aortic knob and descending aorta (arrows). Transaxial black blood half Fourier single-shot turbo spin-echo images (B) and transaxial true fast imaging with steady-state precession images (C) show a dilated descending aorta that also contains a dissection flap (arrowheads).

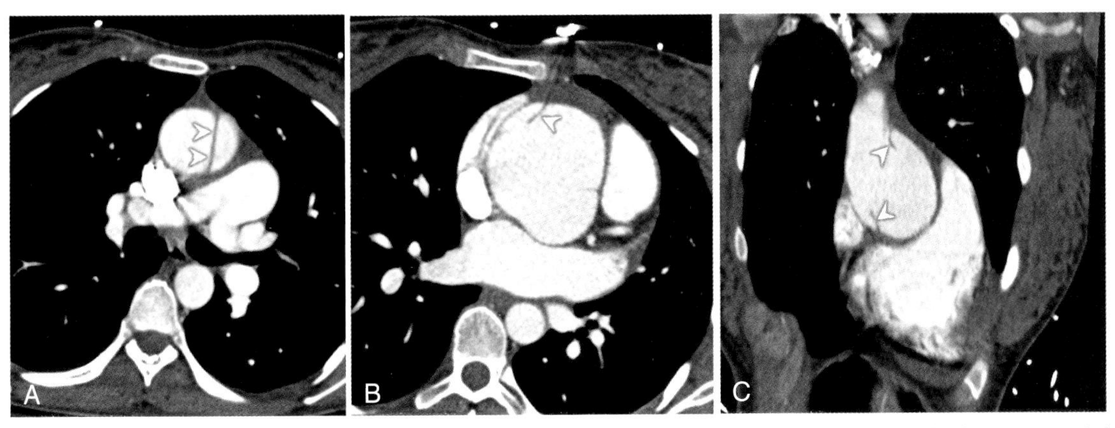


**Fig. 4.3** Aortic dissection. A 23-year-old female with known history of Marfan syndrome and ascending aortic aneurysm develops acute-onset chest pain after a cesarean section. Transaxial images of the postcontrast computed tomography scan at the level of the pulmonary artery (A) and the aortic root (B) and an oblique coronal of the ascending aorta (C) show a dissection flap in the ascending aorta (arrowheads).

The remainder of cases of ACS are attributed to embolism, hypercoagulability, and vasospasm.[34,35]

### Clinical Manifestations

Symptoms of ACS in pregnancy are similar to those seen in nonpregnant patients and include chest discomfort that radiates to the shoulders, jaw, or back. Young women with ACS may have an atypical presentation without chest pain or discomfort but can present with dyspnea, nausea, palpitations, syncope, and cardiac arrest.[38] Treatment of patients with SCAD and ACS is similar to that of the general population and includes revascularization techniques. The mortality rate of SCAD in pregnant or postpartum patients is estimated at 38%.[39]

### Imaging

The modality of choice for patients who develop symptoms of myocardial infarction with highly suggestive findings on laboratory studies and electrocardiogram (ECG) is coronary angiography. Coronary angiography is the first-line diagnostic tool and should be performed as early as possible, as it allows for both diagnosis and possible percutaneous intervention.

In patients with atypical chest pain, equivocal laboratory and ECG findings, and clinical suspicion for ACS or SCAD, a coronary CT of the chest may be considered. Coronary CT can detect and quantify coronary calcification, which correlates with total disease burden.[40] The angiographic portion of the CTA will help identify noncalcified plaque and quantify luminal stenosis.[40] The involved area of myocardial infarction can also sometimes be seen on contrast-enhanced CT as an area of relative hypoenhancement (Fig. 4.4).

CMR can be used to work up suspected infarcts and will show reduced wall motion in the territory of infarction. Postcontrast imaging (reserved for the postpartum patient) will show enhancement that may be subendocardial or transmural (Fig. 4.5). Patients with nontransmural subendocardial enhancement may benefit from revascularization.

Coronary CT of the patients with SCAD will show an intramural hematoma or slow flow in the false lumen appearing as low to intermediate attenuation that results in narrowing or occlusion of the vessel. As opposed to dissection of larger vessels, such as the aorta, when dissection occurs in smaller vessels, a dissection flap is not always appreciated.[37] The proximal segments of the coronary arteries are more commonly affected, and the most common artery affected is the left anterior descending coronary artery in 41% of cases, followed by the right coronary artery, which accounts for 11%.[41] One-third of patients will present with multivessel dissections. CMR is not usually used in the initial workup of patients with suspected SCAD, but may be used to identify myocardial infarction and for follow-up of cardiac function.

## MECHANICAL VALVE THROMBOSIS

Pregnant patients with mechanical valves are at increased risk of thrombosis. The increased risk is secondary to

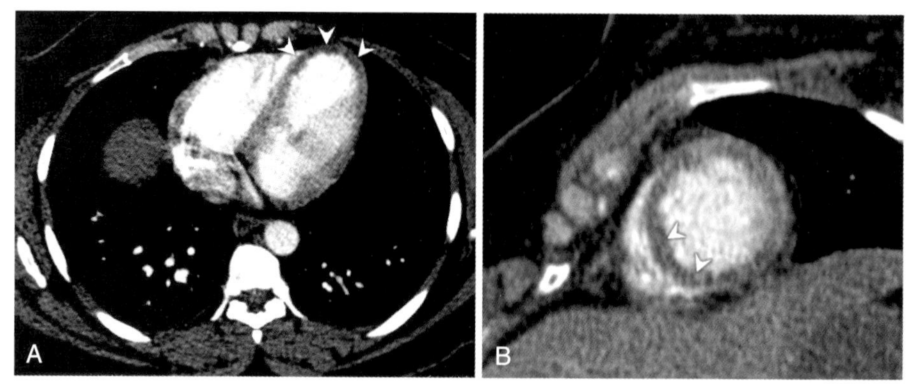


**Fig. 4.4** Myocardial infarction from coronary artery dissection. A 36-year-old female who is 8 weeks pregnant presenting with chest pain, elevated troponin and ST elevation on electrocardiogram. Transaxial image of computed tomography of the chest (A) shows an area of hypoenhancement in the septum and apex (arrowheads) suggestive of ischemia/infarct. A short-axis multiplanar reconstruction (B) shows the area of relative hypoenhancement (arrowheads). The patient underwent a coronary catheterization that confirmed the presence of a dissection in the distal left anterior descending artery (not shown).

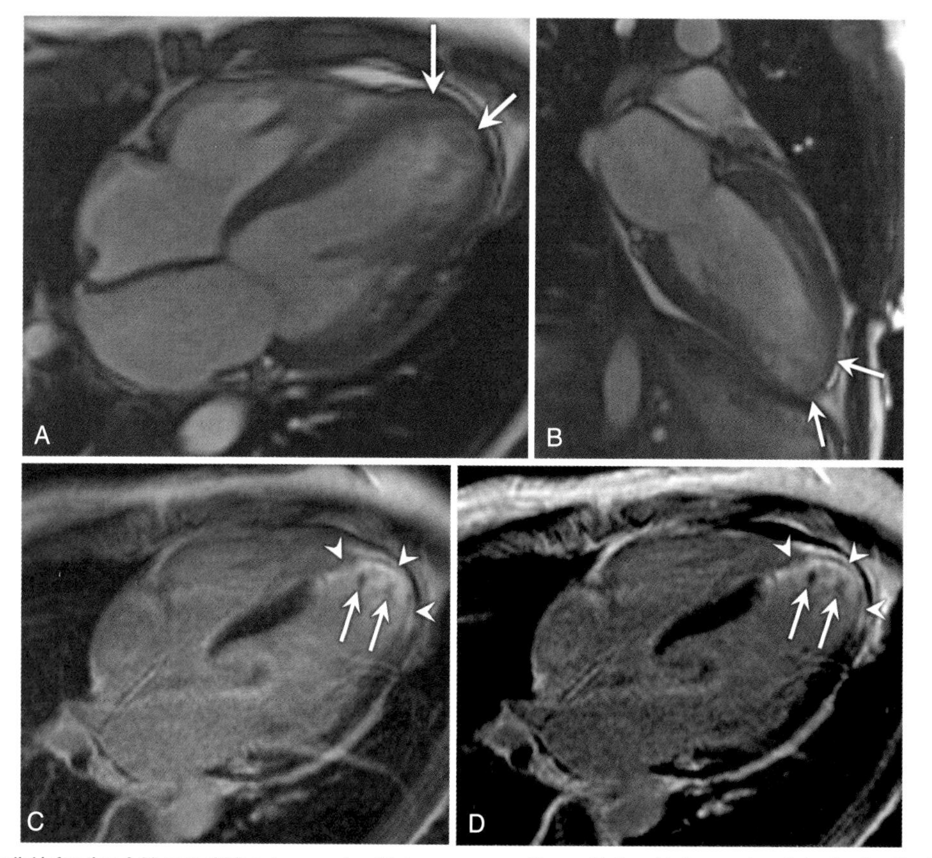


**Fig. 4.5** Myocardial infarction. A 38-year-old female presents with dyspnea on exertion and is found to have reduced ejection fraction 3 months after delivery. Coronary computed tomography angiography (CTA) was performed (not shown) and was negative, and cardiac magnetic resonance imaging was performed a few days later. Four-chamber images (A) and two-chamber long-axis images (B) show thinning, dilatation, and hypokinesis of the left ventricular apex (arrows). Postcontrast magnitude inversion recovery (C) and phase-sensitive inversion recovery (D) images in four-chamber views show transmural subendocardial enhancement (arrowheads) of the apex and the anteroseptal, septal, and inferoseptal wall of the apex. Small nonenhancing foci (arrows) were favored to represent possible areas of microvascular occlusion. The cause of the infarct was believed to be secondary to spontaneous coronary artery dissection, given the normal coronary CTA.

physiologic changes resulting in a hypercoagulable state beginning in early pregnancy and persisting for at least 6 to 12 weeks after delivery.[42] Additionally, even though these patients are on anticoagulation, increased renal clearance and increase volume status due to pregnancy can lead to suboptimal therapeutic levels.[42] In a European study that reviewed more than 2900 pregnant patients with structural heart disease, the 212 patients with mechanical heart valves (MHVs) demonstrated increased mortality (1.4%) and pregnancy loss (18%) compared with patients without mechanical valves.[43] In this series, two of the three deaths were secondary to mechanical valve thrombosis.[43] Thrombotic events were also significantly more common in patients with MHVs, with no difference between aortic or mitral MHV.[43] Bleeding complications, possibly related to anticoagulation, were also more common and occurred typically at the time of delivery.[43]

#### Clinical Manifestations

MHV thrombosis is suspected when a patient develops a new murmur, new symptoms of heart failure, syncope or presyncope, or rarely sudden cardiac death.[44,45] When a patient presents with a new stroke or other thromboembolic events, there should be a high suspicion for this diagnosis.[45]

#### Imaging

Typically, imaging of mechanical valves is initially performed using echocardiography and fluoroscopy.[46,47] Transesophageal echocardiography can provide clues to valve dysfunction, such as increased gradient and the presence of regurgitation. However, evaluation can be somewhat limited on echocardiography due to acoustic shadowing from the MHV. Fluoroscopy allows for assessment of valve motion but not visualization of thrombus. CMR is of limited use for evaluation of the valve, *per se*, due to susceptibility artifact from the MHV.

Gated CT is the optimal modality for evaluation of suspected mechanical prosthetic valve dysfunction, given its spatial and temporal resolution. Despite artifact from the metallic components, diagnostic images can still be obtained.[47] CT with retrospective gating allows for evaluation for leaflet opening and closing angles and evaluation of valve leaflet motion throughout the cardiac cycle. CT with intravenous contrast also allows for visualization of MHV thrombus. Although not always possible to differentiate thrombus from pannus, thrombus tends to have lower attenuation.[48]

## Pulmonary

### PULMONARY EMBOLISM

Pulmonary embolism is a well-known complication occurring in pregnant patients due to hemodynamic and metabolic changes. Pregnant patients are four times more likely to develop pulmonary embolism,[49] and the risk increases to 30 times that of age-matched nonpregnant females.[48] The risk is highest in the third trimester and the immediate postpartum period.

#### Clinical Manifestations

Pulmonary embolism in pregnancy results in clinical findings similar to those of nonpregnant patients. The presentation is often nonspecific, rendering clinical identification difficult. Symptoms may range from no symptoms at all to shock and death. The most common reported symptoms include dyspnea, chest pain, cough, and sweating. As in nonpregnant patients, new and acute-onset dyspnea, chest pain, and hemoptysis should raise clinical suspicion for pulmonary embolism.[50]

#### Imaging

In cases where pulmonary embolism is suspected, a lower extremity Doppler ultrasound should be performed if the patient has lower extremity symptoms.[51] If there is deep vein thrombosis, then further imaging is not usually needed, and the patient can be started on anticoagulation. In patients without lower extremity symptoms, imaging may begin with CT or ventilation-perfusion (V/Q) scintigraphy. A V/Q scan will result in lower maternal breast radiation exposure with no significant difference in fetal dose compared with CT.[52] Given the decreased dose, it is usually recommended to perform a V/Q scan (rather than a CT) in patients with a normal chest radiograph. Patients with abnormalities on chest radiography or equivocal perfusion scintigraphy should proceed with CT pulmonary angiography (CTPA). CTPA will show filling defects within the pulmonary arteries (Fig. 4.6). Infarcts can sometimes be seen and manifest as peripheral wedge-shaped areas of consolidation, often with central lucency (Fig. 4.7). CT may also show findings suspicious for right heart strain, which include dilatation of the right ventricle, bowing of the ventricular septum, and reflux of contrast in the inferior vena cava.

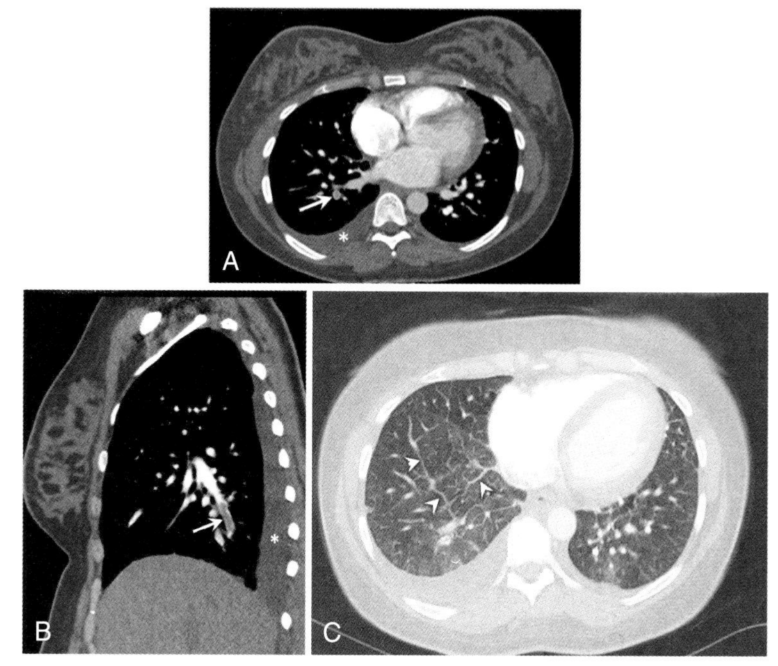


**Fig. 4.6** Pulmonary embolism. A 34-year-old who is 5 days postpartum presents with chest pain and dyspnea. Transaxial (A) and sagittal (B) images in soft tissue window from a contrast-enhanced computed tomography pulmonary angiogram show a filling defect in the right lower lobe pulmonary artery (arrow) consistent with pulmonary embolism. Of note there is also a small right pleural effusion (*). Transaxial image of the chest in lung window (C) shows smooth interlobular septal line thickening (arrowheads) consistent with pulmonary edema, a contributing factor to the patient's dyspnea.

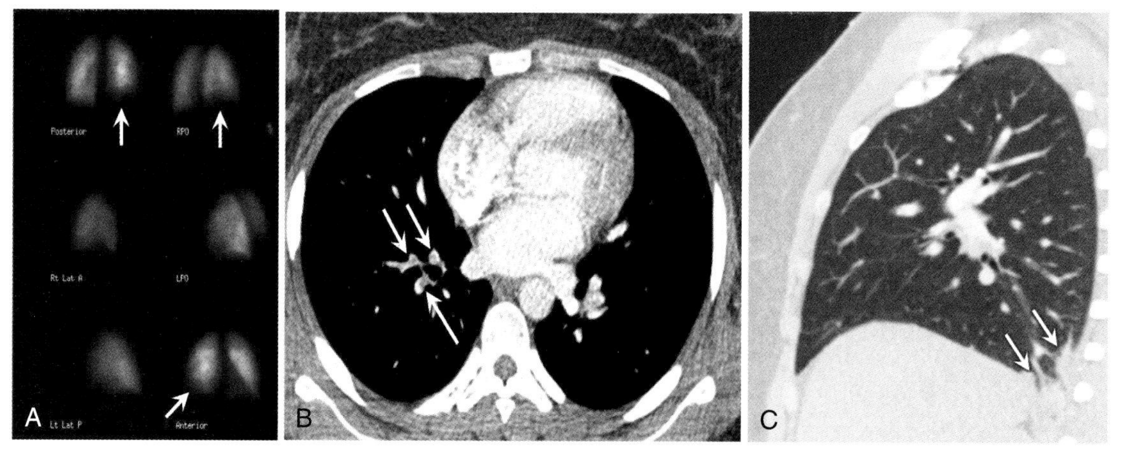


**Fig. 4.7** Pulmonary embolism. A 23-year-old female who is 8 weeks pregnant presents with shortness of breath and elevated D-dimer. A perfusion scan (A) shows a few areas of peripheral photopenia in the right lower lobe (arrows). Transaxial images from the computed tomography pulmonary angiogram (B) shows filling defects (arrows) in the right lower lobe pulmonary arteries consistent with pulmonary emboli. A coronal image of the right lung in lung windows (C) shows peripheral wedge-shaped areas of consolidation representing infarcts (arrows).

Noncontrast CMR with bright-blood techniques can also be considered in select cases in centers with thoracic MR expertise.[53]

## PNEUMONIA AND ASPIRATION

Pneumonia is the most frequent cause of fatal nonobstetric infections in pregnant patients.[54] While the true incidence and mortality are unknown, and there is no evidence to suggest higher rates than in nonpregnant adults, pregnant patients who develop pneumonia are more likely to deliver early and have infants of lower birth weight.[54] Pregnancy is associated with altered cellular immunity, which is believed to occur to protect the fetus from the mother but makes patients more susceptible to community-acquired and viral pneumonias. These alterations are most notable in the second and third trimesters. In addition to changes in immunity, the enlarging uterus produces mass effect on the diaphragm, which can be displaced up to 4 cm superiorly.[54,55] As a result, the ability to clear pulmonary secretions is decreased, which, along with increased fluid within the lungs, leads to increased vulnerability for infection. Pregnant patients are also at increased risk of aspiration, especially in patients with preexisting gastroesophageal reflux disease and increased gastric acidity. Increased progesterone levels results in relaxation of the lower gastroesophageal sphincter and delayed gastric emptying. Additionally, narcotics administered during delivery can cause delayed gastric emptying. Anesthetics administered during cesarean section also place those patients at higher risk of aspiration than those who deliver vaginally.[54,55]

### Clinical Manifestations

A pregnant patient who presents with new-onset cough should be worked up for pneumonia.[56] Symptoms of pneumonia are similar to those seen in nonpregnant patients. Diagnosing pneumonia in pregnant patients is not always straightforward, as there is overlap with symptoms that usually occur due to physiological changes, particularly dyspnea and crepitations on lung auscultation.[56] As such, a delay in diagnosis and even misdiagnosis is not uncommon. The severity and clinical manifestations of aspiration pneumonia depend on the pH and volume of aspiration contents, which result in a chemical pneumonitis that may lead to edema, hypoxia, and sometimes respiratory failure.

### Imaging

Chest radiography will show findings similar to those of nonpregnant patients, with areas of consolidation in bacterial pneumonia (Figs. 4.8 and 4.9). Findings on chest radiography that are indicative of aspiration include lower lobe consolidation (Fig. 4.10). CT of the chest is usually not needed for the diagnosis of pneumonia or aspiration pneumonia. The role of CT is to exclude other causes of the patient's symptoms and to evaluate for complications of pneumonia and aspiration, including cavitary or necrotizing pneumonia, pulmonary abscess, and empyema.

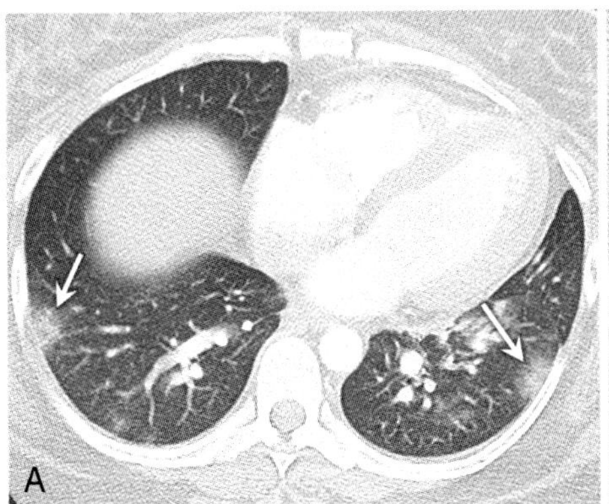


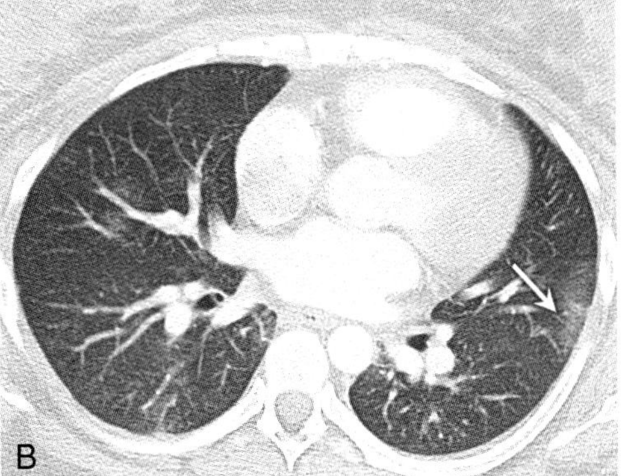


**Fig. 4.8** Viral pneumonia. A 28-year-old female who is 25 weeks pregnant presents with chest pain and elevated D-dimer. Transaxial images of computed tomography of the chest shows multiple peripheral areas of ground glass opacities in both lungs presents (arrows). A nasal polymerase chain reaction swab was performed that returned positive for SARS-CoV-2.

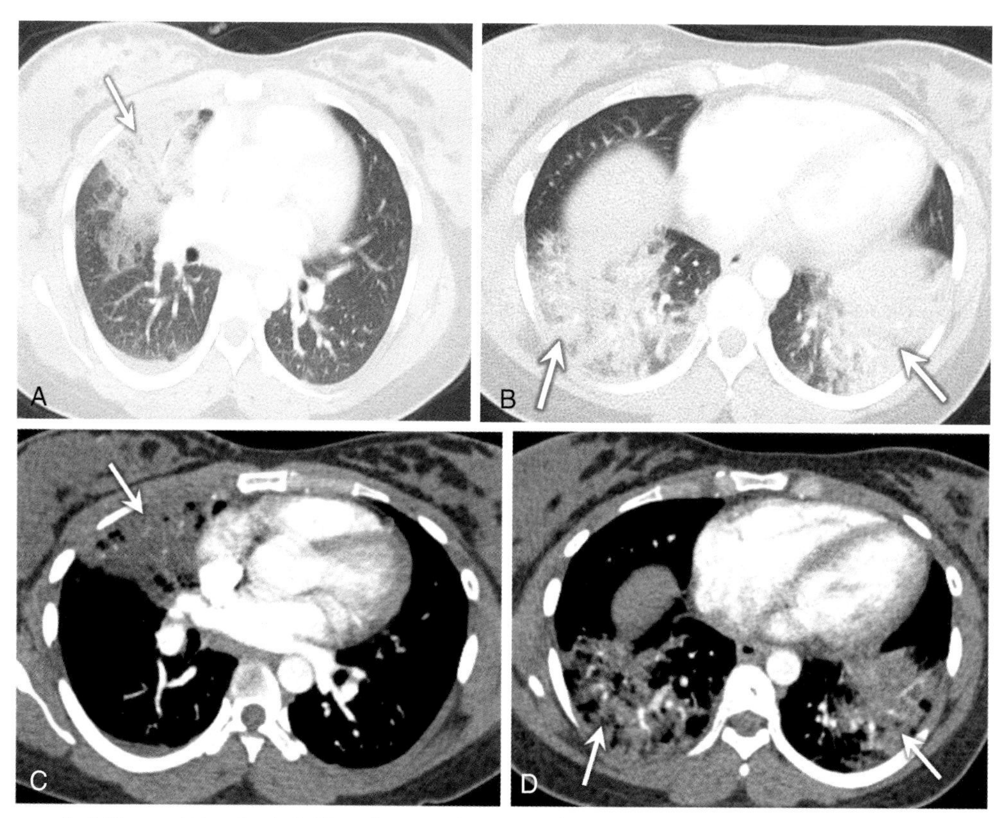


**Fig. 4.9** Pneumonia. A 30-year-old female who is 31 weeks pregnant presents with shortness of breath and pleuritic chest pain. Transaxial images in lung windows (A and B) show multifocal areas of consolidation without enhancement on the soft tissue windows (C and D). The patient had an elevated white blood cell count and was diagnosed with pneumonia. The patient improved with antimicrobial therapy.

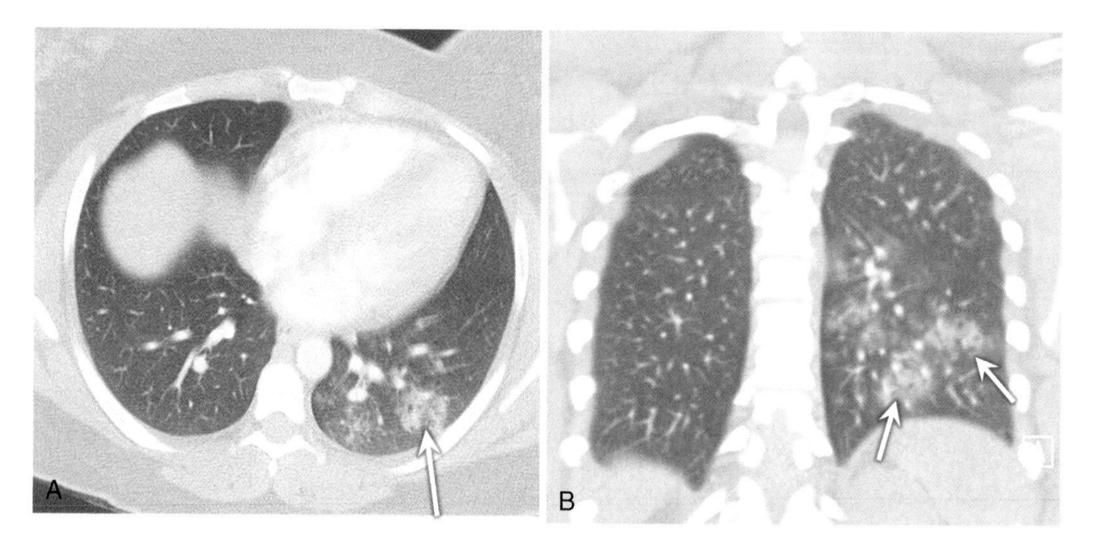


**Fig. 4.10** Aspiration. A 26-year-old female who was 32 weeks pregnant is diagnosed with eclampsia. Transaxial (A) and coronal (B) images in lung window, a few hours after a seizure, show airway centered areas of ground glass opacities (arrows) in the left lower lobe, consistent with aspiration.

## AMNIOTIC FLUID EMBOLISM

Amniotic fluid embolism (AFE) is a rare but severe complication of pregnancy that accounts for 10% of pregnancy-related deaths, with a mortality rate as high as 80%.[57] Risk factors for development of AFE include polyhydramnios, placenta previa, pregnancy-induced hypertension, labor induction, and instrumental vaginal and cesarean delivery.[57] It is believed that after membrane rupture, small tears in the uterine veins and increased pressure gradients during labor result in amniotic fluid entering the maternal venous system. The amniotic fluid travels through the venous system to the pulmonary arteries and is lodged within the small arterioles and capillary bed of the lungs, resulting in transient small vessel occlusion. The breakdown products of the fluid will result in peripheral chemical pneumonitis and an immune cascade that manifests with severe edema, alveolar damage, disseminated intravascular coagulation (DIC), and cardiopulmonary failure.

### Clinical Manifestations

Patients with AFE usually present with abrupt and rapidly progressive symptoms, including shock and symptoms of DIC. These patients may deteriorate rapidly to severe pulmonary edema and cardiopulmonary collapse. Up to one-third of patients will experience a so-called "aura" that precedes the sudden cardiorespiratory failure and can manifest with a sense of sudden doom, chills, nausea, agitation, or altered mental status. DIC results in increased hemorrhage, occurring in more than 80% of patients, most commonly as prolonged uterine bleeding.[58,59]

### Imaging Manifestations

Patients with AFE are rarely imaged, owing to the rapid onset of this severe condition. Findings on chest radiography and CT are similar to those of noncardiogenic pulmonary edema, including bilateral airspace opacities (Fig. 4.11). CT may also show ill-defined centrilobular ground glass nodules (indicative of chemical pneumonitis), usually with a gravity-dependent predominance (Fig. 4.12). Filling defects are rarely seen within the pulmonary arteries. CT can be helpful to exclude other causes of acute respiratory failure such as pulmonary embolism, pneumonia, and aspiration.[41]

## HEREDITARY HEMORRHAGIC TELANGIECTASIA AND ARTERIOVENOUS MALFORMATIONS

Hereditary hemorrhagic telangiectasia is an autosomal dominant disease that results in multiple arteriovenous malformations (AVMs), most commonly in the lung (30%) and liver (30%), followed by the brain (10%–20%).[60] The hemodynamic changes that occur in pregnancy can increase the size and shunting through the AVMs, with hemorrhage being a rare but well-known complication.

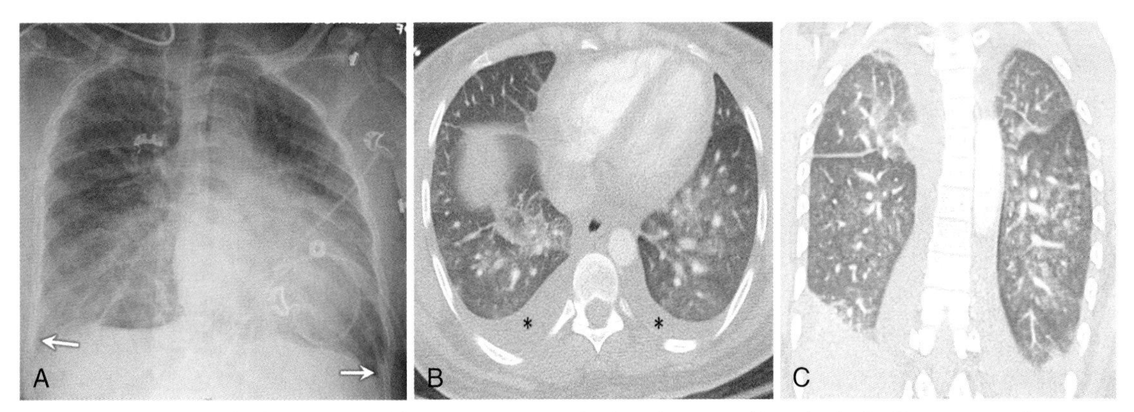


**Fig. 4.11** Amniotic fluid embolization. A 23-year-old postpartum woman develops dyspnea and hypoxia shortly after an emergent cesarean section for premature rupture of membranes and chorioamnionitis. Chest radiography (A) shows increased pulmonary vasculature, bilateral airspace opacities, and blunting of the costophrenic recesses suggesting pleural effusions (arrows) and increased pulmonary vasculature. Transaxial (A) and coronal images (B) of computed tomography of the chest shows diffuse centrilobular ground glass opacities consistent with amniotic fluid embolism. Also note the bilateral pleural effusions (*).

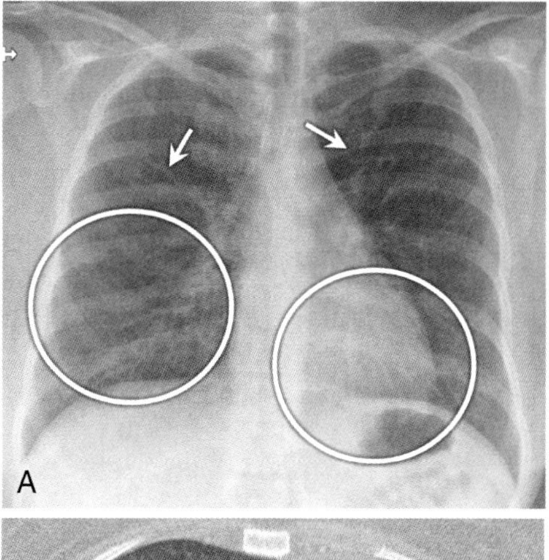


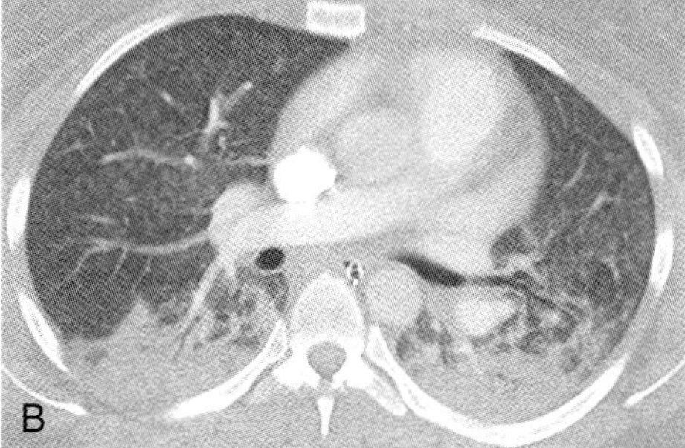


**Fig. 4.12** Amniotic fluid embolism. A 23-year-old female presenting with acute-onset dyspnea and hypoxia after vaginal delivery. Chest radiograph (A) shows patchy, ill-defined opacities in both lungs (circles) and increased vascular markings (arrows). Transaxial image of contrast-enhanced computed tomography in lung window (B) shows centrilobular opacities throughout both lungs suggestive of amniotic fluid embolism.

## Clinical Manifestations

The presence of AVMs in the lung results in right to left vascular shunting that, depending on the size of the shunt, can result rarely in hypoxia.[60] The intrapulmonary shunts also increase the risk of developing paradoxical emboli in these patients who are already at increased risk of venous thromboembolism. On physical examination, telangiectasias can be seen involving the buccal mucosa; involvement of the nasal mucosa can result in recurrent epistaxis.[61] The most serious complication of AVMs is hemorrhage, which can be in the lungs, resulting in hemoptysis, or into the brain, resulting in stroke symptoms. The rate of life-threatening hemorrhage from AVMs is estimated at 1.4% antepartum and peripartum, and 0.6% postpartum.[61] Because the size and symptoms related to AVMs may increase during pregnancy, it is recommended that AVMs be embolized prior to pregnancy, even if the patient is asymptomatic.[60]

## Imaging

CT is usually the modality of choice in patients with known AVMs, given its superior spatial resolution and its ability to create maximum intensity projection images and multiplanar reformats. It is important that the radiologist follow the vessels leading to and from the nidus (Fig. 4.13): a pulmonary AVM should have a feeding artery and a draining vein. Many mimickers of AVMs can be seen on imaging, including granulomas, venovenous collaterals, and meandering veins.

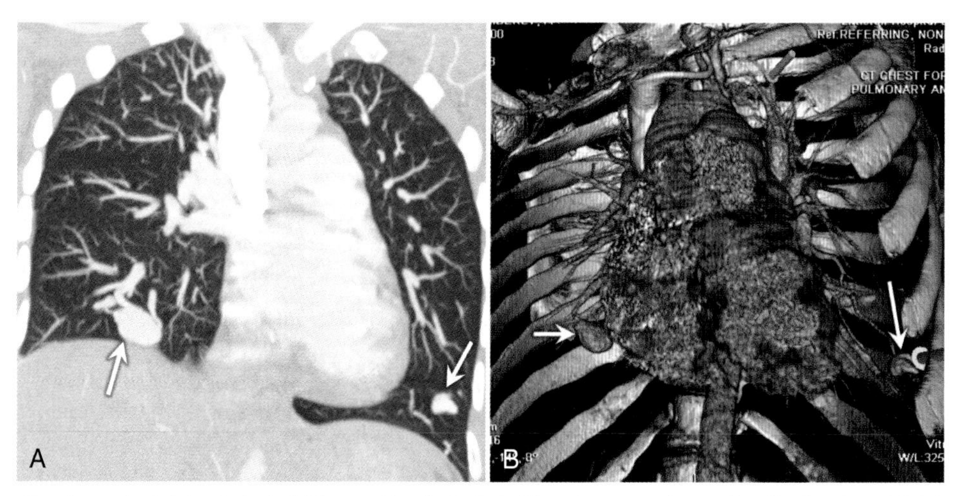


**Fig. 4.13** Hereditary hemorrhagic telangiectasia. A 28-year-old patient who is 27 weeks pregnant presents with altered mental status and seizure. Brain imaging reveals a brain abscess (not shown). Coronal maximum intensity projection images (A) and volume-rendered three-dimensional reconstructions (B) from computed tomography of the chest shows multiple arteriovenous malformations in the bilateral lungs (arrows).

The role of the radiologist is not only to detect the malformations, but also to assess for interval growth and the size of the feeding artery, which when greater than 3 mm is amenable to coil embolization.[62] Patients who develop hemorrhage will show consolidation and ground glass opacification surrounding the arteriovenous malformation in the area of bleeding.

## NONCARDIOGENIC EDEMA

Noncardiogenic edema has been reported with tocolytic therapy given to patients to prevent preterm delivery. Medications include terbutaline, ritodrine, atosiban,[63] calcium channel–blocking tocolytic drugs such as nifedipine and nicardipine,[64,65] and β-adrenoreceptor agonists.[66] The pathogenesis and mechanism of action are not completely understood. Tocolytics are believed to have an affinity for vasopressin receptors, and inhibit antidiuretic hormone effects, which leads to congestive heart failure and hypertension.[67] These agents alter the renin-aldosterone system and result in increased antidiuretic hormone levels, plasma volume, and capillary permeability. Calcium channel blockers also cause precapillary vasodilation, which results in increased hydrostatic pressure in the lungs that in turn leads to capillary leakage in patients who are likely overhydrated and given steroid, resulting in sodium and water retention.[64] The patients most at risk are those with anemia, fluid overload, and multiple gestations. Preeclampsia and eclampsia can also lead to noncardiogenic edema.

### Clinical Manifestations

Patients with noncardiogenic edema will usually develop dyspnea and tachypnea. Depending on the degree of edema, patients may progress to orthopnea, respiratory distress with accessory muscle use, hypoxia, and cyanosis.[63] Physical examination will reveal decreased bilateral breath sounds, as well as crepitations and crackles and lower extremity edema.

### Imaging

Chest radiography and CT will show findings of pulmonary edema. In contrast to PCCM, the cardiac silhouette is of usually of normal size, and pleural effusions are not common (Fig. 4.14). CT has the added benefit of excluding other causes of dyspnea and tachypnea.

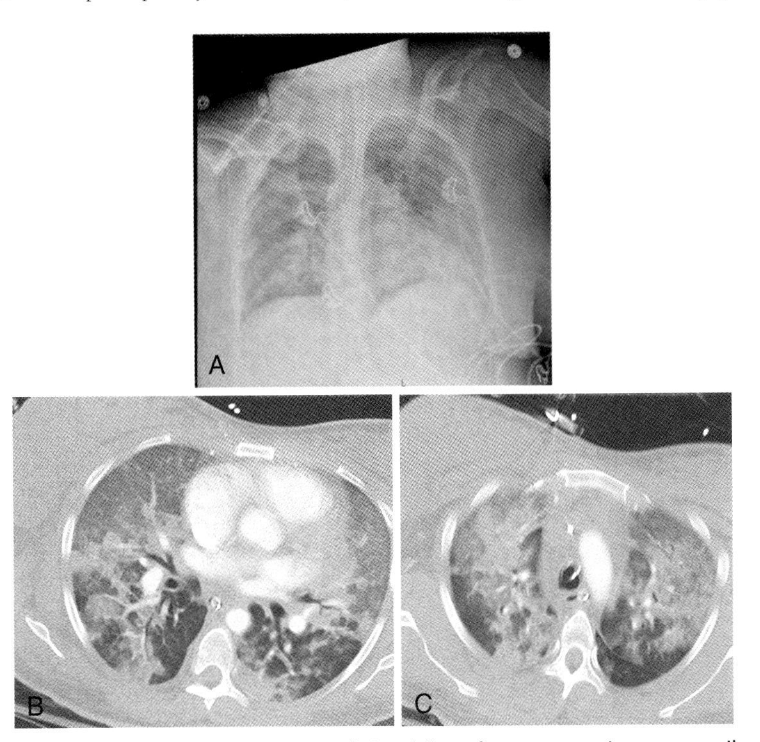


**Fig. 4.14** Noncardiogenic edema. A 29-year-old develops acute respiratory failure after an emergent cesarean section for preeclampsia. Chest radiography (A) shows bilateral and parahilar predominant airspace opacification. Transaxial images of computed tomography of the chest (B and C) performed to rule out pulmonary embolism shows diffuse airspace opacities with lobular sparing. Note the absence of pleural effusions.

## PNEUMOTHORAX AND PNEUMOMEDIASTINUM

Pneumothorax and pneumomediastinum during pregnancy is not common, with risk factors including prolonged labor, pneumonia, and asthma. Most patients are young and primiparous. Primary spontaneous pneumothorax can also occur in young patients and is not usually associated with significant clinical outcomes, unless tension develops.[68] Patients who have a history of pneumothorax who are contemplating pregnancy should be aware that they are at higher risk of recurrence during pregnancy, during delivery, or shortly after delivery, with a recurrence rate of 44%,[69] as opposed to nonpregnant patients, in whom the recurrence rate is approximately 30%.[70] It is speculated that accelerated breathing patterns and repeated Valsalva maneuvers may increase the risk of rupture of small subpleural blebs at the apices.[68] Spontaneous pneumothorax occurred in the first and second trimester in 51% of the cases and in the peripartum period in 49% of the cases.[71]

Pneumomediastinum can occur in postpartum patients with vaginal deliveries. It is also postulated that the prolonged pushing, such as in cases of shoulder dystocia or large fetuses, can lead to pneumomediastinum secondary to Macklin's effect due to increased intraalveolar pressure.[72] Pneumomediastinum can also uncommonly occur secondary to esophageal rupture in pregnant patients with hyperemesis gravidarum in the first trimester or vomiting in late pregnancy and postpartum.[72]

### Clinical Manifestations

Patients with pneumothorax usually report sharp chest pain and, depending on the size of pneumothorax, dyspnea and respiratory distress. Pneumothorax should be in the differential of a pregnant patient with chest pain and dyspnea, especially if there is a history or prior pneumothorax.

Spontaneous pneumomediastinum can result in chest pain, dyspnea, pleuritic chest pain, and odynophagia and dysphagia.[73] Patients with esophageal rupture from hyperemesis gravidarum can present with Mackler's triad in 20% to 45% of cases. The triad includes vomiting, chest pain, and subcutaneous emphysema.[72] Other symptoms of esophageal rupture include severe chest pain, upper abdominal pain, odynophagia, fever, and shock.[73]

### Imaging

Chest radiography can be used to evaluate for both pneumothorax and pneumomediastinum. If esophageal perforation is present, pleural effusions and/or pneumonia are usually present.[72] In cases where an esophageal perforation is suspected, an esophagram with water-soluble contrast can be performed. CT of the chest after oral contrast can also be used to diagnose perforations.[74] CT is more sensitive in detecting pneumomediastinum, as approximately 30% of cases are estimated to be missed on chest radiography.[73]

## Conclusion

Cardiac and pulmonary complications that occur in pregnancy vary in incidence and severity. Because many of these entities may have nonspecific clinical findings that overlap with those of expected physiologic changes during pregnancy, it is imperative that both the clinician and the radiologist maintain a high level of suspicion. Many of these complications demonstrate characteristic findings on imaging, and radiologists can help to promptly provide a diagnosis and guide treatment.

## REFERENCES


1. Creanga AA, Syverson C, Seed K, Callaghan WM. Pregnancy-related mortality in the United States, 2011–2013. *Obstet Gynecol*. 2017;130(2):366.
2. Petersen SE, Aung N, Sanghvi MM, et al. Reference ranges for cardiac structure and function using cardiovascular magnetic resonance (CMR) in Caucasians from the UK Biobank population cohort. *J Cardiovasc Magn Reson*. 2017;19(1):1–19.
3. Okuda Y, Sagami F, Tirone P, Morisetti A, Bussi S, Masters RE. Reproductive and developmental toxicity study of gadobenate dimeglumine formulation (E7155)(3): study of embryo-fetal toxicity in rabbits by intravenous administration. *J toxicological Sci*. 1999;24(Supplement I):79–87.
4. Chen MM, Coakley FV, Kaimal A, Laros RK. Guidelines for computed tomography and magnetic resonance imaging use during pregnancy and lactation. *Obstet Gynecol*. 2008;112(2):333–340.
5. American College of Radiology. ACR–SPR Practice Parameter for theSafe and Optimal Performance of Fetal Magnetic Resonance Imaging (MRI). Accessed May 22, 2021. https://www.acr.org/-/media/ACR/Files/Practice-Parameters/mr-fetal.pdf.
6. Hurwitz LM, Reiman RE, Yoshizumi TT, et al. Radiation dose from contemporary cardiothoracic multidetector CT protocols with an anthropomorphic female phantom: implications for cancer induction. *Radiology*. 2007;245(3):742–750.
7. McCollough CH, Schueler BA, Atwell TD, et al. Radiation exposure and pregnancy: when should we be concerned? *Radiographics*. 2007;27(4):909–917.
8. Otake M, Schull WJ. In utero exposure to A-bomb radiation and mental retardation; a reassessment. *Br J radiology*. 1984;57(677):409–414.

9. Yamazaki JN, Schull WJ. Perinatal loss and neurological abnormalities among children of the atomic bomb: Nagasaki and Hiroshima revisited, 1949 to 1989. *JAMA*. 1990;264(5):605–609.
10. Wieseler KM, Bhargava P, Kanal KM, Vaidya S, Stewart BK, Dighe MK. Imaging in pregnant patients: examination appropriateness. *Radiographics*. 2010;30(5):1215–1229.
11. Colletti PM, Lee KH, Elkayam U. Cardiovascular imaging of the pregnant patient. *Am J Roentgenol*. 2013;200(3):515–521.
12. Pierce T, Hovnanian M, Hedgire S, Ghoshhajra B. Imaging of cardiovascular disease in pregnancy and the peripartum period. *Curr Treat Options Cardiovasc Med*. 2017;19(12):94.
13. Mogos MF, Piano MR, McFarlin BL, Salemi JL, Liese KL, Briller JE. Heart failure in pregnant women: a concern across the pregnancy continuum. *Circ Heart Fail*. 2018;11(1):e004005.
14. Anthony J, Sliwa K. Decompensated heart failure in pregnancy. *Card Fail Rev*. 2016;2(1):20.
15. Sanghavi M, Rutherford JD. Cardiovascular physiology of pregnancy. *Circulation*. 2014;130(12):1003–1008.
16. Jensen D, Webb KA, O'Donnell DE. Chemical and mechanical adaptations of the respiratory system at rest and during exercise in human pregnancy. *Appl Physiol Nutr Metab*. 2007;32(6):1239–1250.
17. Arany Z, Elkayam U. Peripartum cardiomyopathy. *Circulation*. 2016;133(14):1397–1409.
18. Gunderson EP, Croen LA, Chiang V, Yoshida CK, Walton D, Go AS. Epidemiology of peripartum cardiomyopathy: incidence, predictors, and outcomes. *Obstet Gynecol*. 2011;118(3):583–591.
19. Mielniczuk LM, Williams K, Davis DR, et al. Frequency of peripartum cardiomyopathy. *Am J Cardiology*. 2006;97(12): 1765–1768.
20. Brar SS, Khan SS, Sandhu GK, et al. Incidence, mortality, and racial differences in peripartum cardiomyopathy. *Am J Cardiology*. 2007;100(2):302–304.
21. Yancy CW, Jessup M, Bozkurt B, et al. 2013 ACCF/AHA guideline for the management of heart failure: a report of the American College of Cardiology Foundation/American Heart Association Task Force on Practice Guidelines. *J Am Coll Cardiol*. 2013;62(16):e147–e239.
22. Bauersachs J, König T, van der Meer P, et al. Pathophysiology, diagnosis and management of peripartum cardiomyopathy: a position statement from the Heart Failure Association of the European Society of Cardiology Study Group on peripartum cardiomyopathy. *Eur J Heart Fail*. 2019;21(7):827–843.
23. Sliwa K, Hilfiker-Kleiner D, Petrie MC, et al. Current state of knowledge on aetiology, diagnosis, management, and therapy of peripartum cardiomyopathy: a position statement from the Heart Failure Association of the European Society of Cardiology Working Group on peripartum cardiomyopathy. *Eur J Heart Fail*. 2010;12(8):767–778.
24. Ntusi NB, Mayosi BM. Aetiology and risk factors of peripartum cardiomyopathy: a systematic review. *Int J Cardiol*. 2009;131(2):168–179.
25. Srichai MB, Junor C, Rodriguez LL, et al. Clinical, imaging, and pathological characteristics of left ventricular thrombus: a comparison of contrast-enhanced magnetic resonance imaging, transthoracic echocardiography, and transesophageal echocardiography with surgical or pathological validation. *Am Heart J*. 2006;152(1):75–84.
26. Coulon C. Thoracic aortic aneurysms and pregnancy. *La Presse Médicale*. 2015;44(11):1126–1135.
27. Regitz-Zagrosek V, Blomstrom Lundqvist C, Borghi C, et al. ESC Guidelines on the management of cardiovascular diseases during pregnancy: the Task Force on the Management of Cardiovascular Diseases during Pregnancy of the European Society of Cardiology (ESC). *Eur Heart J*. 2011;32(24):3147–3197.
28. Ohki M. Thoracic saccular aortic aneurysm presenting with recurrent laryngeal nerve palsy prior to aneurysm rupture: a prodrome of thoracic aneurysm rupture? *Case Rep Otolaryngology*. 2012;2012:367873.
29. Isselbacher EM. Thoracic and abdominal aortic aneurysms. *Circulation*. 2005;111(6):816–828.
30. Amparo E, Higgins C, Hricak H, Sollitto R. Aortic dissection: magnetic resonance imaging. *Radiology*. 1985;155(2):399–406.
31. Sakamoto I, Sueyoshi E, Uetani M. MR imaging of the aorta. *Radiol Clin North Am*. 2007;45(3):485–497.
32. Litmanovich D, Bankier AA, Cantin L, Raptopoulos V, Boiselle PM. CT and MRI in diseases of the aorta. *Am J Roentgenol*. 2009;193(4):928–940.
33. Bush N, Nelson-Piercy C, Spark P, et al. Myocardial infarction in pregnancy and postpartum in the UK. *Eur J Preventive Cardiology*. 2013;20(1):12–20.
34. Elkayam U, Jalnapurkar S, Barakkat MN, et al. Pregnancy-associated acute myocardial infarction: a review of contemporary experience in 150 cases between 2006 and 2011. *Circulation*. 2014;129(16):1695–1702.
35. Roth A, Elkayam U. Acute myocardial infarction associated with pregnancy. *J Am Coll Cardiol*. 2008;52(3):171–180.
36. Thompson EA, Ferraris S, Gress T, Ferraris V. Gender differences and predictors of mortality in spontaneous coronary artery dissection: a review of reported cases. *J Invasive Cardiol*. 2005;17(1):59–61.
37. Vrints CJ. Spontaneous coronary artery dissection. *Heart*. 2010;96(10):801–808.
38. Canto JG, Rogers WJ, Goldberg RJ, et al. Association of age and sex with myocardial infarction symptom presentation and in-hospital mortality. *JAMA*. 2012;307(8):813–822.
39. Koul AK, Hollander G, Moskovits N, Frankel R, Herrera L, Shani J. Coronary artery dissection during pregnancy and the postpartum period: two case reports and review of literature. *Catheter Cardiovasc Interv*. 2001;52(1):88–94.
40. Bastarrika G, Lee YS, Huda W, Ruzsics B, Costello P, Schoepf UJ. CT of coronary artery disease. *Radiology*. 2009;253(2):317–338.
41. Plowman RS, Javidan-Nejad C, Raptis CA, et al. Imaging of pregnancy-related vascular complications. *Radiographics*. 2017;37(4):1270–1289.
42. Economy KE, Valente AM. Mechanical heart valves in pregnancy: a sticky business. *Am Heart Assoc*. 2015;132(2): 79–81.
43. Van Hagen IM, Roos-Hesselink JW, Ruys TP, et al. Pregnancy in women with a mechanical heart valve: data of the European Society of Cardiology Registry of Pregnancy and Cardiac Disease (ROPAC). *Circulation*. 2015;132(2):132–142.
44. Burke A, Farb A, Sessums L, Virmani R. Causes of sudden cardiac death in patients with replacement valves: an autopsy study. *J Heart Valve Dis*. 1994;3(1):10–16.
45. Dürrleman N, Pellerin M, Bouchard D, et al. Prosthetic valve thrombosis: twenty-year experience at the Montreal Heart Institute. *J Thorac Cardiovascular Surg*. 2004;127(5):1388–1392.

46. Suchá D, Symersky P, Tanis W, et al. Multimodality imaging assessment of prosthetic heart valves. *Circ Cardiovasc Imaging*. 2015;8(9):e003703.
47. Moss AJ, Dweck MR, Dreisbach JG, et al. Complementary role of cardiac CT in the assessment of aortic valve replacement dysfunction. *Open Heart*. 2016;3(2):e000494.
48. Elliott CG. Evaluation of suspected pulmonary embolism in pregnancy. *J Thorac Imaging*. 2012;27(1):3–4.
49. Heit JA, Kobbervig CE, James AH, Petterson TM, Bailey KR, Melton III LJ. Trends in the incidence of venous thromboembolism during pregnancy or postpartum: a 30-year population-based study. *Ann Intern Med*. 2005;143(10):697–706.
50. Gherman RB, Goodwin TM, Leung B, Byrne JD, Hethumumi R, Montoro M. Incidence, clinical characteristics, and timing of objectively diagnosed venous thromboembolism during pregnancy. *Obstet Gynecol*. 1999;94(5):730–734.
51. Leung AN, Bull TM, Jaeschke R, et al. American Thoracic Society documents: an official American Thoracic Society/Society of Thoracic Radiology clinical practice guideline—evaluation of suspected pulmonary embolism in pregnancy. *Radiology*. 2012;262(2):635–646.
52. Ridge CA, McDermott S, Freyne BJ, Brennan DJ, Collins CD, Skehan SJ. Pulmonary embolism in pregnancy: comparison of pulmonary CT angiography and lung scintigraphy. *Am J Roentgenol*. 2009;193(5):1223–1227.
53. Kluge A, Luboldt W, Bachmann G. Acute pulmonary embolism to the subsegmental level: diagnostic accuracy of three MRI techniques compared with 16-MDCT. *Am J Roentgenol*. 2006;187(1):W7–W14.
54. Lim W, Macfarlane J, Colthorpe C. Pneumonia and pregnancy. *Thorax*. 2001;56(5):398–405.
55. Goodnight WH, Soper DE. Pneumonia in pregnancy. *Crit Care Med*. 2005;33(10):S390–S397.
56. Zeldis SM. Dyspnea during pregnancy. Distinguishing cardiac from pulmonary causes. *Clin Chest Med*. 1992;13(4):567–585.
57. Han D, Lee KS, Franquet T, et al. Thrombotic and nonthrombotic pulmonary arterial embolism: spectrum of imaging findings. *Radiographics*. 2003;23(6):1521–1539.
58. Gist RS, Stafford IP, Leibowitz AB, Beilin Y. Amniotic fluid embolism. *Anesth Analg*. 2009;108(5):1599–1602.
59. Clark SL, Hankins GD, Dudley DA, Dildy GA, Porter TF. Amniotic fluid embolism: analysis of the national registry. *Am J Obstet Gynecol*. 1995;172(4):1158–1169.
60. Begbie M, Wallace G, Shovlin C. Hereditary haemorrhagic telangiectasia (Osler-Weber-Rendu syndrome): a view from the 21st century. *Postgrad Med J*. 2003;79(927):18–24.
61. Shovlin C, Sodhi V, McCarthy A, Lasjaunias P, Jackson J, Sheppard M. Estimates of maternal risks of pregnancy for women with hereditary haemorrhagic telangiectasia (Osler–Weber–Rendu syndrome): suggested approach for obstetric services. *BJOG*. 2008;115(9):1108–1115.
62. Narsinh KH, Ramaswamy R, Kinney TB. Management of pulmonary arteriovenous malformations in hereditary hemorrhagic telangiectasia patients. *SemInterventional Radiology*. 2013;30(4):408–412.
63. Fernandez A, Dominguez D, Delgado L. Severe non-cardiogenic pulmonary oedema secondary to atosiban and steroids. *Int J Obstet Anesth*. 2011;20(2):189–190.
64. Abbas OM, Nassar AH, Kanj NA, Usta IM. Acute pulmonary edema during tocolytic therapy with nifedipine. *Am J Obstet Gynecol*. 2006;195(4):e3–e4.
65. Gatault P, Genee O, Legras A, Garot D, Mercier E, Fichet J. Calcium-channel blockers: An increasing cause of pulmonary edema during tocolytic therapy. *Int J Cardiols*. 2008;130(3):e123–e124.
66. de Heus R, Erwich J-JH, van Geijn HP, et al. Adverse drug reactions to tocolytic treatment for preterm labour. Maternal and Fetal effects of Tocolytic. *Drugs*. 2008:35–49.
67. Afschar P, Schöll W, Bader A, Bauer M, Winter R. A prospective randomised trial of atosiban versus hexoprenaline for acute tocolysis and intrauterine resuscitation. *BJOG*. 2004;111(4):316–318.
68. Lal A, Anderson G, Cowen M, Lindow S, Arnold AG. Pneumothorax and pregnancy. *Chest*. 2007;132(3):1044–1048.
69. Terndrup T, Bosco S, McLean E. Spontaneous pneumothorax complicating pregnancy—case report and review of the literature. *J Emerg Med*. 1989;7(3):245–248.
70. Sadikot R, Greene T, Meadows K, Arnold A. Recurrence of primary spontaneous pneumothorax. *Thorax*. 1997;52(9):805–809.
71. Garg R, Sanjay VD, Usman K, Rungta S, Prasad R. Spontaneous pneumothorax: An unusual complication of pregnancy-A case report and review of literature. *Ann Thorac Med*. 2008;3(3):104.
72. Whelan S, Kelly M. Pneumomediastinum following a prolonged second stage of labor–an emphasis on early diagnosis and conservative management: a case report. *J Med Case Rep*. 2017;11(1):1–5.
73. Khoo J, Mahanta VR. Spontaneous pneumomediastinum with severe subcutaneous emphysema secondary to prolonged labor during normal vaginal delivery. *Radiology Case Rep*. 2012;7(3):713.
74. Farhan F, Ruiz DE, Dawn SK, Webb WR, and Gotway MB. Helical CT esophagography for the evaluation of suspected esophageal perforation or rupture. *AJR*, 2004;182(5):1177–1179. .

# Abdominal Emergencies in Cancer and Immunocompromised Patients

Christian B. van der Pol, Rahul Sarkar, Amar Udare, Omar Alwahbi, and Michael N. Patlas

## Outline



## Key Points

- Contrast-enhanced abdomen and pelvis computed tomography is often a more appropriate initial imaging strategy for oncology and immunocompromised patients with acute nonlocalized abdominal pain compared with radiographs, ultrasound, or magnetic resonance imaging.
- Immune checkpoint inhibitors, molecular targeted therapies, and conformal radiation treatment can present with unique complications in the abdomen and pelvis that are not typical of those seen with classic cytotoxic chemotherapy; familiarity with several treatment categories and associated complications may lead the radiologist to the correct diagnosis.
- Several pitfalls when interpreting abdominal imaging in oncology patients include diagnosing disease response or progression without consideration of overall tumor burden elsewhere in the body, mistaking treatment-related changes for acute pathology or worsening malignancy, and using unclear terminology when describing vascular filling defects.

## Introduction

Oncology and immunocompromised patients pose a unique challenge when presenting with abdominal pain in the emergency department. History and physical exam findings can be misleading due to pain medication or a blunted inflammatory response.[1,2] In addition to the more common acute pathologies seen in otherwise healthy patients, cancer and immunocompromised patients can present with abdominal pain directly due to an underlying malignancy, a malignancy-related complication, a complication of immunosuppression, or a treatment-related complication. In this chapter, an approach to these patients is discussed, and acute processes related to a variety of organ systems are reviewed. A comprehensive discussion of treatment-related complications is provided, followed by a review of imaging pitfalls.

## Approach to Cancer and Immunocompromised Patients With Abdominal Pain

Acute abdominal pain is one of the most common complaints of oncology patients presenting to the emergency department, with the gastrointestinal system being the most frequent source.[3,4] Identifying the cause of pain can be challenging, as the clinical presentation may be misleading. While it is possible that pain may be due to uncontrollable cancer progression, all reasonable attempts must be made to ensure there are no reversible sources of pain that are treatable and that, once treated, may improve quality of life.

Contrast-enhanced abdomen and pelvis computed tomography (CT) is usually appropriate for immunocompromised patients with acute nonlocalized abdominal pain, and is a favored initial imaging strategy compared with radiographs, ultrasound, or magnetic resonance imaging (MRI) by the American College of Radiology.[5] Bowel pathologies including obstruction and enterocolitis are common in this population; neutropenic enterocolitis (typhlitis) is the most common cause of pain in neutropenic cancer patients (Fig. 5.1).[6] Other infectious and inflammatory processes of the bowel include opportunistic infections such as *Clostridium difficile* colitis (Fig. 5.2), cytomegalovirus colitis, and treatment-related conditions such as graft-versus-host disease (Fig. 5.3).[7] CT plays an important role in both establishing these diagnoses and excluding other causes of pain. Early initiation of medical treatment may preclude the need for an operation. The threshold to perform CT should therefore be lower for these patients than for the general population. This is particularly true for those with terminal malignancies; cumulative ionizing radiation exposure is unlikely to have any meaningful implication for these patients.

Abdominal radiographs play a limited role in the workup of abdominal pain in the emergency department. Sensitivity of radiographs for the diagnosis of enterocolitis and other acute abdominal pathologies is low, with the majority of radiographs not contributing to management, as shown by Kellow et al.[8] Even more concerning is that, in their study, the majority of patients who had follow-up abdominal imaging after initial normal radiographs were found to have an abnormality, suggesting that abdominal radiographs miss a considerable number of pathologies.

Similar to radiography, ultrasound has a limited role in cancer and immunocompromised patients with generalized abdominal pain. Ultrasound can be

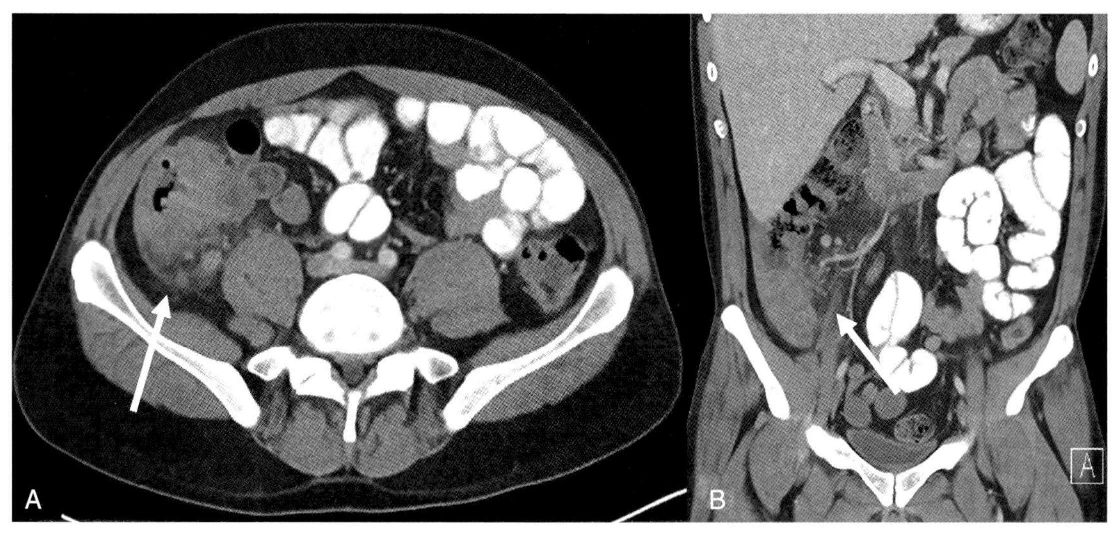


**Fig. 5.1** A 48-year-old male with acute myeloid leukemia and febrile neutropenia. Intravenous and oral contrast-enhanced abdomen and pelvis computed tomography reveals marked inflammation of the cecum in the axial (A) and coronal (B) planes (arrows). The patient was diagnosed with typhlitis.

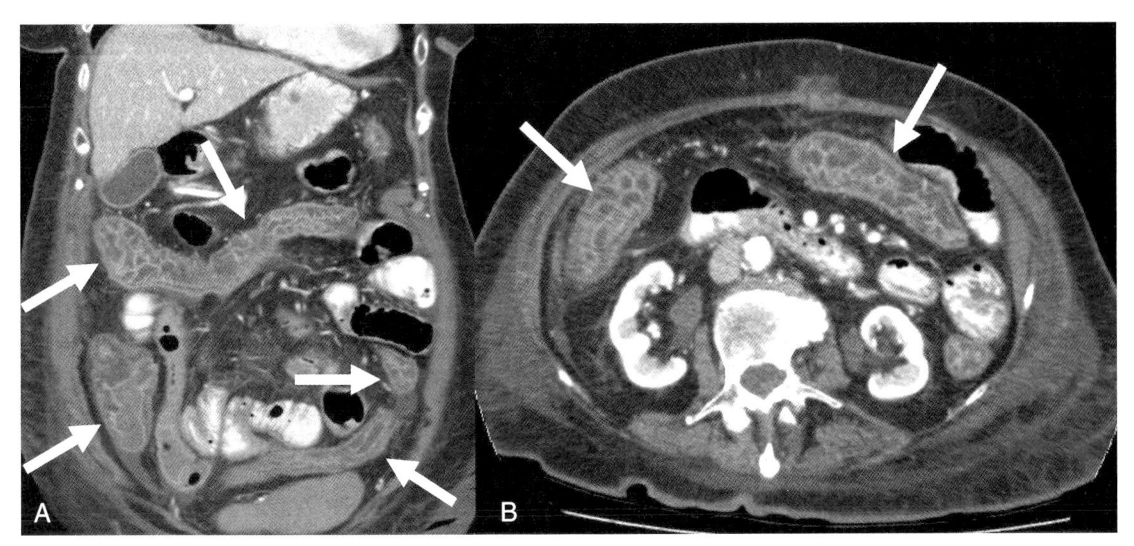


Fig. 5.2 An 85-year-old female who underwent colonic resection for an obstructing rectosigmoid mass. Contrast-enhanced computed tomography reveals diffuse inflammation of the colon characterized by marked wall thickening and mural stratification in the coronal (A) and axial (B) planes (arrows). The patient was diagnosed with pseudomembranous colitis. The thickened colonic folds can resemble an accordion, known as the "accordion sign."

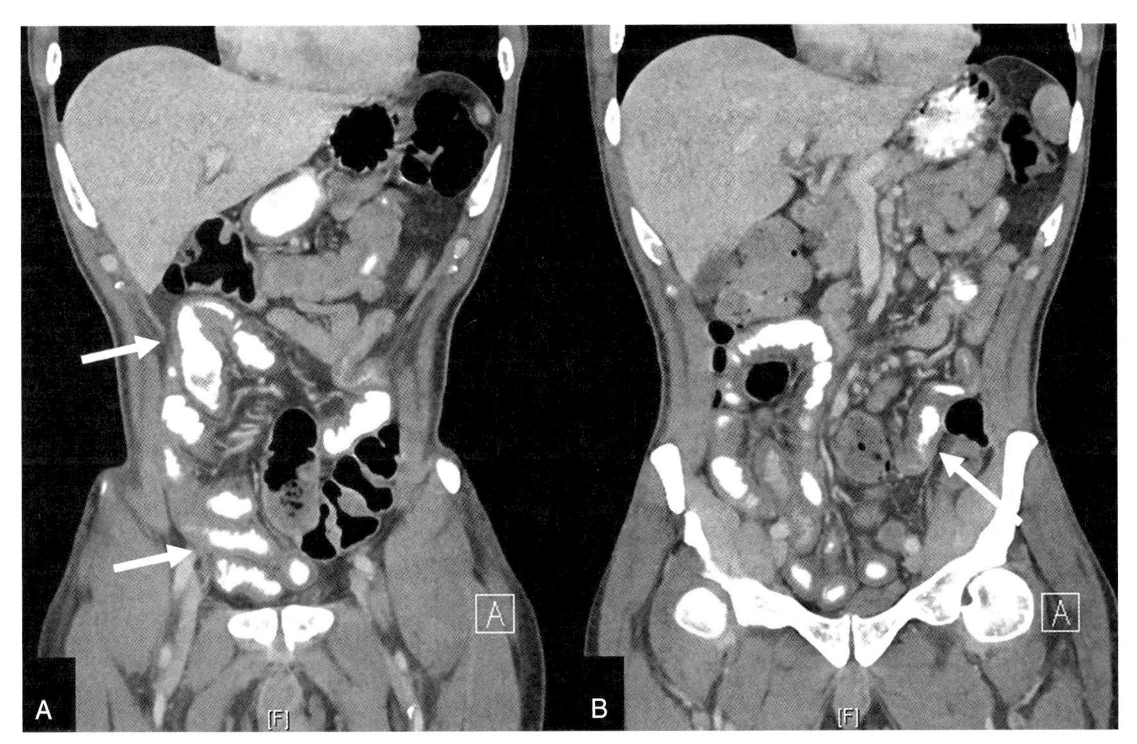


Fig. 5.3 A 49-year-old male with a history of myelodysplastic syndrome, allogeneic hematopoietic stem cell transplant, and abdominal pain. Computed tomography with intravenous and oral contrast reveals diffuse small bowel wall thickening consistent with graft versus host disease (arrows) as shown on two separate coronal images (A and B).

useful in the setting of localized pain, particularly if the presentation is suggestive of acute cholecystitis, as there is limited evidence for the utility of CT for this diagnosis.[9] Ultrasound can also be used for dynamic assessment of the abdomen, for example when assessing abdominal wall hernias, including at prior surgical incision sites or for an adynamic ileus. Another advantage of ultrasound is the lack of ionizing radiation, which is relevant for younger immunocompromised patients without terminal conditions who are likely to experience recurring abdominal pain. Patients with inflammatory bowel disease fit this profile. Ultrasound of the bowel is a highly effective but infrequently utilized tool for patients with Crohn disease and acute abdominal pain.[10] Familiarity with gut signature and the patterns of inflammatory bowel disease seen on ultrasound is recommended for all radiologists involved in the care of emergency department patients.

MRI is not generally performed as an initial imaging technique for patients with acute abdominal pain, with a few exceptions. MRI is accurate for the diagnosis of appendicitis in pregnant patients (Fig. 5.4).[11] Magnetic resonance cholangiopancreatography can be useful for assessment of the biliary system for obstruction or for iatrogenic biliary leaks (using hepatobiliary-specific contrast agent), which may be relevant for patients with prior hepatobiliary interventions where this is a concern.[12]

Radiologists should have a low threshold to image the abdomen and pelvis in cancer and immunocompromised patients, and for most cases CT is a pragmatic starting point. In the next section, vascular complications are explored.

## Vascular Complications

Abdominal malignancies can cause multiple vascular complications from advanced disease stage that can complicate surgical planning and often portend a worse prognosis. Complications include intratumoral hemorrhage, as is commonly seen with large and vascular tumors, bland thrombus formation from

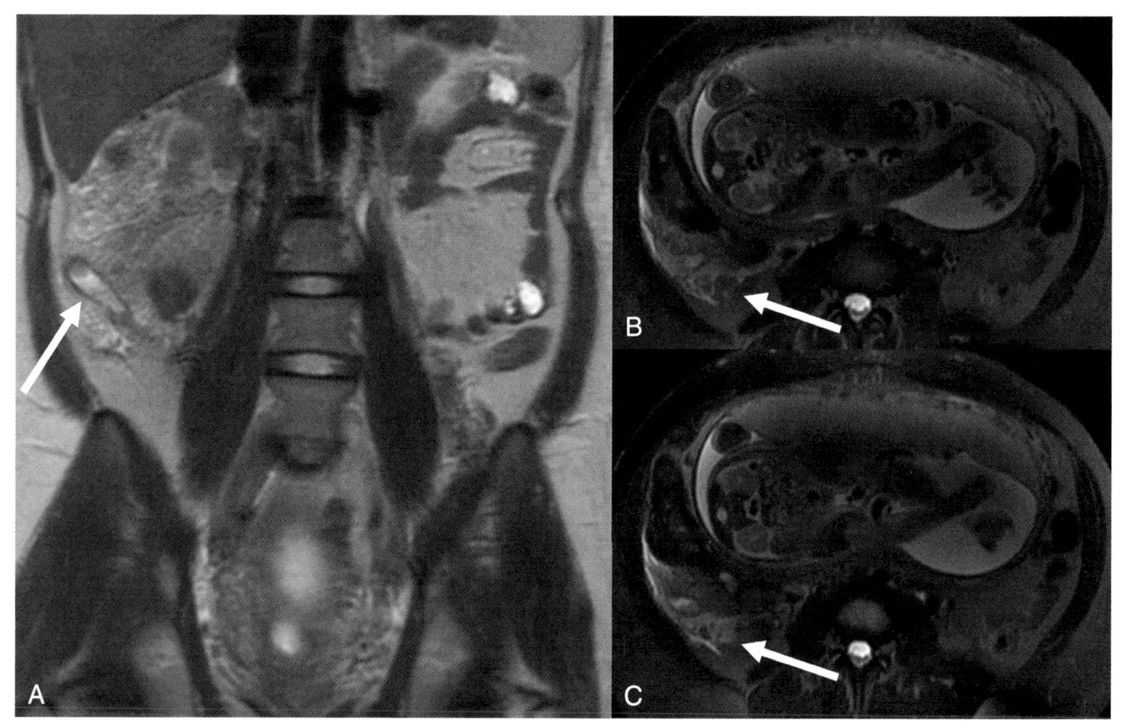


**Fig. 5.4** A 33-year-old pregnant female with acute abdominal pain. Coronal T2-weighted magnetic resonance imaging (A) reveals a dilated fluid-filled appendix in the right lower quadrant (arrow) with extensive surrounding edema, consistent with acute appendicitis. Axial fat-saturated imaging (B and C) confirms extensive periappendiceal edema (arrows).

a hypercoagulable state, and also direct tumor vascular invasion, which can lead to vascular occlusion.[13] Vascular complications can also arise secondary to interventions and treatment, especially with antiangiogenic chemotherapeutic agents.

Abdominal malignancies such as hepatocellular carcinoma (HCC), pancreatic adenocarcinoma, and renal cell carcinoma (RCC) have a propensity to invade and occlude vessels.[13–15] The inferior vena cava (IVC), portal, splanchnic, and pelvic veins are often involved.[16] Vascular occlusion can be secondary to direct tumor invasion (tumor in vein) or secondary to bland thrombus. Although it can be difficult to distinguish tumor from bland thrombus on imaging, vessel expansion, enhancement/arterial flow within the filling defect, contiguity and morphological resemblance to the primary mass, intermediate T2 signal, and diffusion-weighted imaging hyperintensity on MRI favors tumor in vein rather than bland thrombus (Fig. 5.5).[16] Vascular invasion is usually a gradual process allowing for collateral formation; however, rarely, vascular invasion by tumor can cause acute pain or organ infarction secondary to extensive thrombosis or even embolization.[17] Hepatic infarction secondary to tumor in vein is rare given dual hepatic blood supply. However, involvement of the hepatic veins or IVC by hepatic, renal, or adrenal malignancies, or metastatic retroperitoneal lymphadenopathy or primary vascular malignancies, can cause acute Budd-Chiari syndrome.[18–22] In acute Budd-Chiari syndrome, the only findings on imaging may be hepatic venous occlusion and ascites. On contrast-enhanced imaging, there can be patchy decreased enhancement in the peripheral portions of the liver with sparing of the central portion due to its direct venous drainage into the IVC.[23] Pancreatic adenocarcinoma is notorious for vascular invasion, but due to its extensive collateral blood supply pancreatic necrosis secondary to vascular occlusion is rare.[14] Nevertheless, involvement of the splanchnic and splenic veins can cause acute mesenteric ischemia and splenic infarction, respectively.[13,24,25] Acute bowel ischemia can be identified by circumferential

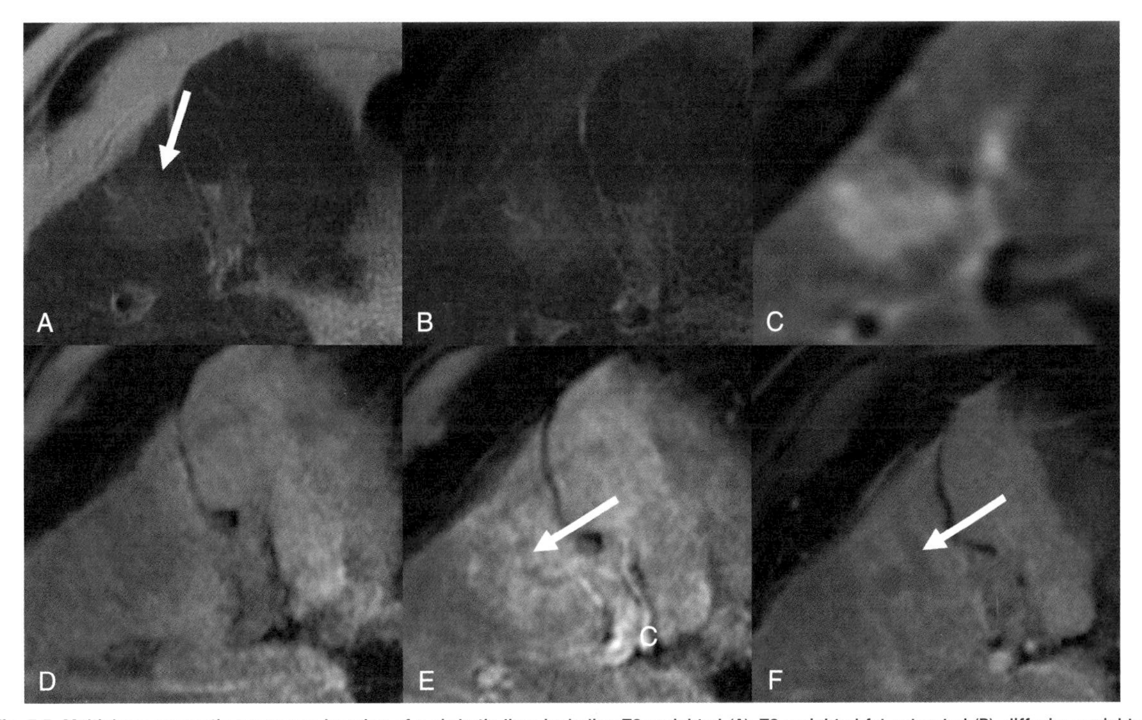


**Fig. 5.5** Multiphase magnetic resonance imaging of a cirrhotic liver including T2-weighted (A), T2-weighted fat-saturated (B), diffusion-weighted imaging (C), T1-weighted fat saturated (D), arterial phase (E), and delayed-phase (F) sequences. A mass in the liver (A, arrow) is inseparable from a portal vein branch that contains a filling defect with arterial enhancement and washout (E and F, arrows), consistent with tumor in vein rather than bland thrombus.

bowel wall thickening with either mural hypoattenuation due to submucosal edema/inflammation or mural hyperattenuation from hemorrhage, and decreased enhancement on postcontrast images.[24] Pneumatosis suggests infarction, which may warrant urgent surgical resection.[24] The spleen is particularly susceptible to acute infarction due to its rich vascularity and exclusive supply by the solitary splenic artery.[14] Splenic infarction can present with acute left upper quadrant pain and is seen on CT as wedge-shaped peripheral hypodensities or diffuse hypoattenuation in severe cases (Fig. 5.6).[14]

Tumor-associated hemorrhage is an important cause of spontaneous hemoperitoneum, commonly seen with hypervascular neoplasms such as HCC, hepatic adenoma, RCC, adrenal pheochromocytoma, adrenocortical carcinoma, and hepatic metastases from melanoma.[13,26,27] HCC is one of the most common causes of spontaneous nontraumatic hemorrhage, with higher incidence in patients with chronic hepatitis B viral infection and those with cirrhosis.[26] HCC rupture carries a poor prognosis, with an overall mortality rate of 24% despite advancements in endovascular treatment.[28] Subcapsular tumors are more prone to hemorrhage, while intraparenchymal tumors can present with acute pain secondary to the tamponade effect of normal adjacent liver parenchyma without significant blood loss.[29] Spontaneous renal and perirenal hemorrhage, also known as Wunderlich syndrome, is reported in 0.3% to 1.4% of RCCs, most commonly the clear cell subtype.[30] Other tumors known to bleed spontaneously include gastrointestinal stromal tumors (GISTs), hepatic angiosarcomas, and hepatic metastases from lung cancer.[29,31] Abdominal tumor hemorrhage can also be iatrogenic from systemic anticoagulation and biopsy.[25] A hyperdense area on noncontrast CT with extravascular contrast blush on the arterial phase that expands on the delayed phase is consistent with active extravasation, for which urgent embolization or surgical management may be needed.[26] The presence of a high-attenuation hematoma abutting an organ can be used to identify the site of hemorrhage and is known as the *sentinel clot sign*.[25] An underlying tumor must be ruled out in all cases presenting with spontaneous nontraumatic hemorrhage, either on follow-up imaging or using subtraction postcontrast MRI (Fig. 5.7).

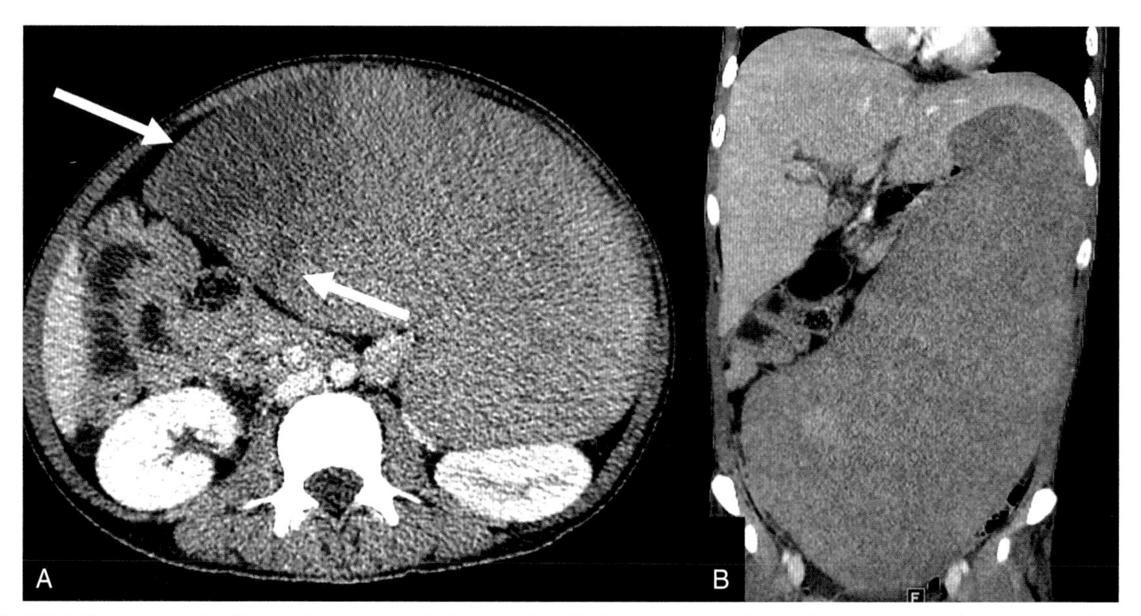


**Fig. 5.6** A 20-year-old male with massive splenomegaly from non-Hodgkin lymphoma on contrast-enhanced computed tomography in the axial (A) and coronal (B) planes. Multiple wedge-shaped hypodense areas (arrows) are present in the spleen consistent with infarcts.

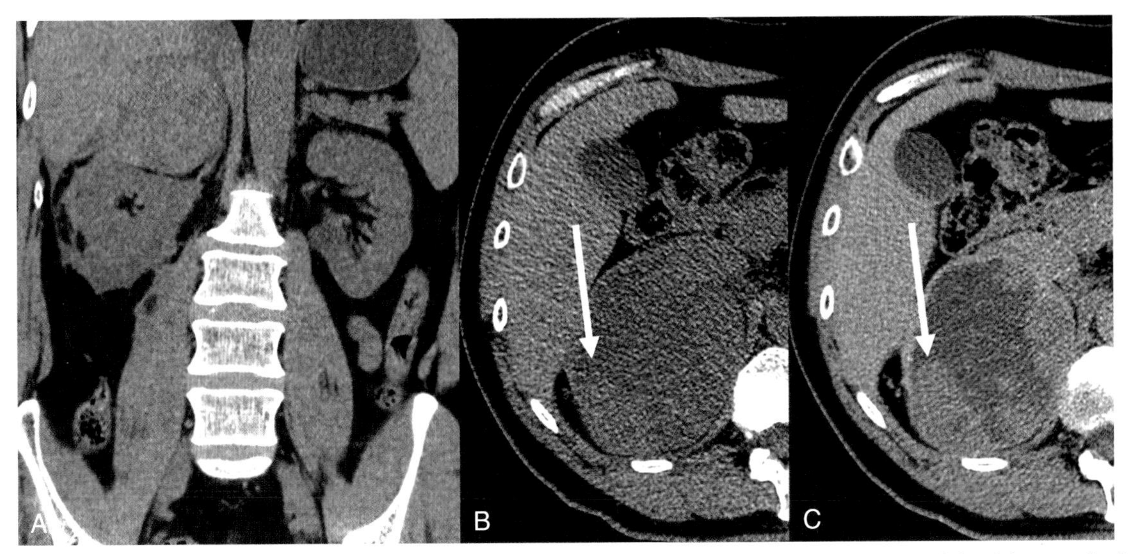


Fig. 5.7 A 58-year-old male with acute abdominal pain. Unenhanced coronal computed tomography (CT) image (A) of the abdomen and pelvis reveals a large right suprarenal fossa heterogeneous mass with hyperdense areas. Acute hemorrhage of the right adrenal gland of unclear etiology was diagnosed. A follow-up CT was performed 3 months later without (B) and with (C) intravenous contrast after a portion of the hematoma had resorbed. Areas of enhancement (arrows) within a right adrenal mass were confirmed, consistent with tumor. The lesion was resected and found to be adrenocortical carcinoma. Deferring follow-up imaging for several weeks can allow for the resorption of hemorrhagic products, which may improve conspicuity of enhancing tumor.

## Tumor and Organ-Specific Complications

Many abdominal malignancies can exert mass effect or invade and obstruct organ systems including the biliary system, urinary system, gastrointestinal tract, vessels, and neurological structures including the spinal cord. Obstruction or compression of these structures can lead to devastating consequences, for example, biliary sepsis, renal failure, bowel obstruction, thrombosis, and paralysis. In addition, all can be associated with debilitating pain. Recognition of these pathologies is critical, as they may be amenable to intervention that can substantially improve quality of life.

### HEPATOBILIARY SYSTEM

Obstruction of the biliary system may result from an intraluminal mass, adjacent tumor mass effect, or invasion. Obstruction may also occur at the extrahepatic or intrahepatic level, such as from pancreatic adenocarcinoma, cholangiocarcinoma, ampullary and periampullary tumors, and also HCC and metastases (Fig. 5.8). Biliary obstruction results in bile stasis and accumulation, which leads to jaundice, hepatic dysfunction, and acute liver failure. Prolonged stasis can act as a nidus for infection, causing cholangitis, hepatic abscess, and sepsis. Obstruction of the common bile duct is typically treated by placement of a biliary stent, usually a removable plastic stent if the obstructing tumor may respond to chemotherapy or radiotherapy. Otherwise, a metallic stent can be considered if survival is expected to be greater than 4 months, as these have better long-term patency.[32] Stents are an option when the biliary system is obstructed at one site; however, multifocal hepatic tumors obstructing multiple separate intrahepatic bile ducts may not be amenable to treatment. Occasionally, more than one percutaneous stent may be inserted, or a combination of stenting and percutaneous drainage may be used, for example, to drain the largest portion of liver in an attempt to lower the serum bilirubin level to initiate chemotherapy for potentially resectable disease to optimize the future liver remnant, or for management of cholangitis or severe pruritis.[33]

Acute pancreatitis is the presenting feature of pancreatic adenocarcinoma in up to 13% of cases and is often associated with a delayed diagnosis.[34,35] Other, less common causes of acute pancreatitis in malignancy include metastases (especially from small cell

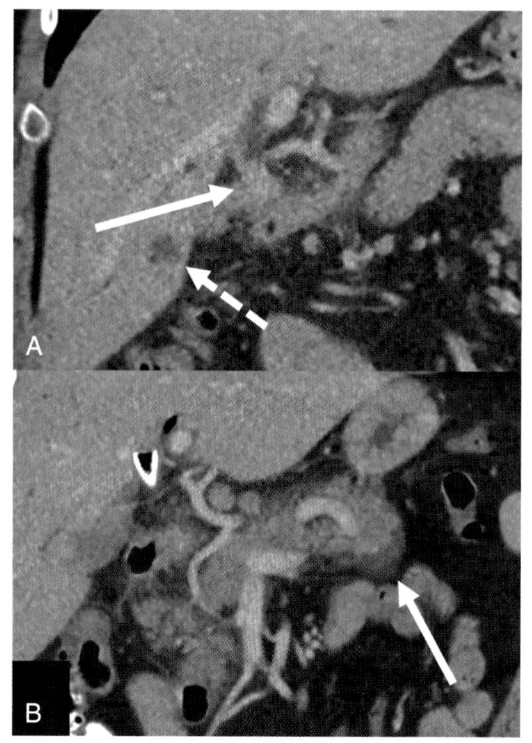


Fig. 5.8 Coronal contrast-enhanced computed tomography showing bile duct dilatation secondary to an obstructing cholangiocarcinoma (A, arrow). A hypodense lesion in the liver (dashed arrow) was suspected to be a metastasis. The patient subsequently underwent endoscopic biliary stent insertion complicated by acute interstitial edematous pancreatitis, as evidenced by peripancreatic fat stranding (B, arrow).

lung cancer), malignant hypercalcemia, chemotherapy-induced pancreatitis (L-asparaginase, ifosfamide, paclitaxel, cisplatin, vinorelbine, cytarabine, tretinoin, sunitinib, and sorafenib), and pancreatitis associated with newer classes of antineoplastic therapies.[13,25,29] On imaging, there can be pancreatic enlargement, peripancreatic fat stranding with or without collections, and pancreatic necrosis similar to other benign causes of pancreatitis. It is imperative to assess for underlying differential parenchymal enhancement and mass effect to rule out a malignant cause. Pancreatic ductal dilatation with a duct to parenchyma ratio of more than 0.34, double duct sign, vascular encasement, vessel deformity, and increased ratio of the superior mesenteric artery to the superior mesenteric vein all suggest an underlying pancreatic adenocarcinoma rather than mass-forming pancreatitis.[36] Alternatively, the duct penetrating sign, characterized by smooth narrowing of the pancreatic duct traversing a mass, suggests an inflammatory mass.[36] Smaller pancreatic lesions can be overlooked due to changes of acute pancreatitis and may only be seen on follow-up imaging.[25,29]

## GENITOURINARY SYSTEM

Malignant obstruction of the urinary system can manifest as unilateral or bilateral hydronephrosis leading to renal failure. Ureteric obstruction may be secondary to intraluminal tumors, external compression, or invasion by retroperitoneal and pelvic malignancy (Fig. 5.9). Common pelvic malignancies directly obstructing ureters include tumors of the cervix, prostate, and urinary bladder, as well as colorectal cancer. Retroperitoneal masses such as retroperitoneal sarcomas, lymphoma, or pathologic lymph nodes, including from prostate and testicular cancers, may also result in obstruction.[25] Primary urothelial malignancy is a concern when there is an intraluminal neoplasm, although metastases can rarely occur here. Ultrasound can be performed to assess for hydronephrosis but is generally inadequate to assess the entire ureter. CT is more ideal for evaluating the extent of tumor involvement of the urinary system.[37] Unilateral obstruction without obstructive symptoms, infection, or a significant drop in the glomerular filtration rate may not require intervention.[38] However, obstruction of both urinary collecting systems, as can occur with invasive cervical carcinoma and other midline pelvic tumors, can lead to renal failure. Urgent urinary diversion using percutaneous nephrostomy or ureteric stents is usually recommended in these cases.[38,39] In cases of bilateral hydronephrosis of unclear etiology, evaluation for an underlying pelvic malignancy obstructing each ureter is essential.[40]

Ovarian torsion can occur as a result of an ovarian mass acting as a lead point. Although benign mature cystic teratomas (dermoids) are the most common cause of ovarian torsion, a malignant tumor causes ovarian torsion in up to 2% of cases.[25,41] In postmenopausal women, torsion can be associated with malignant neoplasms in up to 22% of patients, for whom the diagnosis is more often delayed.[42] Acute ovarian torsion can present with sudden-onset abdominal pain mimicking more common conditions such as acute

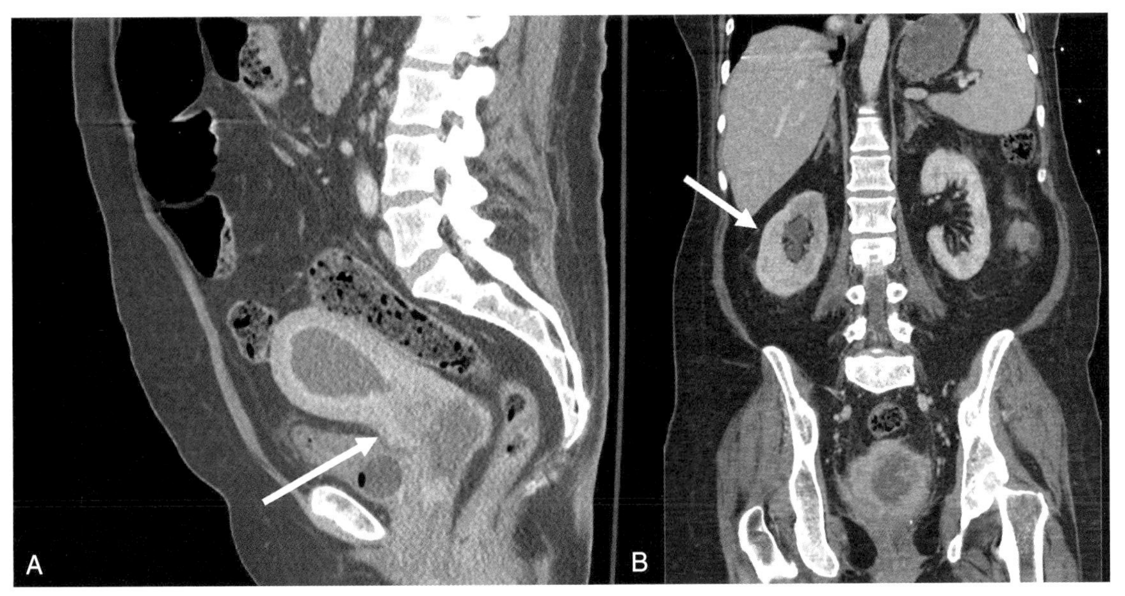


Fig. 5.9 Sagittal contrast-enhanced computed tomography (A) demonstrates an infiltrative cervical mass (arrow) invading the right distal ureter. This was resulting in upstream hydronephrosis and a delayed nephrogram indicating obstructive uropathy (B, arrow).

appendicitis, diverticulitis, tuboovarian abscess, ectopic pregnancy, and a ruptured ovarian cyst.[25] Acute ovarian torsion requires urgent surgical intervention, and imaging plays a crucial role in early diagnosis.[25] Ultrasound can show the presence of an ovarian mass, ovarian enlargement, peripheral ovarian follicles, a twisted vascular pedicle with a whirlpool sign, and free fluid.[43] Additional signs can include subacute hemorrhage and abnormal ovarian enhancement.[43] Ovarian masses can also present with torsion.[43]

## GASTROINTESTINAL TRACT

Malignant obstruction of the gastrointestinal tract can occur anywhere along its length. Obstruction at the level of the esophagus from primary esophageal malignancy, usually adenocarcinoma, can present with progressive dysphagia. Gastric outlet obstruction can be caused by primary gastric adenocarcinoma, metastatic disease, or direct invasion by hepatobiliary malignancies. Small bowel obstruction can be due to both malignant and benign small bowel tumors, with involvement by metastatic disease more common than small bowel primary neoplasms, usually from serosal deposits in peritoneal carcinomatosis.[44] Primary small bowel tumors include adenocarcinoma, GIST, carcinoid tumors, and also small bowel lymphoma.[45] Large bowel obstruction is often due to a primary adenocarcinoma. Treatment for bowel obstruction by malignancy is usually surgical diversion or resection depending on the treatment plan and oncologic stage.[46]

## VASCULAR SYSTEM

Tumor can directly invade vessels or contribute toward bland thrombus formation, owing to prothrombotic properties. Some tumors may arise from the vessel walls, such as sarcomas and hemangiopericytomas.

## NERVOUS SYSTEM

Spinal cord compression by tumor may require urgent diagnosis and radiation treatment or decompressive surgery. Many malignancies can result in cord compression, including those arising from the spine, as well as metastases.[37] MRI should be performed for any tumor suspected to be within the spinal canal that may require directed management. Assessment of the spinal canal can be performed on nondedicated examinations of the abdomen and pelvis in oncology patients presenting with back pain or neurological symptoms.

## Treatment-Related Complications

Cancer patients undergoing treatment represent a unique population requiring special attention to treatment-related aspects of their medical history, including the specific treatment agents and modalities used, as well as the treatment timeline, in order to recognize and distinguish adverse treatment-related effects from other pathologies that can present with overlapping imaging findings. While imaging features of toxicities relating to classical cytotoxic chemotherapy and external-beam radiotherapy are well established, novel treatments including molecular targeted therapies (MTTs), immune checkpoint inhibitors (ICIs), and three-dimensional conformal radiation delivery methods such as stereotactic body radiation therapy (SBRT) have emerged as effective options with more favorable but less intuitive toxicity profiles, making the task of image interpretation in patients on these treatments more complex.[47,48] The imaging findings of the more commonly encountered treatment complications, and a few selected treatment-specific complications of high clinical significance, are reviewed in order to facilitate a pragmatic systems-based approach to assessing acute abdominal imaging studies in cancer patients (Table 5.1).

### PULMONARY TREATMENT-RELATED COMPLICATIONS

Assessment of the lung bases on abdominal CT should be performed to assess for ground glass opacities or areas of consolidation suggestive of pneumonitis. The most observed pattern is that of interstitial pneumonitis, though any pattern of lung injury can be observed, with other common patterns including organizing pneumonia, nonspecific interstitial pneumonia, hypersensitivity pneumonitis, and acute interstitial pneumonia.[49,50] Pneumonitis can be seen with almost any treatment, with notable examples from each category including bleomycin and methotrexate (conventional chemotherapy), tyrosine kinase inhibitors targeting the estimated glomerular filtration rate (eGFR) and mammalian target of rapamycin (mTOR) pathways (MTTs), and anti–CTLA-4 therapies such as ipilimumab (ICIs).[47] Management of pneumonitis associated with chemotherapy may involve discontinuation of treatment and/or administration of steroids. Radiation-induced pneumonitis usually presents with localized opacities appearing between 1 and 6 months after treatment, with subsequent contraction and volume loss progressing to fibrosis.[51] The pattern may correspond to a geographic radiation port in traditional

**TABLE 5.1 Treatment and Side Effects in the Abdomen and Pelvis on Imaging**

| Treatment Type | Example | Side Effects |
|---|---|---|
| Immune checkpoint inhibitors | Atezolizumab, durvalumab, ipilimumab, nivolumab, pembrolizumab | Pancreatitis, pneumonitis, segmental colitis associated with diverticulosis, enteritis/colitis |
| Anti-VEGF molecular targeted therapies | Bevacizumab, pazopanib, sorafenib, sunitinib, ziv-aflibercept | Arterial thromboembolic events, bowel perforation, tumor-bowel fistula |
| Nonantiangiogenic molecular targeted therapies | Cetuximab, crizotinib, erlotinib, everolimus, palbociclib | Enteritis/colitis, hepatic steatosis, pancreatitis |
| Classic cytotoxic chemotherapy | Bleomycin, cyclophosphamide, cisplatin, fluorouracil, gemcitabine, methotrexate, oxaliplatin, vincristine | Enteritis/colitis, hemorrhagic cystitis, hepatic steatosis, nephrotoxicity |
| Radiation | Brachytherapy, traditional external beam radiation, stereotactic body radiation therapy | Cystopathy, enteropathy, insufficiency fractures, pneumonitis |

*VEGF*, Vascular endothelial growth factor.

external-beam techniques or have a more complex irregular shape in SBRT; correlation with radiotherapy planning can be useful in uncertain cases.

## HEPATOBILIARY TREATMENT-RELATED COMPLICATIONS

Hepatotoxicity is associated with several chemotherapeutic agents and demonstrates nonspecific imaging findings including hepatomegaly, periportal edema, and hepatic steatosis. Although steatosis is a common finding in the general population, typically without acute clinical significance, new steatosis in cancer patients can represent treatment-induced steatohepatitis, which may limit detection of hepatic metastases.[52] Notable agents associated with hepatic steatosis include irinotecan and oxaliplatin (conventional), EGFR tyrosine kinase inhibitors (MTTs), and tamoxifen (hormonal).[47,49] Radiation-induced liver disease can present with similar imaging findings in either a geographic distribution or a more irregular pattern, depending on the use of three-dimensional conformal techniques, with findings often resolving after 6 months or progressing to fibrosis in some patients.[53]

In patients undergoing stem cell transplantation, findings of hepatomegaly, gallbladder wall thickening, and ascites should raise concern for the possibilities of hepatic venoocclusive disease (VOD)/sinusoidal obstruction syndrome (allogenic or autologous stem cell transplant) or acute hepatic graft-versus-host disease (GVHD) (allogenic only).[54] Ultrasound findings supporting a diagnosis of VOD include narrowed hepatic veins, decreased/reversed portal venous flow, monophasic hepatic vein waveforms, and increased hepatic arterial resistive indices (>0.8). Findings overlap with acute GVHD, which should be favored in allogenic stem cell transplant patients with associated bowel findings because enteric disease usually exists concurrently.

Chemotherapy-induced biliary sclerosis was first described in the context of intraarterial therapy and manifests with biliary strictures, often preferentially affecting central intrahepatic bile ducts with relative sparing of the peripheral ducts compared with sclerosing cholangitis, although imaging features can overlap. Immunotherapy-associated damage to bile ducts can also be seen, though imaging findings typically more closely resemble nonspecific findings of hepatitis, often without frank biliary strictures.[55]

Pancreatitis is a less common but important toxicity associated with certain agents, with MTTs (e.g., sorafenib) and ICIs representing notable examples.[50,56] Although the primary role of imaging is for assessment of complications, the radiologist may be the first to suggest this diagnosis.

## GASTROINTESTINAL TREATMENT-RELATED COMPLICATIONS

Together, acute colitis and enteritis represent the most common treatment-related toxicities across all agents, although the underlying mechanisms and associated imaging findings can vary.[47,49,50] While typical findings of small bowel wall thickening with or without adjacent fat stranding and bowel dilatation may be present, newer MTTs and ICIs often demonstrate more subtle imaging findings, with the primary abnormality often being diffusely fluid-filled bowel indicative of a mucosal colitis. Despite the more subtle findings, this can represent a treatment-limiting toxicity that can explain a presentation of diarrhea and abdominal pain. ICI-related colitis may manifest as a diffuse pancolitis, or as a distinct segmental colitis associated with diverticulosis (SCAD), with the latter demonstrating imaging appearances that are typically identical those of acute diverticulitis in the general population (Fig. 5.10). The latter distinction is important, as management of SCAD often requires the use of both steroids and antibiotics.

Anti-vascular endothelial growth factor targeted therapies are associated with rare but potentially life-threatening presentations. Bowel perforation and tumor-bowel fistula formation can both be preceded by pneumatosis, with frank perforation typically showing pneumoperitoneum, free fluid, and sometimes organized collections. Tumor-bowel fistula represents an important underreported complication that can present as a complex solid/cystic mass, sometimes with clear communication of gas and liquid between bowel and an adjacent tumor.[57] Importantly, radiologists play a role in the prevention of these complications by identifying sites of concerning serosal disease in patients on anti-VEGF treatments, sometimes prompting a change in treatment strategy for high-risk patients.

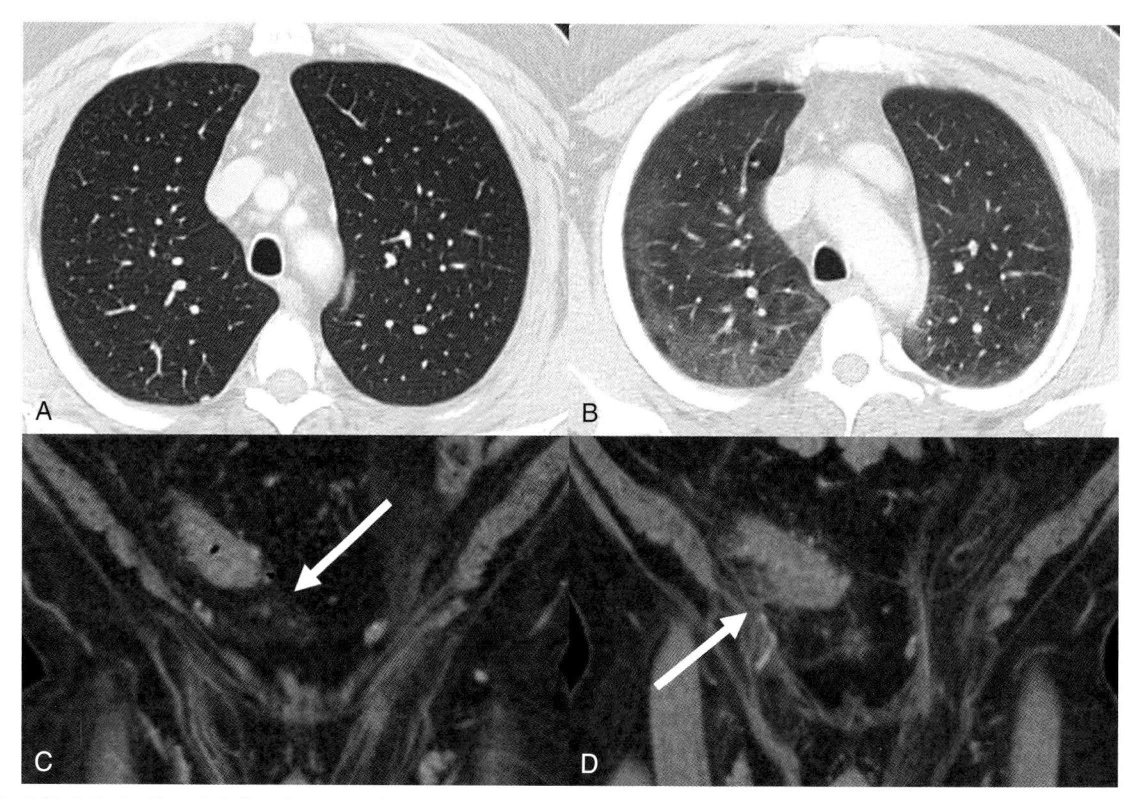


**Fig. 5.10** Patient with metastatic melanoma on immune checkpoint inhibitor therapy. Axial chest computed tomography (CT) (A and B) reveals pulmonary ground glass opacities at the lung bases (B) consistent with pneumonitis. Coronal contrast-enhanced CT images (C and D) demonstrate pericolonic fat stranding surrounding colonic diverticula (white arrows) consistent with segmental colitis associated with diverticulosis. These findings resolved after combined steroids and antibiotic therapy.

Neutropenic colitis and infectious colitis can both be seen in patients with neutropenia from any treatment modality, including cytotoxic chemotherapies and stem cell transplants.[54] Imaging features and distribution overlap between the two entities, but predominantly cecal involvement should raise suspicion for neutropenic colitis (typhlitis) in these patients. Infectious colitis in the patients can be polymicrobial and include opportunistic fungal infections requiring broad-spectrum treatment.

Bowel dilatation may reflect obstruction or adynamic ileus in treated cancer patients, with obstruction more commonly seen in patients who have undergone radiotherapy or patients with serosal disease treated with any agent resulting in fibrosis, and adynamic ileus seen more commonly with conventional agents associated with neurotoxicity to the autonomic nervous system (e.g., vincristine).[49] Identification of a discrete transition point is important in identifying a possible mechanical obstruction.

## GENITOURINARY TREATMENT-RELATED COMPLICATIONS

Hemorrhagic cystitis is a recognized complication of certain conventional agents, including cyclophosphamide and ifosfamide,[58] and demonstrates overlapping features with radiation cystopathy. Imaging findings include diffuse bladder wall thickening/nodularity, with intraluminal debris or clots sometimes seen on ultrasound. Infectious cystitis may be associated with a greater degree of perivesicular stranding and should be considered in neutropenic patients.

Renal failure may be a result of treatment-related renal injury or post-renal obstruction. Nephrotoxicity is associated with MTTs and ICIs, but is most commonly associated with conventional agents such as cisplatin, methotrexate, and cyclophosphamide/ifosfamide.[49] The main role of imaging is to exclude a postrenal obstructive cause, which can be due to treatment related ureteric strictures including those associated with radiation fibrosis.[53] Nonobstructive nephrotoxicity may have no imaging manifestation, though diffusely increased renal cortical echogenicity may be seen on ultrasound evaluation.

Fistulas may form between pelvic organs including the bladder, rectum, and vagina as a result of treatment-related complications in patients undergoing treatment for gynecologic malignancies, including those treated with radiation therapy (particularly brachytherapy) and those on anti-VEGF therapies such as bevacizumab.[47,53] Intracavitary contrast (fluoroscopic/CT cystogram, rectal or vaginal contrast) can improve sensitivity for fistula tract detection (Fig. 5.11).

## VASCULAR TREATMENT-RELATED COMPLICATIONS

Although cancer predisposes to an inherently hypercoagulable state, certain conventional agents such as gemcitabine and cisplatin have been associated with superimposed increased risk of venous thromboembolic events. Pancreatic cancer patients being treated with gemcitabine may be at particularly high risk, given the excessive hypercoagulable state associated with pancreatic cancer.[59] Venous extremity ultrasound should be performed for any clinical suspicion of deep vein thrombus, but cross-sectional abdominal images should also be screened for any evidence of thrombus formation in the systemic or portal veins, as well the visualized portions of the pulmonary arteries.

Unlike most other agents, anti-VEGF targeted therapies are associated with an increased risk of arterial thromboembolic events, and patients being treated with these agents should be assessed for associated imaging manifestations on abdominal pelvic CT exams, including direct evidence of arterial thrombus, secondary features of arterial mesenteric ischemia, and end-organ infarcts.[47]

In patients presenting with clinical signs and symptoms of bleeding, or unexplained decreased hemoglobin, careful assessment for imaging features of bleeding is required. Significant intratumoral hemorrhage can occur in hypervascular tumors, either spontaneously or secondary to treatment-induced tumor changes, with a notable example being GIST treated with c-Kit targeted therapies.[60] Patients on anti-VEGF targeted therapies may present with hemorrhage at sites independent of tumor involvement.

## ABNORMAL FLUID ACCUMULATION

Presentations of abdominal distention with associated imaging findings of ascites, or shortness of breath associated with underlying pleural effusions, can relate to disease progression or reflect a manifestation of treatment-related cardiovascular, hepatic, or renal toxicity,

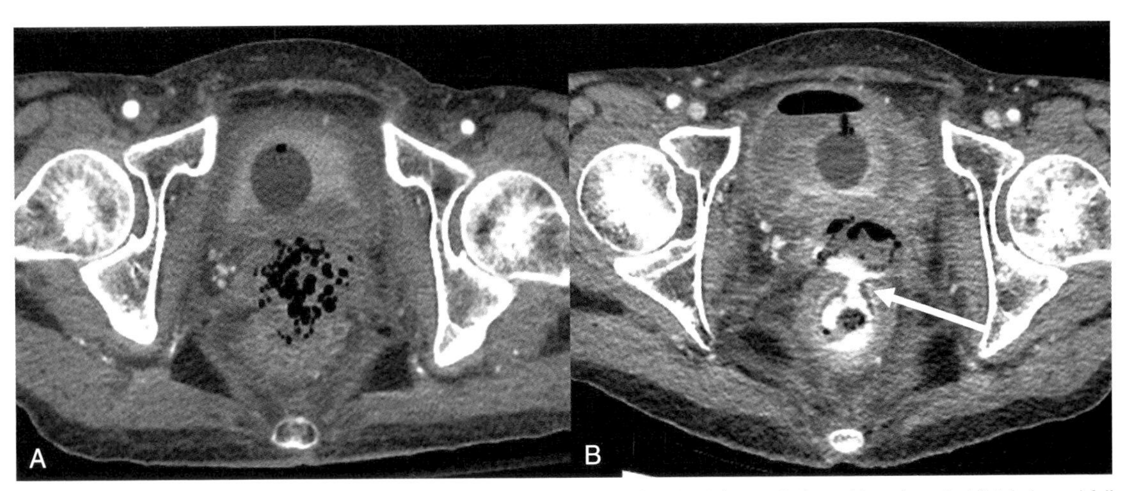


**Fig. 5.11** Posttreatment computed tomography scans without (A) and with (B) rectal contrast demonstrate a wide rectovaginal fistula (arrow) following multimodal treatment of cervical cancer that included bevacizumab (an anti-vascular endothelial growth factor therapeutic) and brachytherapy. The urinary bladder contains air secondary to a Foley catheter.

as outlined above.[61] Some agents are associated with specific forms of fluid overload, for example pleural effusions in dasatinib therapy and pericardial effusions in imatinib therapy.

### OSSEOUS TREATMENT-RELATED COMPLICATIONS

Treatment-induced reduction in bone density can result in the development of pathologic fractures that may result in acute pain that is not always clinically apparent as being of osseous origin. Some commonly used agents are associated with a global reduction in bone density, of which aromatase inhibitors are a notable example.[47] Radiotherapy results in fatty marrow replacement and a localized reduction in bone density that can predispose to pathologic fractures near the treatment site, particular in the spine and other weight-bearing regions. Identification of fractures and associated sites of neurological impingement is important to explain a potential source of pain, as well as other neurological symptoms that might otherwise be incorrectly attributed to treatment-related neuropathy.

## Pitfalls for Radiologists to Avoid

Oncology and immunocompromised patients pose several challenges when presenting with acute symptoms. Malignancy can masquerade as a benign process and vice versa. The radiologist must strike a balance between sensitivity and specificity when suggesting diagnoses, which should be guided by the likelihood of each pathology and also by management implications.

In oncology patients, treatment-related changes can resemble acute pathologies and worsening malignancy. The best defense against this pitfall is establishing the patient's treatment history and gaining familiarity with expected posttreatment changes. Localized treatments such as percutaneous ablation (e.g., microwave, radiofrequency, cryoablation, irreversible electroporation, and others) are becoming more common.[62] Coagulation necrosis in the treatment zone created by thermal ablation, for example, can resemble infarction, acute hemorrhage, or a new lesion on cross-sectional imaging (Fig. 5.12). Systemic therapies can have a similar effect. GISTs treated

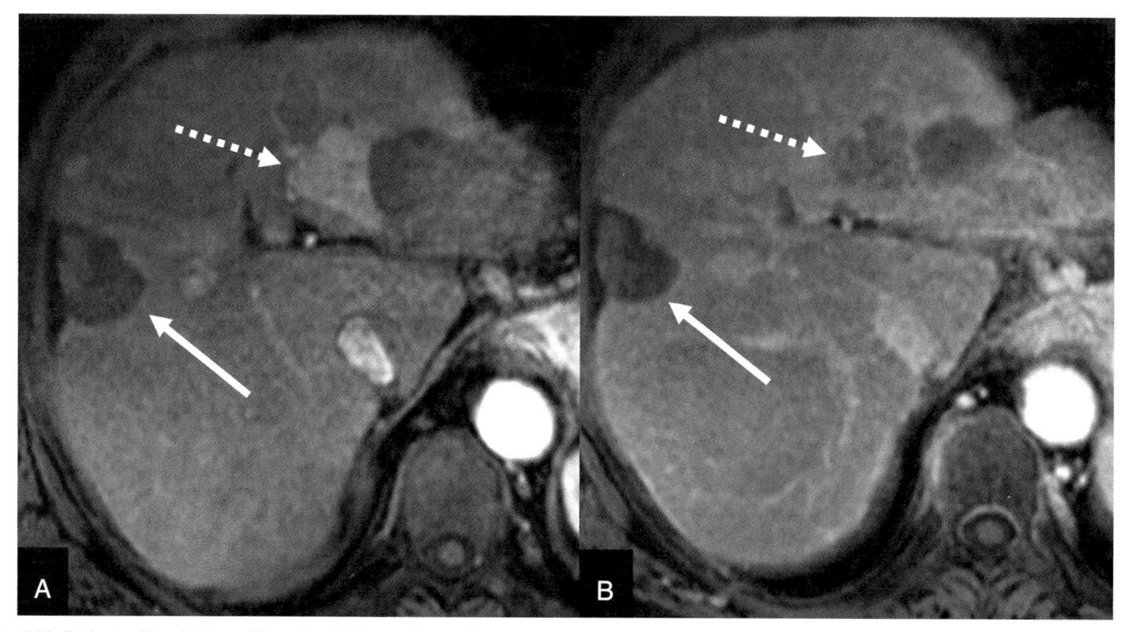


**Fig. 5.12** Patient with a history of hepatocellular carcinoma imaged on magnetic resonance imaging in the axial plane in the late arterial (A) and delayed (B) phases. A new hypoenhancing area in the right hepatic lobe (A and B, solid arrow) could raise concern for a new liver lesion. Note this does not enhance; this was a site of percutaneous ablation. An arterially enhancing mass (A, dashed arrow) with washout (B, dashed arrow) fulfilled Liver Imaging Reporting and Data System (LI-RADS) LR-5 criteria, diagnostic of hepatocellular carcinoma.

with competitive tyrosine kinase receptor inhibitors frequently undergo internal hemorrhage, necrosis, and myxoid degeneration.[63] In some cases, this can lead to a GIST increasing in size despite responding to treatment.[64] Pseudoprogression of liver metastases treated with MTT describes a similar phenomenon by which antiangiogenic drugs result in newly apparent hypoenhancing liver lesions.[65] While new lesions suggest progression, these lesions may have been unnoticed on the pretreatment scan due to enhancement characteristics similar to adjacent hepatic parenchyma. Comparing extrahepatic disease response to changes seen in the liver may tip off the radiologist (Table 5.2). Similarly, metastases can increase in size and number soon after initiating ICI treatment in a minority of patients, usually evident by week 12 after initiating treatment with a trend toward treatment response after week 16, also known as "pseudoprogression."[48] Follow-up imaging is critical to determine if the size increase is a transient phenomenon.

Benign pneumatosis is a consideration for patients with bowel wall gas that can be seen in oncology and immunocompromised patients. This has many potential causes, including steroids and chemotherapy. The absence of portal venous gas on imaging and the lack of findings concerning for intestinal ischemia on clinical history, physical exam, and bloodwork may help the radiologist recognize this diagnosis (Fig. 5.13).[66]

Worsening tumor can resemble acute benign pathologies. Necrotic tumor, for example, can resemble a drainable abscess. It is important to entertain this possibility, as a catheter placed into a necrotic tumor for drainage may remain in place until death.[67] Aneurysmal bowel dilatation, which can mimic an abscess or bowel obstruction, can be seen with lymphoma, GIST, and metastases such as from melanoma.[68] Infiltrative tumor can result in peritumoral fat stranding, which can mimic inflammatory change. One such example is pancreas adenocarcinoma, which often has poorly defined margins and can resemble

**TABLE 5.2 Common Abdominal and Pelvic Imaging Pitfalls in Oncology Patients**

| Pitfall | Example | Tip to Avoid Pitfall |
|---|---|---|
| Treatment-related change mistaken for acute pathology or worsening malignancy | • Newly apparent breast cancer liver metastases that have responded to treatment ("pseudoprogression")<br>• Transient increased size of metastases on immune checkpoint inhibitors ("pseudoprogression")<br>• Percutaneous ablation zone mistaken for a metastasis<br>• Benign pneumatosis of the bowel wall mistaken for ischemia | • Clarify treatment history<br>• Familiarize with expected treatment-related changes, including those related to intravascular therapies and percutaneous ablations<br>• Compare region of concern to malignancy behavior elsewhere in the body and get follow-up imaging |
| Misinterpretation due to limitations of imaging technique | • Flow artifact from mixing of contrast-enhanced and unenhanced blood mistaken for thrombus<br>• Hematoma, collection, or cyst mistaken for enhancing tumor on single-phase | • Recognize contrast timing<br>• Enhancement cannot be established using a single-phase scan |
| Unclear terminology | • "Tumor thrombus"<br>• Classification of malignancy as "progressive disease" or "partial response" when not assessing all of the tumor burden in the body<br>• Not applying response criteria correctly | • Use "bland thrombus," "tumor in vein," or "filling defect"<br>• Familiarize with tumor response criteria terminology and avoid using these terms on nonrestaging exams |

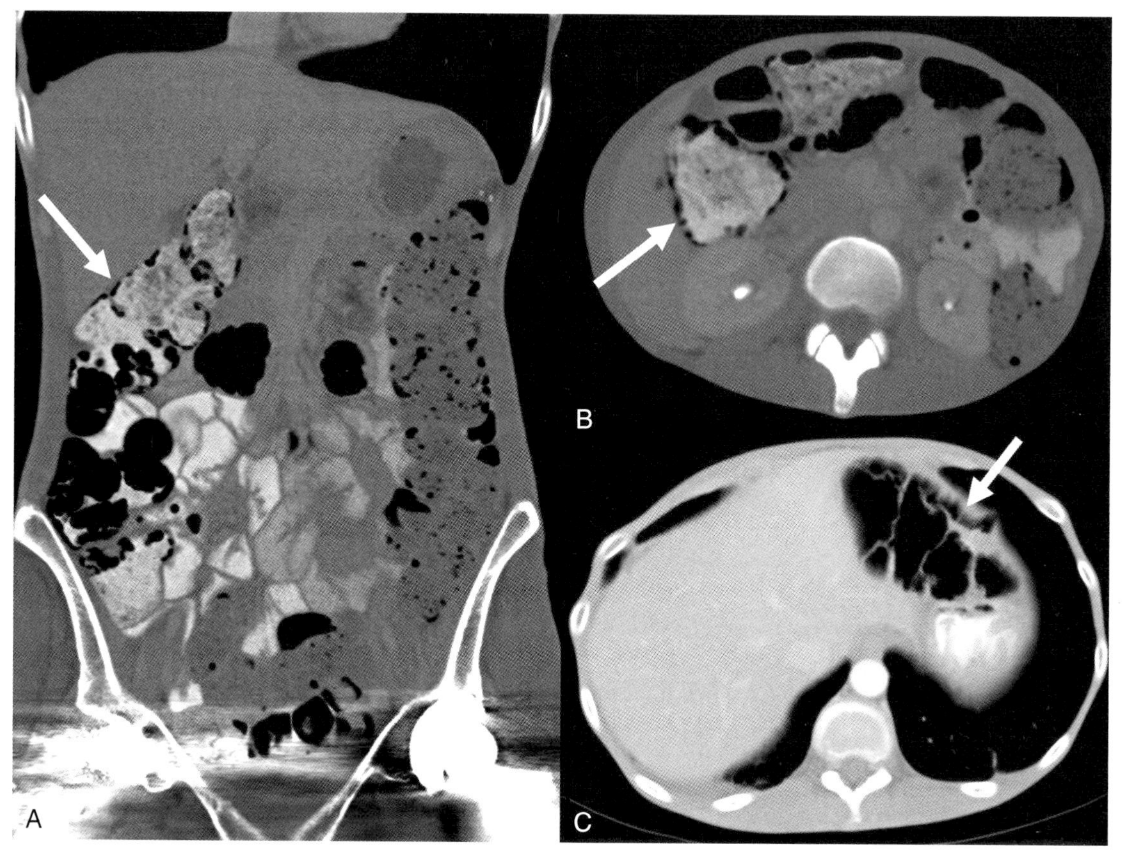


**Fig. 5.13** A 29-year-old female with systemic lupus erythematosus and abdominal pain. Computed tomography in the coronal (A) and axial planes (B and C) reveals multiple cyst-like lucencies in the bowel wall consistent with pneumatosis cystoides coli (arrows). This diagnosis may be suspected when other signs of ischemic bowel are absent, such as portal venous gas, bowel wall edema, and peritonitis on physical exam.

acute pancreatitis. Spontaneous intraabdominal hemorrhage may be benign; however, an underlying ruptured neoplasm is always a consideration. For these cases, recommending repeat multiphase imaging should be considered once sufficient time has passed for the hematoma to have decreased in size or resolved.

Many benign pathologies can resemble tumor. This would include inflammatory and infectious etiologies such as inflammatory bowel disease, endometriosis, and intraabdominal tuberculosis. Benign lesions can undergo acute complications resembling malignancy; one such example is a ruptured ovarian mature cystic teratoma, which can result in fat lobules throughout the peritoneal space (Fig. 5.14).

The imaging technique and its limitations are important considerations when assessing these patients. The identification of enhancing tumor requires multiphase imaging when using CT or MRI; this is important for differentiating complex fluid from solid tissue. Recognition of the phase of enhancement is critical. A frequent pitfall is reporting flow artifact as intravascular filling defects when insufficient time has lapsed to obtain adequate contrast opacification of the vascular structure in question.

Certain terms should be avoided when reporting abdominal imaging in patients with cancer, as they can be misleading. "Tumor thrombus" is one such term that can leave referring physicians confused as to whether or not the patient needs anticoagulation. Instead, "tumor in vein" and "bland thrombus" each provide a clearer description of the underlying pathologic process. If unclear if an intravascular structure

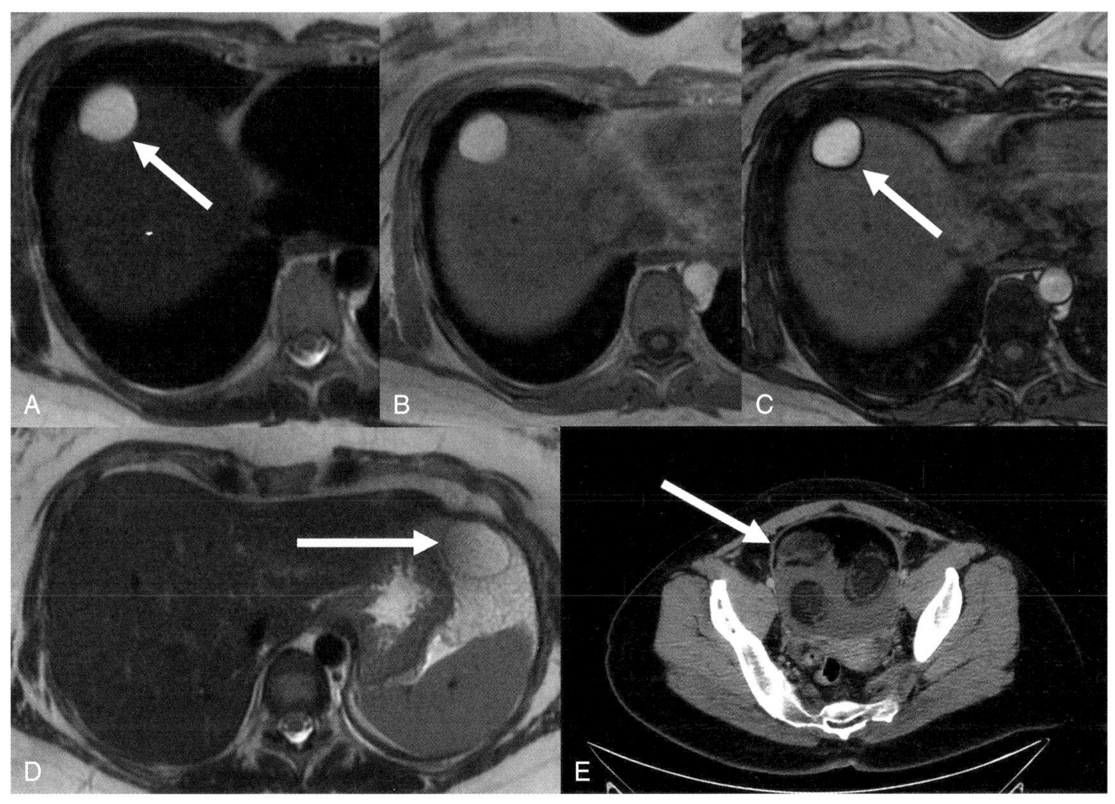


**Fig. 5.14** A 31-year-old female with pelvic pain and a history of motor vehicle collision 1 month earlier. Magnetic resonance imaging reveals a T2-hyperintense lesion in the liver abutting the capsule (A, arrow) with high T1-signal (B) that persists on out-of-phase imaging with black boundary artifact (C, arrow), consistent with fat. Pure fat lesions were present elsewhere in the abdomen, including in the omentum (D, arrow). These were secondary to a ruptured ovarian dermoid, as evidenced by a large fat-containing pelvic mass on computed tomography (E, arrow).

is tumor or bland thrombus, then consider reporting simply as a "filling defect."

In addition to diagnosing acute pathology, restaging of malignancy is often a component of the interpretation of these exams. It is important to avoid terms used in response evaluation criteria such as the Response Evaluation Criteria in Solid Tumors (RECIST) 1.1 unless reporting specifically for a clinical trial or as part of the patient's restaging protocol.[69] Radiologists often get a glimpse of multisystem disease in a single body region that may not be representative of the overall disease status. For example, if a patient has a new brain metastasis, which would of course not be identified on abdominal imaging, the disease status would be "progressive disease" regardless of what is found in the abdomen using RECIST 1.1.[69] Reporting the abdominal imaging as "stable" or "partial response" would be misleading. Therefore, terms such as "improved" are recommended instead of "partial response," "unchanged" rather than "stable," and "worsening" instead of "progressive disease."

## Conclusion

Abdominal imaging of oncology and immunocompromised patients poses unique challenges for the radiologist and can also involve the detection of several unique pathologies. This chapter provided an approach to these patients, a review of pathologies frequently seen in these patients, and pitfalls to avoid.

## REFERENCES

1. Ranji SR, Goldman LE, Simel DL, Shojania KG. Do opiates affect the clinical evaluation of patients with acute abdominal pain? *JAMA*. 2006;296(14):1764–1774.
2. Ilgen JS, Marr AL. Cancer emergencies: the acute abdomen. *Emerg Med Clin North Am*. 2009;27(3):381–399.

3. Swenson KK, Rose MA, Ritz L, Murray CL, Adlis SA. Recognition and evaluation of oncology-related symptoms in the emergency department. *Ann Emerg Med*. 1995;26(1):12–17.
4. Sadik M, Ozlem K, Huseyin M, AliAyberk B, Ahmet S, Ozgur O. Attributes of cancer patients admitted to the emergency department in one year. *World J Emerg Med*. 2014;5(2):85–90.
5. Expert Panel on Gastrointestinal Imaging Scheirey CD, Fowler KJ, Therrien JA, Kim DH, Al-Refaie WB, et al. ACR Appropriateness Criteria(®) acute nonlocalized abdominal pain. *J Am Coll Radiol*. 2018;15(11S):S217–S231.
6. Scott-Conner CE, Fabrega AJ. Gastrointestinal problems in the immunocompromised host. A review for surgeons. *Surg Endosc*. 1996;10(10):959–964.
7. Badgwell BD, Cormier JN, Wray CJ, Borthakur G, Qiao W, Rolston KV, et al. Challenges in surgical management of abdominal pain in the neutropenic cancer patient. *Ann Surg*. 2008;248(1):104–109.
8. Kellow ZS, MacInnes M, Kurzencwyg D, Rawal S, Jaffer R, Kovacina B, et al. The role of abdominal radiography in the evaluation of the nontrauma emergency patient. *Radiology*. 2008;248(3):887–893.
9. Kiewiet JJ, Leeuwenburgh MM, Bipat S, Bossuyt PM, Stoker J, Boermeester MA. A systematic review and meta-analysis of diagnostic performance of imaging in acute cholecystitis. *Radiology*. 2012;264(3):708–720.
10. Muradali D, Goldberg DR. US of gastrointestinal tract disease. *Radiographics*. 2015;35(1):50–68.
11. Kave M, Parooie F, Salarzaei M. Pregnancy and appendicitis: a systematic review and meta-analysis on the clinical use of MRI in diagnosis of appendicitis in pregnant women. *World J Emerg Surg*. 2019;14:37.
12. Melamud K, LeBedis CA, Anderson SW, Soto JA. Biliary imaging: multimodality approach to imaging of biliary injuries and their complications. *Radiographics*. 2014;34(3):613–623.
13. Morani AC, Hanafy AK, Marcal LP, Subbiah V, Le O, Bathala TK, et al. Imaging of acute abdomen in cancer patients. *Abdom Radiol (NY)*. 2020;45(8):2287–2304.
14. Heller MT, Khanna V. Cross-sectional imaging of acute abdominal conditions in the oncologic patient. *Emerg Radiol*. 2011;18(5):417–428.
15. Rohatgi S, Howard SA, Tirumani SH, Ramaiya NH, Krajewski KM. Multimodality Imaging of Tumour Thrombus. *Can Assoc Radiol J*. 2015;66(2):121–129.
16. LeGout JD, Bailey RE, Bolan CW, Bowman AW, Chen F, Cernigliaro JG, et al. Multimodality imaging of abdominopelvic tumors with venous invasion. *Radiographics*. 2020;40(7):2098–2116.
17. Wong M, See JY, Sufyan W, Diddapur RK. Splenic infarction. A rare presentation of anaplastic pancreatic carcinoma and a review of the literature. *JOP*. 2008;9(4):493–498.
18. Schraut WH, Chilcote RR. Metastatic Wilms' tumor causing acute hepatic-vein occlusion (Budd-Chiari syndrome). *Gastroenterology*. 1985;88(2):576–579.
19. Carbonnel F, Valla D, Menu Y, Lecompte Y, Belghiti J, Rueff B, et al. Acute Budd-Chiari syndrome as first manifestation of adrenocortical carcinoma. *J Clin Gastroenterol*. 1988;10(4):441–444.
20. Moreira V, Aller R, De Luis DA, San Roman AL, Ferreiro A. Fulminant acute Budd-Chiari syndrome stemming from an adrenal tumor. *J Clin Gastroenterol*. 1997;24(2):110–112.
21. Ciancio G, Soloway M. Renal cell carcinoma invading the hepatic veins. *Cancer*. 2001;92(7):1836–1842.
22. Sherid M, Samo S, Suliaman S, Gaziano JH. Acute fulminant form of Budd-Chiari syndrome secondary to inferior vena cava sarcoma: a case report and review of the literature. *J Gastrointest Cancer*. 2013;44(4):472–476.
23. Brancatelli G, Vilgrain V, Federle MP, Hakime A, Lagalla R, Iannaccone R, et al. Budd-Chiari syndrome: spectrum of imaging findings. *Am J Roentgenology*. 2007;188(2):W168–W176.
24. Horton KM, Fishman EK. Multi-detector row CT of mesenteric ischemia: can it be done? *Radiographics*. 2001;21(6):1463–1473.
25. Tirumani SH, Ojili V, Gunabushanam G, Chintapalli KN, Ryan JG, Reinhold C. MDCT of abdominopelvic oncologic emergencies. *Cancer imaging: Off Publ Int Cancer Imaging Soc*. 2013;13(2):238–252.
26. Lubner M, Menias C, Rucker C, Bhalla S, Peterson CM, Wang L, et al. Blood in the belly: CT findings of hemoperitoneum. *Radiographics*. 2007;27(1):109–125.
27. Udare A, Agarwal M, Siegelman E, Schieda N. CT and MR imaging of acute adrenal disorders. *Abdom Radiology*. 2021;46(1):290–302.
28. Schwarz L, Bubenheim M, Zemour J, Herrero A, Muscari F, Ayav A, et al. Bleeding recurrence and mortality following interventional management of spontaneous HCC rupture: results of a multicenter European study. *World J Surg*. 2018;42(1):225–232.
29. Kogut MJ, Bastawrous S, Padia S, Bhargava P. Hepatobiliary oncologic emergencies: imaging appearances and therapeutic options. *Curr Probl Diagnostic Radiology*. 2013;42(3):113–126.
30. Diaz JR, Agriantonis DJ, Aguila J, Calleros JE, Ayyappan AP. Spontaneous perirenal hemorrhage: what radiologists need to know. *Emerg Radiol*. 2011;18(4):329–334.
31. Casillas VJ, Amendola MA, Gascue A, Pinnar N, Levi JU, Perez JM. Imaging of nontraumatic hemorrhagic hepatic lesions. *Radiographics*. 2000;20(2):367–378.
32. Expert Panel on Interventional Radiology Fairchild AH, Hohenwalter EJ, Gipson MG, Al-Refaie WB, Braun AR, et al. ACR Appropriateness Criteria(®) radiologic management of biliary obstruction. *J Am Coll Radiol*. 2019;16(5S):S196–S213.
33. Kim JH. Endoscopic stent placement in the palliation of malignant biliary obstruction. *Clin Endosc*. 2011;44(2):76–86.
34. Köhler H, Lankisch PG. Acute pancreatitis and hyperamylasaemia in pancreatic carcinoma. *Pancreas*. 1987;2(1):117–119.
35. Kimura Y, Kikuyama M, Kodama Y. Acute pancreatitis as a possible indicator of pancreatic cancer: the importance of mass detection. *Intern Med*. 2015;54(17):2109–2114.
36. Wolske KM, Ponnatapura J, Kolokythas O, Burke LMB, Tappouni R, Lalwani N. Chronic pancreatitis or pancreatic tumor? a problem-solving approach. *RadioGraphics*. 2019;39(7):1965–1982.
37. Guimaraes MD, Bitencourt AG, Marchiori E, Chojniak R, Gross JL, Kundra V. Imaging acute complications in cancer patients: what should be evaluated in the emergency setting? *Cancer imaging: Off Publ Int Cancer Imaging Soc*. 2014;14:18.
38. Allen DJ, Longhorn SE, Philp T, Smith RD, Choong S. Percutaneous urinary drainage and ureteric stenting in malignant disease. *Clin Oncol (R Coll Radiol)*. 2010;22(9):733–739.
39. Nariculam J, Murphy DG, Jenner C, Sellars N, Gwyther S, Gordon SG, et al. Nephrostomy insertion for patients with bilateral ureteric obstruction caused by prostate cancer. *Br J Radiol*. 2009;82(979):571–576.

40. Organ M, Norman RW. Acute reversible kidney injury secondary to bilateral ureteric obstruction. *Can Urol Assoc J*. 2011;5(6):392–396.
41. Huang C, Hong M-K, Ding D-C. A review of ovary torsion. *Ci Ji Yi Xue Za Zhi*. 2017;29(3):143–147.
42. Eitan R, Galoyan N, Zuckerman B, Shaya M, Shen O, Beller U. The risk of malignancy in post-menopausal women presenting with adnexal torsion. *Gynecol Oncol*. 2007;106(1):211–214.
43. Duigenan S, Oliva E, Lee SI. Ovarian Torsion: Diagnostic Features on CT and MRI with pathologic correlation. *Am J Roentgenology*. 2012;198(2):W122–W131.
44. Silva AC, Pimenta M, Guimaraes LS. Small bowel obstruction: what to look for. *Radiographics*. 2009;29(2):423–439.
45. Iacobellis F, Perillo A, Iadevito I, Tanga M, Romano L, Grassi R, et al. Imaging of oncologic emergencies. *SemUltrasound, CT, MR*. 2018;39(2):151–166.
46. Ripamonti CI, Easson AM, Gerdes H. Management of malignant bowel obstruction. *Eur J Cancer*. 2008;44(8):1105–1115.
47. Krajewski KM, Braschi-Amirfarzan M, DiPiro PJ, Jagannathan JP, Shinagare AB. Molecular targeted therapy in modern oncology: imaging assessment of treatment response and toxicities. *Korean J Radiol*. 2017;18(1):28–41.
48. Wang GX, Kurra V, Gainor JF, Sullivan RJ, Flaherty KT, Lee SI, et al. Immune checkpoint inhibitor cancer therapy: spectrum of imaging findings. *Radiographics*. 2017;37(7):2132–2144.
49. Torrisi JM, Schwartz LH, Gollub MJ, Ginsberg MS, Bosl GJ, Hricak H. CT findings of chemotherapy-induced toxicity: what radiologists need to know about the clinical and radiologic manifestations of chemotherapy toxicity. *Radiology*. 2011;258(1):41–56.
50. Nishino M, Hatabu H, Hodi FS. Imaging of cancer immunotherapy: current approaches and future directions. *Radiology*. 2019;290(1):9–22.
51. Larici AR, del Ciello A, Maggi F, Santoro SI, Meduri B, Valentini V, et al. Lung abnormalities at multimodality imaging after radiation therapy for non-small cell lung cancer. *Radiographics*. 2011;31(3):771–789.
52. Fernandez FG, Ritter J, Goodwin JW, Linehan DC, Hawkins WG, Strasberg SM. Effect of steatohepatitis associated with irinotecan or oxaliplatin pretreatment on resectability of hepatic colorectal metastases. *J Am Coll Surg*. 2005;200(6):845–853.
53. Maturen KE, Feng MU, Wasnik AP, Azar SF, Appelman HD, Francis IR, et al. Imaging effects of radiation therapy in the abdomen and pelvis: evaluating “innocent bystander” tissues. *Radiographics*. 2013;33(2):599–619.
54. del Campo L, Leon NG, Palacios DC, Lagana C, Tagarro D. Abdominal complications following hematopoietic stem cell transplantation. *Radiographics*. 2014;34(2):396–412.
55. Kim KW, Ramaiya NH, Krajewski KM, Jagannathan JP, Tirumani SH, Srivastava A, et al. Ipilimumab associated hepatitis: imaging and clinicopathologic findings. *Invest N Drugs*. 2013;31(4):1071–1077.
56. Tirumani SH, Fairchild A, Krajewski KM, Nishino M, Howard SA, Baheti AD, et al. Anti-VEGF molecular targeted therapies in common solid malignancies: comprehensive update for radiologists. *Radiographics*. 2015;35(2):455–474.
57. Tirumani SH, Baez JC, Jagannathan JP, Shinagare AB, Ramaiya NH. Tumor-bowel fistula: what radiologists should know. *Abdom Imaging*. 2013;38(5):1014–1023.
58. Lawson M, Vasilaras A, De Vries A, Mactaggart P, Nicol D. Urological implications of cyclophosphamide and ifosfamide. *Scand J Urol Nephrol*. 2008;42(4):309–317.
59. Campello E, Ilich A, Simioni P, Key NS. The relationship between pancreatic cancer and hypercoagulability: a comprehensive review on epidemiological and biological issues. *Br J Cancer*. 2019;121(5):359–371.
60. Tirumani SH, Baheti AD, Tirumani H, O’Neill A, Jagannathan JP. Update on gastrointestinal stromal tumors for radiologists. *Korean J Radiol*. 2017;18(1):84–93.
61. Keraliya AR, Rosenthal MH, Krajewski KM, Jagannathan JP, Shinagare AB, Tirumani SH, et al. Imaging of fluid in cancer patients treated with systemic therapy: chemotherapy, molecular targeted therapy, and hematopoietic stem cell transplantation. *AJR Am J Roentgenol*. 2015;205(4):709–719.
62. Hinshaw JL, Lubner MG, Ziemlewicz TJ, Lee Jr. FT, Brace CL. Percutaneous tumor ablation tools: microwave, radiofrequency, or cryoablation: what should you use and why? *Radiographics*. 2014;34(5):1344–1362.
63. Choi H, Charnsangavej C, de Castro Faria S, Tamm EP, Benjamin RS, Johnson MM, et al. CT evaluation of the response of gastrointestinal stromal tumors after imatinib mesylate treatment: a quantitative analysis correlated with FDG PET findings. *AJR Am J Roentgenol*. 2004;183(6):1619–1628.
64. Tirkes T, Hollar MA, Tann M, Kohli MD, Akisik F, Sandrasegaran K. Response criteria in oncologic imaging: review of traditional and new criteria. *Radiographics*. 2013;33(5):1323–1341.
65. Shinagare AB, Jagannathan JP, Krajewski KM, Ramaiya NH. Liver metastases in the era of molecular targeted therapy: new faces of treatment response. *AJR Am J Roentgenol*. 2013;201(1):W15–W28.
66. Ho LM, Paulson EK, Thompson WM. Pneumatosis intestinalis in the adult: benign to life-threatening causes. *AJR Am J Roentgenol*. 2007;188(6):1604–1613.
67. Mueller PR, White EM, Glass-Royal M, Zeman RK, Saini S, Silverman SG, et al. Infected abdominal tumors: percutaneous catheter drainage. *Radiology*. 1989;173(3):627–629.
68. Maizlin ZV, Brown JA, Buckley MR, Filipenko D, Barnard SA, Wong X, et al. Case of the season: aneurysmal dilatation of the small bowel (not only lymphoma). *Semin Roentgenol*. 2006;41(4):248–249.
69. Eisenhauer EA, Therasse P, Bogaerts J, Schwartz LH, Sargent D, Ford R, et al. New response evaluation criteria in solid tumours: revised RECIST guideline (version 1.1). *Eur J Cancer*. 2009;45(2):228–247.

Chapter 6

# Nontraumatic Abdominal Emergencies in Pregnant Patients

Reza Salari, Daniel R. Ludwig, and Vincent M. Mellnick

## Outline



## Key Points

- Normal physiological changes of pregnancy often interfere with clinical evaluation of pathological causes of abdominal pain.
- Imaging, particularly ultrasound, and increasingly magnetic resonance, plays a critical role in evaluation of abdominal pain in pregnancy.
- Various processes can lead to abdominal pain, with management strategies ranging from medical therapy to emergent surgeries.
- Familiarity with the imaging appearance of these processes is crucial in directing timely and effective care.

## Introduction

Abdominal pain is a common symptom in pregnancy that results from a variety of causes ranging from normal physiological changes to serious conditions that require prompt diagnosis and treatment. Vague abdominal pain, nausea, and vomiting are frequent complaints during a normal pregnancy. Furthermore, physiologic leukocytosis, displacement of bowel and the appendix by the gravid uterus, and loss of guarding in the case of peritonitis can limit the typical clinical clues for surgical causes of abdominal pain.[1–4] Therefore, imaging plays a crucial role in identifying potential surgical causes of abdominal pain and directing timely and effective care.

In the pregnant patient, imaging modalities that do not expose the patient to ionizing radiation are strongly preferred, specifically ultrasound and magnetic resonance imaging (MRI). Ultrasound is by far the most used imaging technique in pregnancy, especially for evaluating fetal health and obstetric complications.[5–7] It is also typically the first-line technique for evaluating suspected gallbladder and renal pathologies.[8–10] However, normal physiological changes in pregnancy, along with gravid uterus and bowel gas, can potentially limit its use for evaluating deeper structures such as the bowel and appendix. MRI without intravenous contrast has been increasingly used in evaluation of abdominal pain in pregnancy due to lack of ionizing radiation, superb resolution of anatomical details, and the ability to depict various causes of abdominal pain in pregnancy, especially in the evaluation of suspected appendicitis.[11–15] Gadolinium-based intravenous contrast is avoided in pregnancy, as it crosses the placenta and is associated with adverse fetal outcomes.[16]

The causes of abdominal pain in pregnancy can be divided into four main categories: gastrointestinal, hepatobiliary, genitourinary, and obstetric causes. In the following sections, we discuss the common causes of abdominal pain and review the spectrum of imaging findings in each category (Table 6.1).

**TABLE 6.1 Typical Imaging Findings of the Common Causes of Nontraumatic Abdominal Pain During Pregnancy**

| Category | Imaging Findings |
|---|---|
| **Gastrointestinal** | |
| Acute appendicitis | Appendiceal distention, wall thickening, fluid-filled appendix, surrounding soft tissue stranding, free fluid, appendicolith |
| Inflammatory bowel disease | Bowel wall thickening, submucosal edema, perienteric stranding, terminal ileal involvement, penetrating disease |
| Small bowel obstruction | Dilated fluid-filled small bowel loops with a transition point |
| Diverticulitis | Diverticula, colonic wall thickening, surrounding fat stranding |
| Epiploic appendagitis | Edema and fat stranding surrounding a fat-intensity mass adjacent to the colon |
| **Hepatobiliary** | |
| Cholelithiasis | Gallstones, typically with posterior acoustic shadowing on US |
| Acute cholecystitis | Gallbladder distention and wall thickening, pericholecystic fluid, gallstones |
| Acute pancreatitis | Focal or diffuse pancreatic edema, restricted diffusion, surrounding fat stranding |
| HELLP syndrome | Hepatomegaly, hepatic necrosis and intra- and extrahepatic hematoma |
| **Genitourinary** | |
| Nephrolithiasis | Echogenic foci with shadowing and twinkle artifact (ultrasound) or T2 hypointense calculus (MRI) |
| Acute pyelonephritis | Imaging is frequently normal, ultrasound may show collecting system debris or reduced vascularity in uncomplicated cases, abscess |
| Ovarian torsion | Asymmetrically enlarged ovary, peripheralization of follicles, stromal edema, twisted vascular pedicle |
| Leiomyoma degeneration | Edema (increased T2 signal on MRI), hemorrhage (increased T1 signal on MRI) |
| Pelvic inflammatory disease | Hydrosalpinx, tubo-ovarian abscess |
| Endometriosis | T1-hyperintense and T2-hypointense masses typically involving the adnexa, hemoperitoneum |
| **Obstetric** | |
| Ectopic pregnancy | Lack of intrauterine gestational sac, adnexal mass, free fluid in the pelvis |
| Uterine rupture | Focal myometrial defect, extrusion of the pregnancy products, hemoperitoneum |

*HELLP*, Hemolysis, elevated liver enzymes, and low platelet count; *US*, ultrasound; *MRI*, magnetic resonance imaging.

## Gastrointestinal Pathologies

### ACUTE APPENDICITIS

Appendicitis is the most common nonobstetric cause of emergency surgery in the pregnant patient, complicating approximately 1 per 1000 pregnancies.[17–19] Early diagnosis of appendicitis is of paramount importance, as delayed diagnosis can lead to serious maternal and fetal complications, including up to 36% fetal loss in the case of perforation.[20]

Although ultrasound may be used in the initial evaluation of suspected appendicitis, it is limited by a high nonvisualization rate.[21] MRI has emerged as the preferred modality due to its nonionizing nature and high sensitivity and specificity of 94% and 97%, respectively.[22] The MRI protocol can be optimized for safe and fast examination, which also allows for evaluation of other potential causes of abdominal pain.[15] MRI findings of acute appendicitis include appendiceal distension (≥8 mm), wall thickening, fluid-filled appendix, surrounding soft tissue stranding/free fluid, and presence of appendicolith (Fig. 6.1).[15] The normal appendix can be greater than 8 mm in diameter, and therefore size should be used in conjunction with other features to suggest appendicitis.[23]

The appendix may not always be visualized on MRI, but the lack of an abnormal appendix and inflammatory change in the right lower quadrant has a high negative predictive value and should be interpreted as negative rather than indeterminate.[24]

### INFLAMMATORY BOWEL DISEASE

Inflammatory bowel disease affects women of childbearing age, and pregnancy itself may be a risk factor in disease exacerbations.[25] The presenting symptoms include abdominal pain, diarrhea, and potentially fever. MRI findings of active inflammation include bowel wall thickening, submucosal edema, and perienteric stranding, most frequently involving the distal and terminal ileum.[26] MRI can also show potential complications such as bowel obstruction, fistulization, abscess formation, and perforation (Fig. 6.2).

### SMALL BOWEL OBSTRUCTION

Small bowel obstruction in pregnancy has similar etiologies to that in nonpregnant patients, most frequently due to adhesions from prior surgery. Other etiologies include hernias, intussusception, and volvulus, particularly in patients with prior gastric bypass surgeries.[27] The clinical presentation of early small bowel obstruction can be subtle or masked by physiologic findings and symptoms of pregnancy.[28,29] Although computed tomography in general is the preferred modality for the diagnosis of small bowel obstruction,[30] MRI without contrast should be strongly considered in the pregnant patient with suspected small bowel obstruction if the patient is clinically stable. In small bowel obstruction, MRI shows dilated fluid-filled loops of small bowel upstream of the transition point and depicts potential complications such as closed-loop configuration, peritonitis, or perforation (Fig. 6.3).

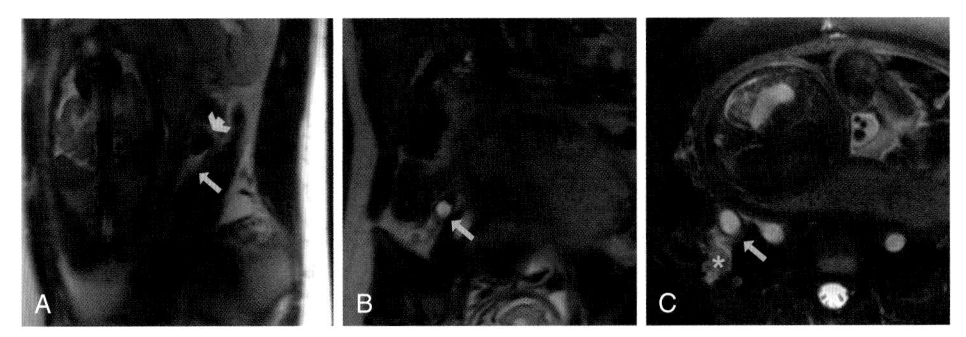


**Fig. 6.1** Acute appendicitis in an 18-year-old pregnant woman at 30 weeks' gestation who presented with right lower quadrant abdominal pain. Sagittal and coronal T2-weighted magnetic resonance (MR) images (A and B) demonstrate dilated appendix (arrows) with an obstructing appendicolith (arrowhead). T2-weighted fat-suppressed MR image (C) shows adjacent fat stranding and small amount of free fluid (asterisk). The patient subsequently underwent laparoscopic appendectomy, which confirmed acute appendicitis.

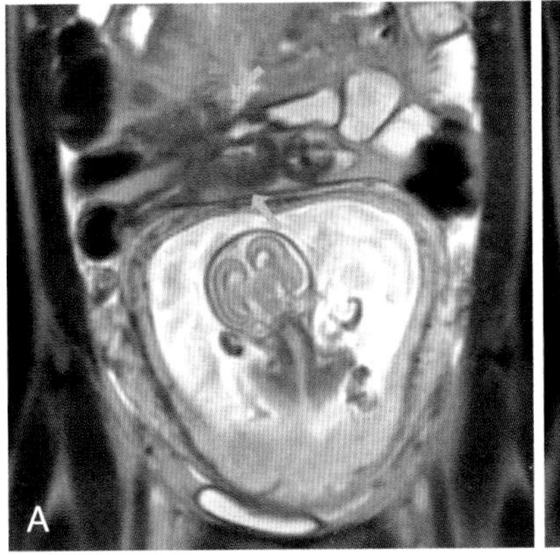


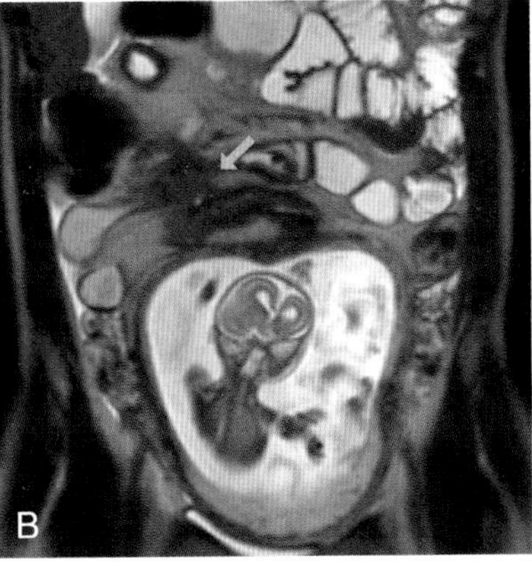


**Fig. 6.2** Terminal ileitis and enteroenteric fistula in a 16-year-old pregnant woman with history of Crohn's disease at 16 weeks' gestation who presented with right lower quadrant abdominal pain. Coronal T2-weighted magnetic resonance images (A and B) demonstrate marked wall thickening of terminal ilium (arrows in A), consistent with terminal ileitis, with tethering of two loops of terminal ilium (arrow in B) indicative of chronic entero-enteric fistulization.

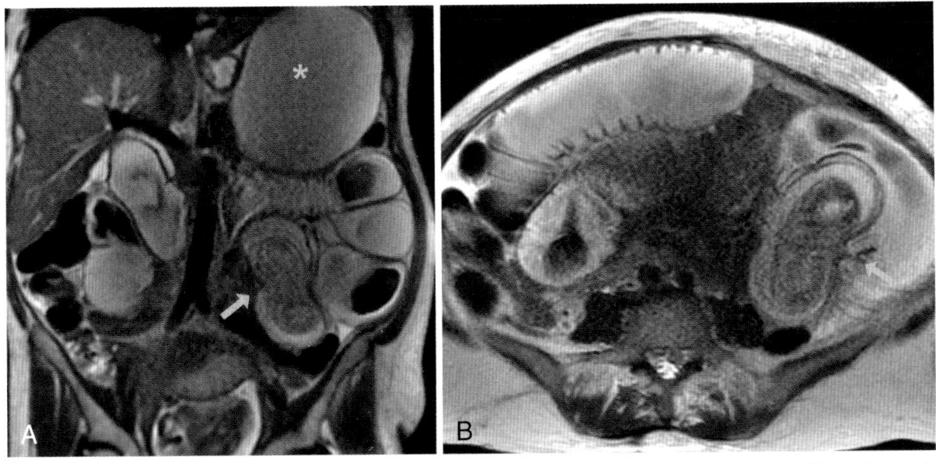


**Fig. 6.3** Small bowel obstruction secondary to jejunojejunal intussusception in a 36-year-old pregnant woman at 28 weeks' gestation with prior history of Roux-en-Y gastric bypass who initially presented with abdominal pain. Coronal (A) and axial (B) T2-weighted magnetic resonance images demonstrate marked distention of both Roux and pancreaticobiliary limbs, including the excluded stomach (asterisk). There is jejunojejunal intussusception (arrows) leading to small bowel obstruction, which was confirmed at surgery.

### DIVERTICULITIS

Diverticulitis is relatively rare in younger patients and presents with similar symptoms to nonpregnant patients, namely left lower quadrant pain and fever.[31] MRI shows colonic wall thickening and surrounding fat stranding and also depicts potential complications such as perforation and abscess formation (Fig. 6.4).[32]

### EPIPLOIC APPENDAGITIS

Epiploic appendagitis is a form of intraperitoneal focal fat necrosis resulting from epiploic appendage infarction due to torsion or spontaneous venous thrombosis.[33] This is a relatively rare and self-limiting entity, but the symptoms can mimic other abdominopelvic pathologies, in particular acute diverticulitis. MRI shows edema and fat stranding surrounding a small fat-intensity mass adjacent to the colon (Fig. 6.5).

## Hepatobiliary Pathologies

### GALLSTONE DISEASE

Pregnancy promotes gallstone formation through various mechanisms, including bile supersaturation and

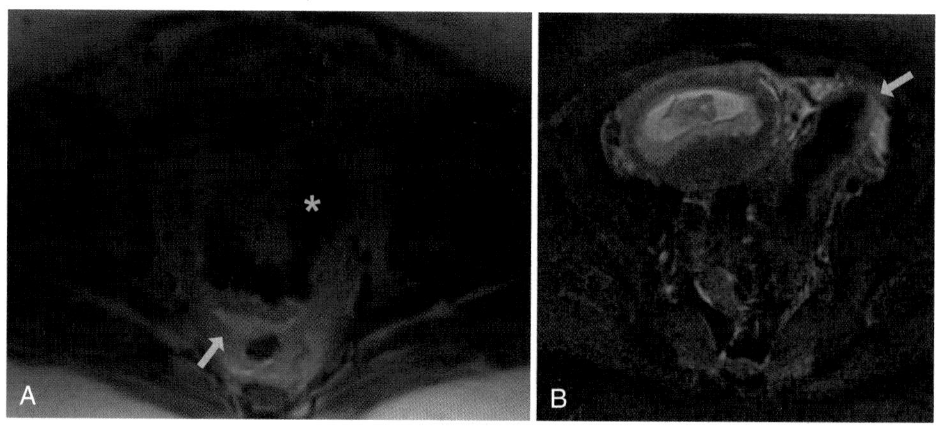


**Fig. 6.4** Diverticulitis in a 37-year-old pregnant woman in her first trimester who presented with lower abdominal pain. Axial T2-weighted magnetic resonance (MR) image of the pelvis (A) demonstrates diverticulosis (asterisk) and free fluid in the pelvis (arrow). Axial T2-weighted fat-suppressed MR image (B) demonstrates sigmoid colon thickening with adjacent edema (arrow), consistent with uncomplicated diverticulitis. This patient was managed conservatively.

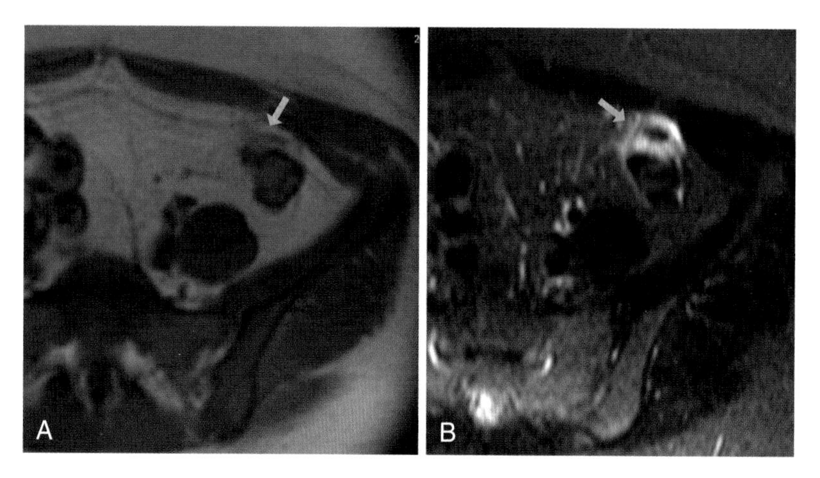


**Fig. 6.5** Epiploic appendagitis in a 21-year-old pregnant woman at 12 weeks' gestation presenting with left lower quadrant abdominal pain. Axial T1-weighted magnetic resonance image (A) demonstrates fat stranding anterior to distal descending colon (arrow). T2-weighted fat-suppressed image (B) demonstrates adjacent edema (arrow). Note that the stranding surrounds a lesion that parallels the signal intensity of fat on all imaging sequences. This was managed conservatively.

delayed gallbladder emptying.[34–37] A prospective study showed new gallstones in nearly 8% of pregnant women by the third trimester.[38] If symptomatic, they present similarly to those in nonpregnant patients, with intermittent postprandial right upper quadrant or epigastric pain. Ultrasound is the modality of choice in evaluation of suspected gallbladder pathologies[8] and typically shows mobile echogenic gallstones with posterior acoustic shadowing (Fig. 6.6).

Acute cholecystitis occurs in 1 per 1600 pregnancies and, after appendicitis, is the second most common nonobstetric cause for surgery during pregnancy.[37] Patients with acute cholecystitis typically present with right upper quadrant pain, nausea/vomiting, fever, and leukocytosis. Imaging findings of cholecystitis include gallbladder distension, cholelithiasis, gallbladder wall thickening, and pericholecystic fluid (Fig. 6.7).

Choledocholithiasis typically occurs after a gallstone passes into the common bile duct and may lead to biliary obstruction. Though both ultrasound and magnetic resonance cholangiopancreatography (MRCP) may depict choledocholithiasis, MRCP has higher sensitivity owing to its superior ability to visualize the distal bile duct, which may be obscured by bowel gas on ultrasound. Gallstones visualized in the common bile duct are diagnostic of choledocholithiasis and are often associated with upstream biliary ductal dilation due to obstruction.[39,40]

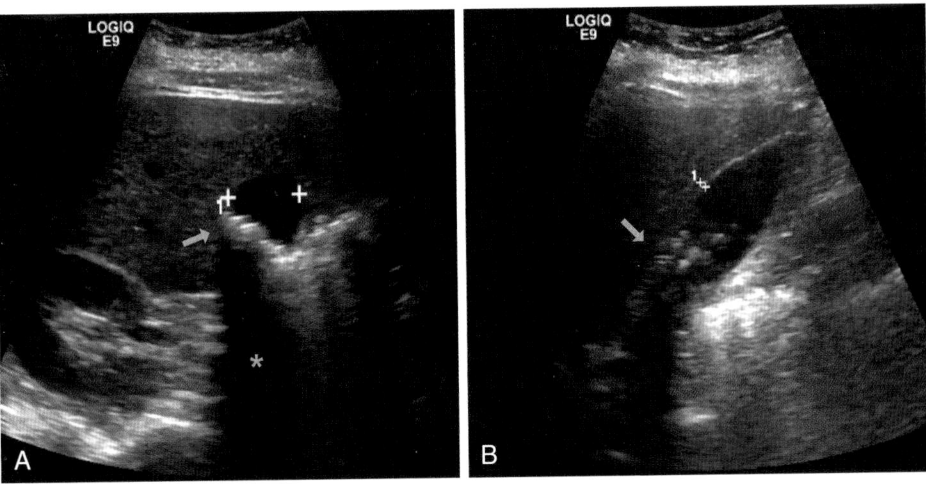


**Fig. 6.6** Cholelithiasis in a 30-year-old pregnant woman at 32 weeks' gestation who presented with right upper quadrant pain. Grayscale ultrasound images (A and B) demonstrate a nondistended gallbladder with multiple stones (arrows) and posterior acoustic shadowing (asterisk in A). Sonographic Murphy sign was negative.

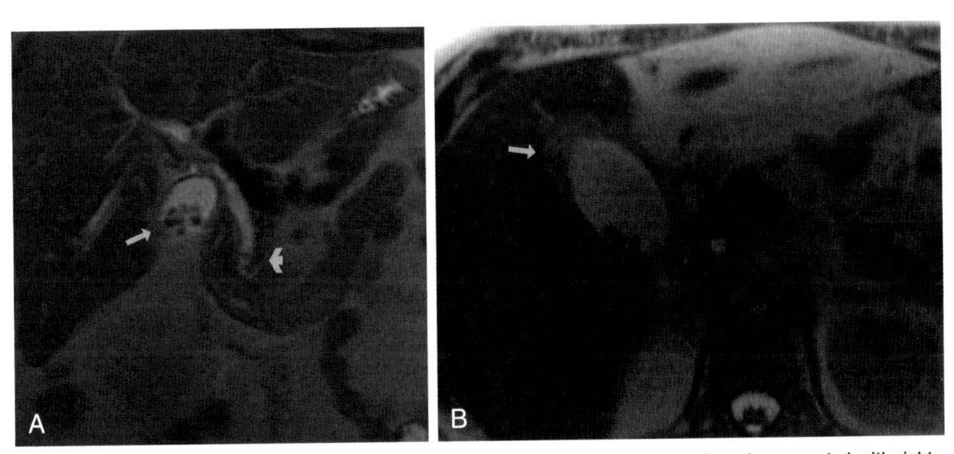


**Fig. 6.7** Cholecystitis and choledocholithiasis in a 34-year-old pregnant woman at 24 weeks' gestation who presented with right upper quadrant abdominal pain. Coronal T2-weighted magnetic resonance (MR) image (A) demonstrates multiple gallstones in the gallbladder (arrow) as well as in the common bile duct (arrowhead). Axial T2-weighted MR image (B) shows gallbladder wall thickening (arrow). This patient subsequently underwent laparoscopic cholecystectomy, which confirmed acute gangrenous cholecystitis. Hospital course was complicated by preterm delivery on postoperative day 1.

## ACUTE PANCREATITIS

Gallstone pancreatitis is the most common cause of acute pancreatitis in pregnancy, resulting from obstruction of the pancreatic duct at the level of ampulla.[41] Patients with acute pancreatitis typically present with severe epigastric pain and elevated lipase. MRI can be used to evaluate for potential causes and complications. Typical imaging findings include focal or diffuse pancreatic edema, restricted diffusion, surrounding fat stranding, and possible necrosis or fluid collection (Fig. 6.8).[42]

## HEMOLYSIS, ELEVATED LIVER ENZYMES, AND LOW PLATELET COUNT SYNDROME

Hemolysis, elevated liver enzymes, and low platelet count (HELLP) syndrome is a rare but serious

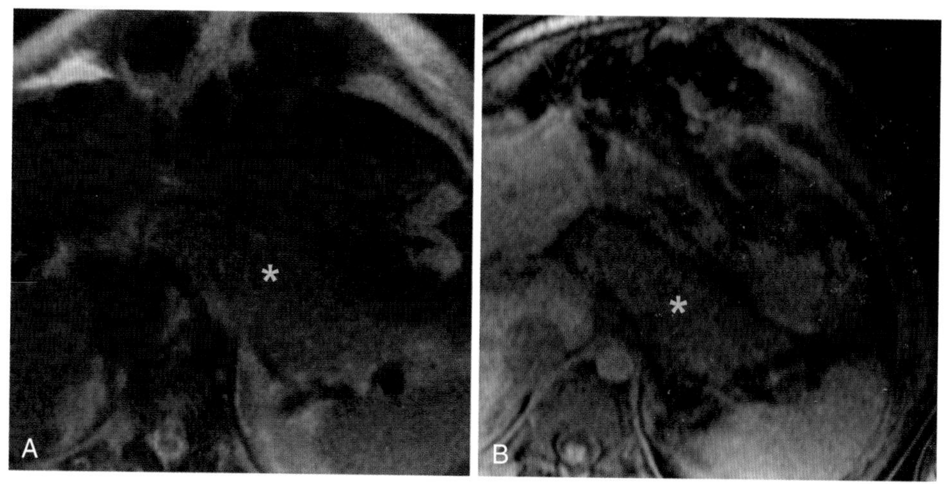


**Fig. 6.8** Acute pancreatitis in a 21-year-old pregnant woman at 34 weeks' gestation who presented with upper abdominal pain and elevated lipase. Axial T2-weighted magnetic resonance (MR) image (A) demonstrates diffuse enlargement of the pancreas (asterisk). There is also uniformly decreased intrinsic T1 signal intensity of the pancreas on axial T1-weighted MR image (B). No gallstone was identified, and the etiology was idiopathic. This patient was managed conservatively.

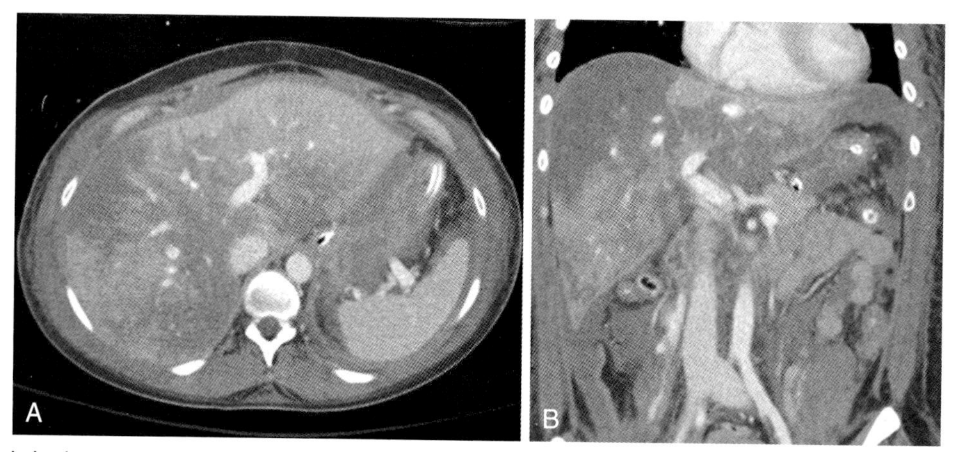


**Fig. 6.9** Hemolysis, elevated liver enzymes, and low platelet count (HELLP) syndrome in a 29-year-old pregnant woman at 29 weeks' gestation status post emergent cesarean section. Patient initially presented with abdominal pain, markedly elevated liver enzymes, and thrombocytopenia, which were further complicated by disseminated intravascular coagulation. Axial and coronal (A and B) computed tomography images on postoperative day 1 demonstrate diffuse areas of hypoenhancement, consistent with hepatic necrosis.

complication of pregnancy that occurs in 1 in 1500 pregnancies,[43] typically in the late third trimester or early postpartum period. Imaging features of HELLP syndrome include hepatomegaly, hepatic necrosis, and intra- and extrahepatic hematoma (Fig. 6.9).[44] Up to 40% of cases with HELLP syndrome are complicated by disseminated intravascular coagulation, which may lead to multiorgan dysfunction.[45] The definitive treatment for HELLP syndrome is delivery.[45]

## Genitourinary Pathologies

### NEPHROLITHIASIS

Renal colic is relatively rare during pregnancy (1 in 1500 pregnancies).[46] The common presentation symptoms include flank pain and hematuria. Ultrasound remains the modality of choice in evaluating patients with suspected nephrolithiasis, and readily shows hydronephrosis, renal calculi, and elevated resistive index, which

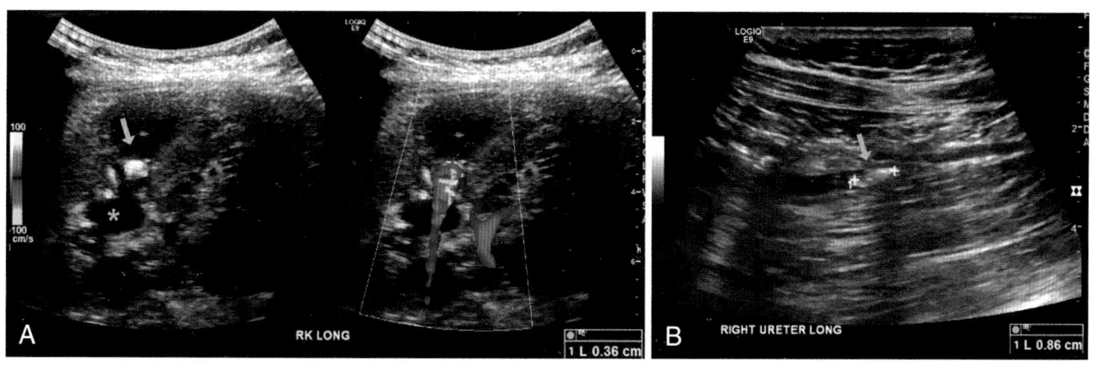


**Fig. 6.10** Obstructing nephrolithiasis in a 22-year-old pregnant woman at 10 weeks' gestation who presented with right-sided abdominal pain. Grayscale and color Doppler images of the right kidney (A) demonstrate a 4-mm caliceal stone in the upper pole (arrow) with associated twinkle artifact on color Doppler and mild hydronephrosis (asterisk). Grayscale ultrasound image of the proximal right ureter (B) demonstrates a 9-mm obstructing stone in the proximal right ureter (arrow) with mild upstream hydroureter. Patient was initially managed by ureteral stent placement, followed by lithotripsy 4 weeks later.

results from increased resistance to diastolic flow in the setting of obstruction (Fig. 6.10). Ultrasound, however, has decreased sensitivity and specificity in pregnancy (74% and 67%, respectively) due to the high frequency of physiologic hydronephrosis related to compression by the gravid uterus.[46] MRI can be used to demonstrate obstructive nephrolithiasis as evidenced by abrupt change in the ureteral caliber and presence of an obstructing stone. On MRI, physiologic hydronephrosis is characterized by smooth tapering of the mid to distal ureter, while in contrast obstructive hydronephrosis is characterized by abrupt change in the ureteral caliber upstream to the obstructing T2-hypointense calculus.

## ACUTE PYELONEPHRITIS

Acute pyelonephritis is the most serious form of urinary tract infection and complicates 1% to 2% of all pregnancies.[47] Patients typically present with flank pain, bacteriuria, and systemic signs of infection. Acute pyelonephritis is primarily a clinical diagnosis, although imaging is used to evaluate for potential complications such as abscess formation and to identify associated urinary tract anomalies. Though ultrasound is frequently normal, it can show debris in the collecting system and reduced vascularity in up to 25% of acute pyelonephritis cases (Fig. 6.11).[48]

## OVARIAN TORSION

Ovarian torsion is a gynecologic emergency and occurs secondary to partial or complete twist of the ovary around its vascular pedicle, leading to vascular compromise and eventually hemorrhagic infarction. It is relatively rare in spontaneous pregnancies (1–5 in 10,000) but occurs much more frequently in the setting of assisted ovarian stimulation, reaching 16% in this context.[49] Torsion in the context of an underlying ovarian mass typically occurs during the mid to late first trimester[50]; however, torsion can also occur without an underlying mass. Presenting symptoms typically include acute, sharp pelvic pain that can overlap with other pathologies such as appendicitis.

Ultrasound is the preferred modality for evaluation of torsion and often shows asymmetric enlargement of the ovary, peripherally displaced follicles, displacement of the uterus to the torsed side, and free fluid in the pelvis. Similar findings are seen on MRI, which also shows ovarian edema with increased stromal T2 signal (Fig. 6.12).

## UTERINE LEIOMYOMA

Uterine leiomyomas, also known as fibroids, are the most common gynecologic neoplasm, with a lifetime incidence of approximately 70% in the general population.[51] They often enlarge during pregnancy due to maternal hormones, may outgrow their blood supply or degenerate secondary to venous thrombosis or rupture of intramural arteries,[52] or a pedunculated fibroid may torse on its stalk, all of which may precipitate acute abdominal pain. On MRI, fibroids typically have low T1 and T2 signal intensity. However, degenerating fibroids

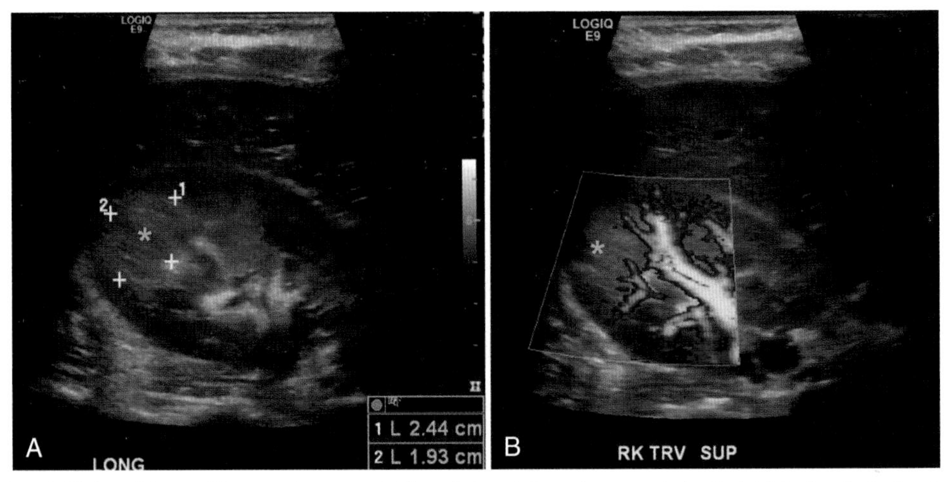


**Fig. 6.11** Pyelonephritis in a 17-year-old pregnant woman at 14 weeks' gestation who presented with right flank pain, leukocytosis, and urine analysis positive for infection. Grayscale ultrasound image of the right kidney (A) demonstrates a small ill-defined iso- to mildly hyperechoic area in the upper pole of the right kidney (asterisk). Power Doppler ultrasound image (B) demonstrates lack of Doppler signal in this region, consistent with focal pyelonephritis. Patient was subsequently placed on appropriate antimicrobial therapy.

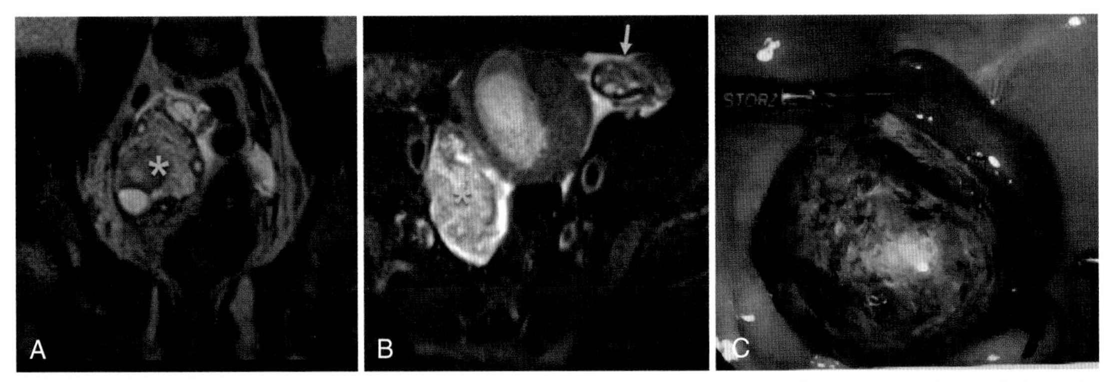


**Fig. 6.12** Ovarian torsion in a 26-year-old pregnant woman at 9 weeks' gestation who presented with right lower quadrant abdominal pain. Coronal (A) and axial fat-suppressed (B) T2-weighted magnetic resonance images show enlarged and edematous right ovary (asterisks) with stromal edema and peripheralized follicles. Note the normal left ovary (arrow in B). This patient underwent laparoscopic surgery that showed a torsed ischemic right ovary (C), which was successfully detorsed.

can have increased T2 signal due to cystic or myxoid degeneration or increased T1 signal due to blood products from hemorrhagic degeneration (Fig. 6.13).

## PELVIC INFLAMMATORY DISEASE

Pelvic inflammatory disease (PID) is an infection involving the upper genital tract and ranges from cervicitis to hydrosalpinx and tubo-ovarian abscess.[53] PID can cause pelvic pain mimicking other pathologies and may also increase the risk of pregnancy-related complications such as ectopic pregnancy by a factor of seven.[54] The imaging findings in the early stages of disease are often subtle and nonspecific, while more advance cases can show hydrosalpinx, pyosalpinx, and tubo-ovarian abscess (Fig. 6.14).

## ENDOMETRIOSIS

Endometriosis is a chronic condition characterized by functional endometrial-like tissue outside of the uterus.[55] It is a rare condition in pregnancy, as it is typically associated with infertility, and symptomatic cases often improve during pregnancy.[56] MRI is the modality

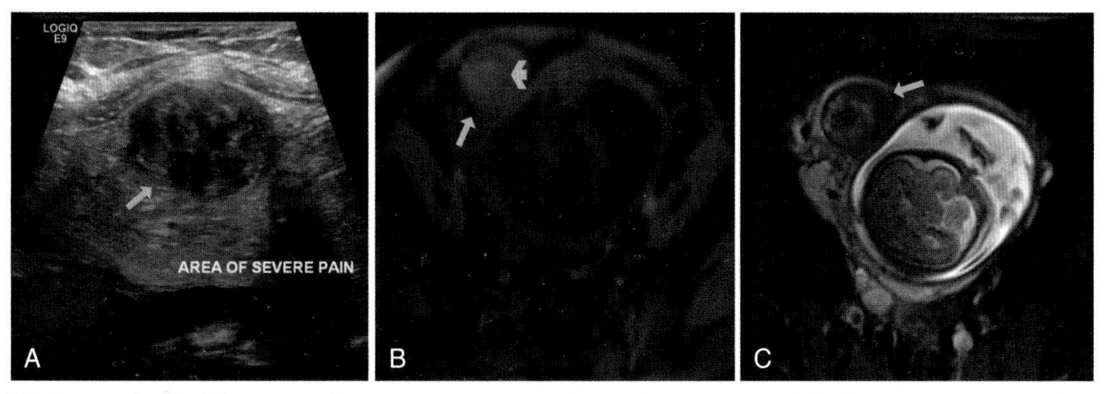


**Fig. 6.13** Degenerating fibroid in a 29-year-old pregnant woman at 24 weeks' gestation who presented with right lower quadrant abdominal pain. Grayscale ultrasound image (A) shows a mixed-echogenicity mass at the area of maximum tenderness, likely arising from the uterus. Axial T1-weighted magnetic resonance (MR) image (B) demonstrates a uterine fibroid (arrow) with internal T1-hyperintensity (arrowhead), consistent with hemorrhage. Axial T2-weighted MR image (C) shows internal edema within the fibroid (arrow) and surrounding fluid.

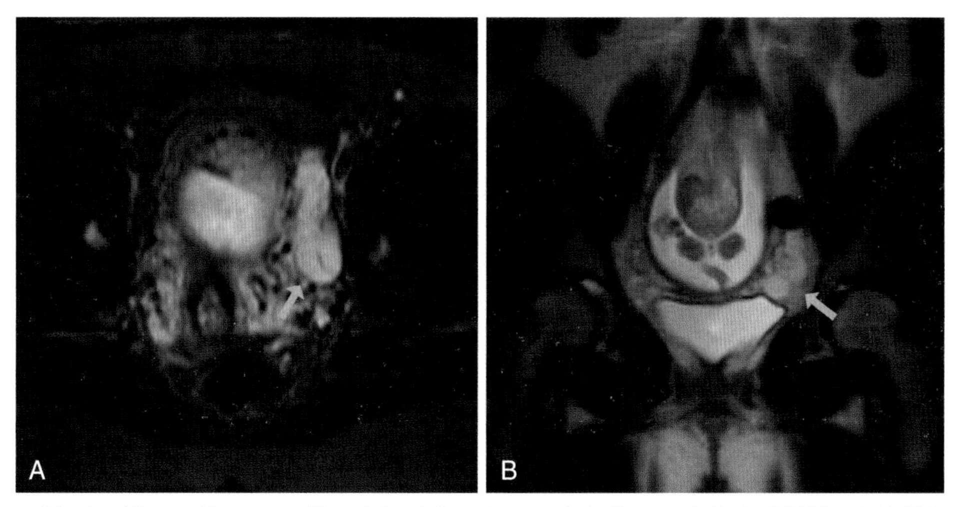


**Fig. 6.14** Hydrosalpinx in a 29-year-old woman at 17 weeks' gestation who presented with abdominal pain. Axial T2-weighted fat-suppressed (A) and coronal T2-weighted (B) magnetic resonance images demonstrate a tubular fluid-filled structure (arrows) in the region of left adnexa, consistent with hydrosalpinx.

of choice for evaluation of endometriosis and demonstrates hemorrhagic masses in the pelvis and hemoperitoneum. Adnexal endometriosis (endometriomas) is common and is characterized by T1-hyperintense and T2-hypointense (T2 "shading") masses secondary to recurrent hemorrhages (Fig. 6.15).[57]

## Obstetrics Pathologies

### ECTOPIC PREGNANCY

Ectopic pregnancy is referred to as implantation of the fertilized egg outside of the uterine cavity, with approximately 95% cases occurring in the fallopian tubes.[58] It affects up to 2% of pregnancies and remains the leading cause of maternal mortality during the first trimester.[59] The incidence of ectopic pregnancy has been increasing over the past few decades, in part due to PIDs and use of assisted reproductive techniques.[58,60,61] The presentation symptoms typically include abdominal pain and vaginal bleeding, though it may initially present as mild spotting.[62]

Ultrasound plays a crucial role in evaluation of ectopic pregnancy and can confirm an intrauterine pregnancy. An intrauterine gestational sac should

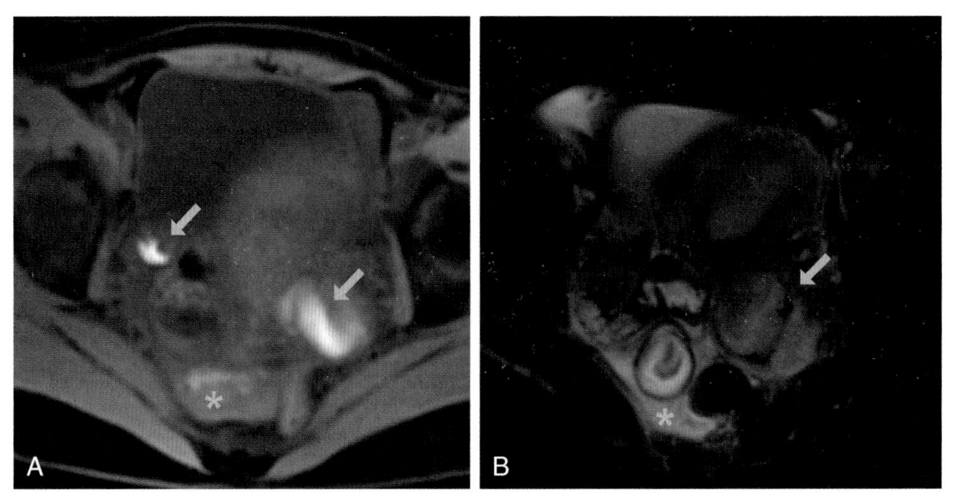


**Fig. 6.15** Endometriosis in a 39-year-old pregnant woman status post *in vitro* fertilization at 6 weeks' gestation who presented with lower abdominal pain. Axial T1-weighted fat-suppressed magnetic resonance image (A) demonstrates multiple T1 hyperintensities in the pelvis (arrows) with corresponding hypointense signal intensity on T2-weighted fat-suppressed image (B). There is intermediate T1 signal intensity fluid in the pelvis, consistent with hemoperitoneum (asterisks).

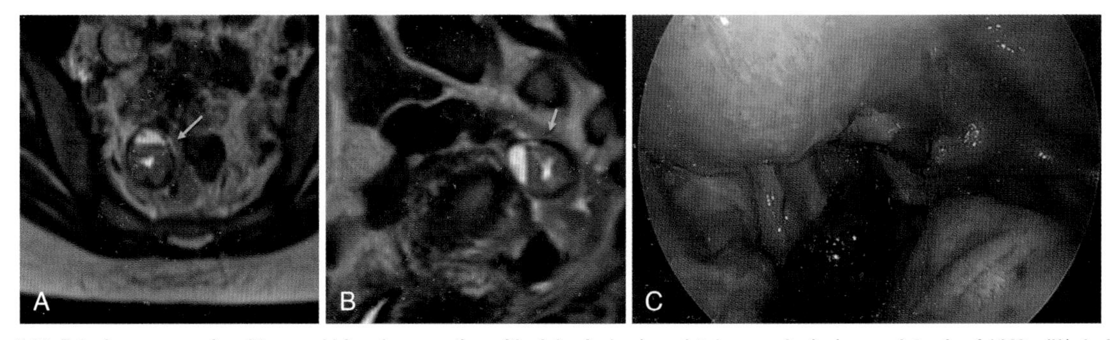


**Fig. 6.16** Ectopic pregnancy in a 35-year-old female presenting with abdominal pain and β–human chorionic gonadotropin of 1440 mIU/mL. Axial and sagittal T2-weighted images (A and B) demonstrate a complex thick-walled lesion in the right adnexa (arrows) without an intrauterine gestational sac, consistent with ectopic pregnancy. This was confirmed at surgery (C).

typically be visible on transvaginal ultrasound by 5 to 5.5 weeks' gestational age when the β–human chorionic gonadotropin levels are greater than 1500 to 2000 mIU/mL.[58,63–65] Sonographic findings of ectopic pregnancy include lack of intrauterine gestational sac, adnexal mass (especially if complex or ring-like) and free fluid in the pelvis (hemoperitoneum). Similar findings can also be seen on MRI (Fig. 6.16).

Heterotopic pregnancy, a coexisting intrauterine and ectopic pregnancy, is rare but can occur up to 1% of pregnancies using assisted reproductive techniques.[66,67] Therefore, care must be taken in evaluating the entire pelvis regardless of the presence of intrauterine pregnancy.

## UTERINE RUPTURE

Uterine rupture is a rare but potentially catastrophic complication of the pregnancy and is associated with high rates of maternal and fetal mortality. In the nontraumatic setting, predisposing factors often include focal uterine wall weakness from prior surgery such as cesarean section or myomectomy, and congenital uterine anomalies.[68–70]

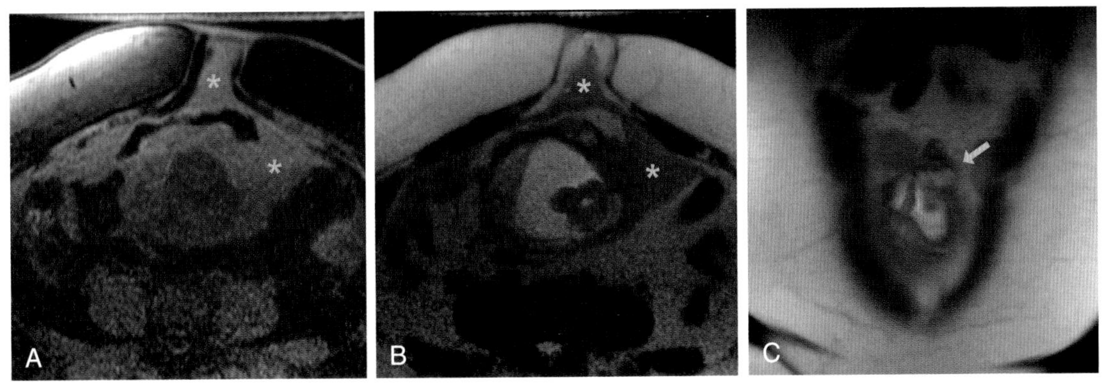


**Fig. 6.17** Atraumatic uterine rupture in a 36-year-old pregnant woman at 17 weeks' gestation who presented with abdominal pain. Axial T1-weighted fat-suppressed (A) and T2-weighted (B) magnetic resonance (MR) images demonstrate periuterine and free intraperitoneal hemorrhage (asterisks). Coronal T2-weighted MR image (C) demonstrated focal discontinuity in the uterine fundus (arrow). This was confirmed at the time of surgery.

The presenting symptoms typically include severe abdominal pain with possible hemodynamic compromise. Ultrasound or MRI, if performed, may show a focal myometrial defect, extrusion of the pregnancy products into the peritoneal cavity, and hemoperitoneum (Fig. 6.17).

## Conclusion

Abdominal pain is a common but nonspecific symptom in pregnancy, with etiologies ranging from normal physiological changes to life-threatening conditions. Typical clinical clues for early diagnosis of surgical causes of abdominal pain are rather limited in pregnancy, and therefore imaging plays a critical role in timely identification of potential causes of abdominal pain. The choice of the imaging modality is usually directed by initial clinical suspicion. Ultrasound, and increasingly MRI without intravenous contrast, are employed in the workup of abdominal pain in pregnancy due to their nonionizing nature. In particular, MRI is the modality of choice when gastrointestinal pathologies such as acute appendicitis are suspected in a pregnant patient, and has the advantage of simultaneous assessment of alternative causes of abdominal pain. Considering the spectrum of pathological causes of abdominal pain in pregnancy, familiarity with their imaging appearance is crucial in directing timely and effective care.

## REFERENCES


1. Cappell MS, Friedel D. Abdominal pain during pregnancy. *Gastroenterol Clin North Am*. 2003;32(1):1–58.
2. Mayer IE, Hussain H. Abdominal pain during pregnancy. *Gastroenterol Clin North Am*. 1998;27(1):1–36.
3. Oto A, Srinivasan PN, Ernst RD, et al. Revisiting MRI for appendix location during pregnancy. *AJR Am J Roentgenol*. 2006;186(3):883–887.
4. Wu V, Armson BA. Appendicitis in pregnancy: clinical presentation and perinatal outcome. *J SOGC*. 1999;21(14):1328–1333.
5. Andreotti RF, Lee SI, Allison SOD, et al. ACR appropriateness criteria® acute pelvic pain in the reproductive age group. *Ultrasound Q*. 2011;27(3):205–210.
6. Brown DL, Packard A, Maturen KE, et al. ACR appropriateness criteria® first trimester vaginal bleeding. *J Am Coll Radiol*. 2018;15(5, Supplement):S69–S77.
7. Shipp TD, Poder L, Feldstein VA, et al. ACR appropriateness criteria® second and third trimester vaginal bleeding. *J Am Coll Radiol*. 2020;17(11, Supplement):S497–S504.
8. Yarmish GM, Smith MP, Rosen MP, et al. ACR appropriateness criteria right upper quadrant pain. *J Am Coll Radiol*. 2014;11(3):316–322.
9. Coursey CA, Casalino DD, Remer EM, et al. ACR Appropriateness criteria® acute onset flank pain--suspicion of stone disease. *Ultrasound Q*. 2012;28(3):227–233.
10. Nikolaidis P, Dogra VS, Goldfarb S, et al. ACR appropriateness criteria® acute pyelonephritis. *J Am Coll Radiol*. 2018;15(11):S232–S239.
11. Oh KY, Gilfeather M, Kennedy A, et al. Limited abdominal MRI in the evaluation of acute right upper quadrant pain. *Abdom Imaging*. 2003;28(5):643–651.
12. Vu L, Ambrose D, Vos P, Tiwari P, Rosengarten M, Wiseman S. Evaluation of MRI for the diagnosis of appendicitis during pregnancy when ultrasound is inconclusive. *J Surg Res*. 2009;156(1):145–149.
13. Israel GM, Malguria N, McCarthy S, Copel J, Weinreb J. MRI vs. ultrasound for suspected appendicitis during pregnancy. *J Magn Reson Imaging*. 2008;28(2):428–433.

14. Pedrosa I, Levine D, Eyvazzadeh AD, Siewert B, Ngo L, Rofsky NM. MR imaging evaluation of acute appendicitis in pregnancy. *Radiology*. 2006;238(3):891–899.
15. Ludwig DR, Tsai R, Raptis DA, Mellnick VM. MRI evaluation of the pregnant patient with suspected appendicitis: imaging considerations and alternative explanations for abdominal and pelvic pain. *Emergency Imaging of Pregnant Patients. Edited by Patlas MN, Katz DS and Scaglione M*. Springer; 2020:87–109.
16. Fraum TJ, Ludwig DR, Bashir MR, Fowler KJ. Gadolinium-based contrast agents: A comprehensive risk assessment. *J Magn Reson Imaging*. 2017;46(2):338–353.
17. Tracey M, Fletcher HS. Appendicitis in pregnancy. *Am Surg*. 2000;66(6):555–559. discussion 559-560.
18. Abbasi N, Patenaude V, Abenhaim HA. Management and outcomes of acute appendicitis in pregnancy-population-based study of over 7000 cases. *BJOG Int J Obstet Gynaecol*. 2014;121(12):1509–1514.
19. Aptilon Duque G, Mohney S. Appendicitis in pregnancy. StatPearls. Updated August 10, 2021. Accessed May 13, 2021. http://www.ncbi.nlm.nih.gov/books/NBK551642/
20. Babaknia A, Parsa H, Woodruff JD. Appendicitis during pregnancy. *Obstet Gynecol*. 1977;50(1):40.
21. Lehnert BE, Gross JA, Linnau KF, Moshiri M. Utility of ultrasound for evaluating the appendix during the second and third trimester of pregnancy. *Emerg Radiol*. 2012;19(4):293–299.
22. Duke E, Kalb B, Arif-Tiwari H, et al. A systematic review and meta-analysis of diagnostic performance of MRI for evaluation of acute appendicitis. *AJR Am J Roentgenol*. 2016;206(3):508–517.
23. Willekens I, Peeters E, Maeseneer MD, Mey Jde. The normal appendix on CT: does size matter? *PLoS ONE*. 2014;9(5):e96476.
24. Tsai R, Raptis C, Fowler KJ, Owen JW, Mellnick VM. MRI of suspected appendicitis during pregnancy: interradiologist agreement, indeterminate interpretation and the meaning of non-visualization of the appendix. *Br J Radiol*. 2017;90(1079):20170383.
25. Hatch Q, Champagne BJ, Maykel JA, et al. The impact of pregnancy on surgical Crohn disease: an analysis of the Nationwide Inpatient Sample. *J Surg Res*. 2014;190(1):41–46.
26. Kaushal P, Somwaru AS, Charabaty A, Levy AD. MR enterography of inflammatory bowel disease with endoscopic correlation. *RadioGraphics*. 2017;37(1):116–131.
27. Gonzalez-Urquijo M, Zambrano-Lara M, Patiño-Gallegos JA, Rodarte-Shade M, Leyva-Alvizo A, Rojas-Mendez J Pregnant patients with internal hernia after gastric bypass: a single-center experience. Surg Obes Relat Dis. 2021;17(7):1344–1348.
28. Wax JR, Pinette MG, Cartin A. Roux-en-Y gastric bypass-associated bowel obstruction complicating pregnancy–an obstetrician's map to the clinical minefield. *Am J Obstet Gynecol*. 2013;208(4):265–271.
29. Webster P, Bailey M, Wilson J, Burke D. Small bowel obstruction in pregnancy is a complex surgical problem with a high risk of fetal loss. *Ann R Coll Surg Engl*. 2015;97(5):339–344.
30. Chang KJ, Marin D, Kim DH, et al. ACR appropriateness criteria® suspected small-bowel obstruction. *J Am Coll Radiol*. 2020;17(5, Supplement):S305–S314.
31. Longo SA, Moore RC, Canzoneri BJ, Robichaux A. Gastrointestinal conditions during pregnancy. *Clin Colon Rectal Surg*. 2010;23(2):80–89.
32. Heverhagen JT, Ishaque N, Zielke A, et al. Feasibility of MRI in the diagnosis of acute diverticulitis: initial results. *Magma N Y N*. 2001;12(1):4–9.
33. Rao PM, Rhea JT, Wittenberg J, Warshaw AL. Misdiagnosis of primary epiploic appendagitis. *Am J Surg*. 1998;176(1):81–85.
34. Maringhini A. Biliary sludge and gallstones in pregnancy: incidence, risk factors, and natural history. *Ann Intern Med*. 1993;119(2):116.
35. Valdivieso V, Covarrubias C, Siegel F, Cruz F. Pregnancy and cholelithiasis: pathogenesis and natural course of gallstones diagnosed in early puerperium. *Hepatology*. 1993;17(1):1–4.
36. Augustin G. Acute biliary tract diseases. In: Augustin G, ed. *Acute Abdomen During Pregnancy*.: Springer International Publishing; 2014:45–90.
37. Schwulst SJ, Son M. Management of gallstone disease during pregnancy. *JAMA Surg*. 2020;155(12):1162.
38. Ko CW, Beresford SAA, Schulte SJ, Matsumoto AM, Lee SP. Incidence, natural history, and risk factors for biliary sludge and stones during pregnancy. *Hepatology*. 2005;41(2):359–365.
39. Singh A, Mann HS, Thukral CL, Singh NR. Diagnostic accuracy of MRCP as compared to ultrasound/CT in patients with obstructive jaundice. *J Clin Diagn Res JCDR*. 2014;8(3):103–107.
40. Chen W, Mo J-J, Lin L, Li C-Q, Zhang J-F. Diagnostic value of magnetic resonance cholangiopancreatography in choledocholithiasis. *World J Gastroenterol*. 2015;21(11):3351–3360.
41. Mali P. Pancreatitis in pregnancy: etiology, diagnosis, treatment, and outcomes. *Hepatobiliary Pancreat Dis Int*. 2016;15(4):434–438.
42. Sandrasegaran K, Heller MT, Panda A, Shetty A, Menias CO. MRI in acute pancreatitis. *Abdom Radiol N Y*. 2020;45(5):1232–1242.
43. Haram K, Svendsen E, Abildgaard U. The HELLP syndrome: Clinical issues and management. A Review. *BMC Pregnancy Childbirth*. 2009;9(1):8.
44. Nunes JO, Turner MA, Fulcher AS. Abdominal imaging features of HELLP syndrome: A 10-year retrospective review. *Am J Roentgenol*. 2005;185(5):1205–1210.
45. Aloizos S, Seretis C, Liakos N, et al. HELLP syndrome: Understanding and management of a pregnancy-specific disease. *J Obstet Gynaecol*. 2013;33(4):331–337.
46. Blanco LT, Socarras MR, Montero RF, et al. Renal colic during pregnancy: Diagnostic and therapeutic aspects. Literature review. *Cent Eur J Urol*. 2017;70(1):93–100.
47. Jolley JA, Wing DA. Pyelonephritis in pregnancy: an update on treatment options for optimal outcomes. *Drugs*. 2010;70(13):1643–1655.
48. Craig WD, Wagner BJ, Travis MD. Pyelonephritis: radiologic-pathologic review. *RadioGraphics*. 2008;28(1):255–276.
49. Hasson J, Tsafrir Z, Azem F, et al. Comparison of adnexal torsion between pregnant and nonpregnant women. *Am J Obstet Gynecol*. 2010;202(6):536.e1–536.e6.
50. Grendys EC, Barnes WA. Ovarian cancer in pregnancy. *Surg Clin North Am*. 1995;75(1):1–14.
51. Styer AK, Rueda BR. The epidemiology and genetics of uterine leiomyoma. *Best Pract Res Clin Obstet Gynaecol*. 2016;34:3–12.
52. Murase E, Siegelman ES, Outwater EK, Perez-Jaffe LA, Tureck RW. Uterine leiomyomas: histopathologic features, MR imaging findings, differential diagnosis, and treatment. *RadioGraphics*. 1999;19(5):1179–1197.
53. Revzin MV, Mathur M, Dave HB, Macer ML, Spektor M. Pelvic inflammatory disease: multimodality imaging approach with clinical-pathologic correlation. *RadioGraphics*. 2016;36(5):1579–1596.
54. Soper DE. Pelvic inflammatory disease. *Obstet Gynecol*. 2010;116(2 Part 1):419–428.
55. Petresin J, Wolf J, Emir S, Müller A, Boosz AS. Endometriosis-associated maternal pregnancy complications – case report and literature review. *Geburtshilfe Frauenheilkd*. 2016;76(8):902–905.

56. Leone Roberti Maggiore U, Ferrero S, Mangili G, et al. A systematic review on endometriosis during pregnancy: diagnosis, misdiagnosis, complications and outcomes. *Hum Reprod Update*. 2016;22(1):70–103.
57. Siegelman ES, Oliver ER. MR imaging of endometriosis: ten imaging pearls. *RadioGraphics*. 2012;32(6):1675–1691.
58. Walker JJ. Ectopic pregnancy. *Clin Obstet Gynecol*. 2007;50(1):89–99.
59. Sivalingam VN, Duncan WC, Kirk E, Shephard LA, Horne AW. Diagnosis and management of ectopic pregnancy. *J Fam Plann Reprod Health Care*. 2011;37(4):231–240.
60. Chang J, Elam-Evans LD, Berg CJ, et al. Pregnancy-related mortality surveillance–United States, 1991–1999. *MMWR Surveill Summ*. 2003;52(2):1–8.
61. Panelli DM, Phillips CH, Brady PC. Incidence, diagnosis and management of tubal and nontubal ectopic pregnancies: a review. *Fertil Res Pract*. 2015;1(1):15.
62. Alkatout I, Honemeyer U, Strauss A, et al. Clinical diagnosis and treatment of ectopic pregnancy. *Obstet Gynecol Surv*. 2013;68(8):571–581.
63. Barnhart K, Mennuti MT, Benjamin I, Jacobson S, Goodman D, Coutifaris C. Prompt diagnosis of ectopic pregnancy in an emergency department setting. *Obstet Gynecol*. 1994;84(6):1010–1015.
64. Shalev E, Yarom I, Bustan M, Weiner E, Ben-Shlomo I. Transvaginal sonography as the ultimate diagnostic tool for the management of ectopic pregnancy: experience with 840 cases. *Fertil Steril*. 1998;69(1):62–65.
65. Levine D. Ectopic pregnancy. *Radiology*. 2007;245(2):385–397.
66. Barrenetxea G, Barinaga-Rementeria L, Lopez de Larruzea A, Agirregoikoa JA, Mandiola M, Carbonero K. Heterotopic pregnancy: two cases and a comparative review. *Fertil Steril*. 2007;87(2):417 e9-417.e15j.
67. Wu Z, Zhang X, Xu P, Huang X. Clinical analysis of 50 patients with heterotopic pregnancy after ovulation induction or embryo transfer. *Eur J Med Res*. 2018;23(1):17.
68. Savukyne E, Bykovaite-Stankeviciene R, Machtejeviene E, Nadisauskiene R, Maciuleviciene R. Symptomatic uterine rupture: a fifteen year review. *Medicina (Mex)*. 2020;56(11):574.
69. Ravasia DJ, Brain PH, Pollard JK. Incidence of uterine rupture among women with müllerian duct anomalies who attempt vaginal birth after cesarean delivery. *Am J Obstet Gynecol*. 1999;181(4):877–881.
70. Turner MJ. Uterine rupture. *Best Pract Res Clin Obstet Gynaecol*. 2002;16(1):69–79.

Chapter 7

# Abdominal Trauma in Pregnant Patients

Daniel D. Friedman, Neeraj Lalwani, Vincent M. Mellnick, and Malak Itani

## Outline



## Key Points

- The primary objective during early management of pregnant female trauma patients is maternal stabilization, given that maternal survival will optimize the chances of fetal survival.
- The risk of fetal harm due to ionizing radiation should not be of concern if there is any risk to the mother's life. Exposure of less than 50 mGy does not increase the risk of anomalies, and almost every diagnostic imaging that uses ionizing radiation will fall safely below this level.
- Placental abruption is the most common cause of fetal death in cases of trauma where the mother survives. Imaging findings include retroplacental hemorrhage, bleeding into the amniotic fluid, and ingested fetal blood from the amniotic fluid.
- Increased blood volume causes late presentation of hemorrhagic shock in pregnant patients. Enlargement and displacement of organs, as well as increased pelvic blood flow, are the basic physiologic changes that affect the patterns of injury with abdominal trauma in the pregnant patient.

## Introduction

Diagnostic imaging of the pregnant trauma patient is among the most important and challenging clinical scenarios that emergency and trauma radiologists may encounter in their practice. With an estimated incidence of 5% to 7% across all pregnancies, trauma is both the leading cause of nonobstetric maternal mortality[1–3] and a significant cause of fetal loss.[4–6] Moreover, pregnant patients face a higher risk of suffering severe abdominal injuries than do nonpregnant patients due to the excellent perfusion of the uterus and placenta, as well as lack of room for soft-tissue distention, which increases the risk of injury to large veins.[7,8] Blunt mechanisms of trauma are overwhelmingly more common than penetrating trauma, with motor vehicle collisions accounting for nearly 50% of cases.[3,9] Falls (25%) and assaults including domestic violence (18%) also account for significant percentages of cases, while gunshot wounds, the most common cause of penetrating trauma, account for 4% of cases.[9]

Pregnant patients are susceptible to the same spectrum of injuries as nonpregnant victims of trauma.[10] While there is no evidence that serious traumatic injuries, taken together, are associated with a higher mortality rate during pregnancy,[4] specific injuries such as pelvic and acetabular fractures are associated with increased maternal mortality due to increased blood flow to the pelvis, and the risk of secondary coagulopathy if amniotic fluid enters maternal circulation.[8,11]

Conversely, bowel injuries are less frequently reported among pregnant women in both blunt and penetrating trauma, presumably due to the protection conferred by the gravid uterus.[12,13] When pregnant women die as a result of trauma, the most common causes are head injuries and hemorrhagic shock.[14,15]

As the severity of the maternal injury increases, the risk of fetal loss rises commensurately, such that an Injury Severity Score (ISS) greater than 25 was associated with a fetal loss rate of 50% in one large study.[16] In nearly all cases, maternal death leads to fetal death.[17] In pregnant women who survive, placental abruption is the most common cause of pregnancy loss.[7,16,18] Fetal loss can also occur following relatively minor maternal injuries,[4] with cases of fetal death reported following insignificant trauma (i.e., ISS = 1).[19]

## Clinical Management of the Pregnant Trauma Patient

The management of the pregnant trauma patient begins with the standard techniques that would be used to care for any trauma patient, including attention to the airway, breathing, and circulation.[10] The primary objective during the critical early management is maternal stabilization, given that maternal survival will optimize the chances of fetal survival.[20] Pregnant women after 20 weeks of gestation should be placed in the 30-degree left lateral decubitus position, which helps avoid systemic hypotension due to compression of the aorta and inferior vena cava by the gravid uterus.[21,22] As the emergency team evaluates a pregnant trauma patient, it is important to consider the normal physiologic changes of pregnancy, including increased blood volume, increased heart rate, and decreased systolic and diastolic blood pressure.[4,21] Physiologic hypervolemia of pregnancy (with up to a 50% increase in total blood volume) and associated vasoconstriction may falsely indicate a stable hemodynamic state and may mask the typical signs of hemorrhage until a significant fraction of blood volume is lost.[21] If classical signs and symptoms of hypovolemic shock are present (typically seen with blood loss of 15%–30% or class II hemorrhage), the rate of fetal mortality can reach up to 80%.[14] A blood loss of 0% to 15% (class I hemorrhage) may be the best window for early intervention. Capillary filling time of more than 3 seconds may be an early indicator to assess signs of early hypovolemic shock, although it may be completely normal in patients in late pregnancy until they lose 15% of their blood volume.[23]

Once the mother is stable, evaluation of the fetus can proceed. Bedside obstetric ultrasonography should be done early on to determine fetal heart condition, viability, gestational age, presentation, and amniotic fluid volume.[4,10,24] For a viable pregnancy (i.e., fetal age between 22 and 24 weeks), continuous external fetal monitoring and tocometry are the most effective way to evaluate uterine activity and to identify signs of placental abruption, including fetal tachycardia or bradycardia, a nonreassuring fetal tracing, or fetal death.[24] Pregnancies that are not viable, i.e., before 20 weeks of gestation, can be sufficiently assessed by intermittent Doppler auscultation of the fetal heart rate.[25,26]

## Imaging of the Pregnant Trauma Patient

### GENERAL PRINCIPLES

The potential benefits of imaging the pregnant trauma patient are threefold: (1) early diagnosis of maternal injuries to allow proactive and aggressive treatment of injuries, (2) avoidance of nonobstetric laparotomy to avoid the risk of preterm labor, and (3) guidance of surgical technique when necessary to address all known maternal injuries in an efficient and effective manner[20] (Fig. 7.1). To accomplish these goals, the initial imaging evaluation often requires a multimodal approach consisting of ultrasound, conventional radiography, computed tomography (CT), and angiography.[10] While ultrasound is free of ionizing radiation, its value for detecting injuries, including active arterial bleeding, in pregnant women is limited.[10] Therefore, conventional radiography and CT remain indispensable for imaging pregnant women in the setting of major trauma despite the use of ionizing radiation in these examinations.[4,20,24] Magnetic resonance imaging (MRI), while considered safe during pregnancy, is typically not feasible or practical in the acute setting, given prolonged scanning times during which the patient will be removed from the acute care setting.[10,24]

### ULTRASOUND

Although it has not been fully validated in pregnant patients, a focused abdominal sonography for

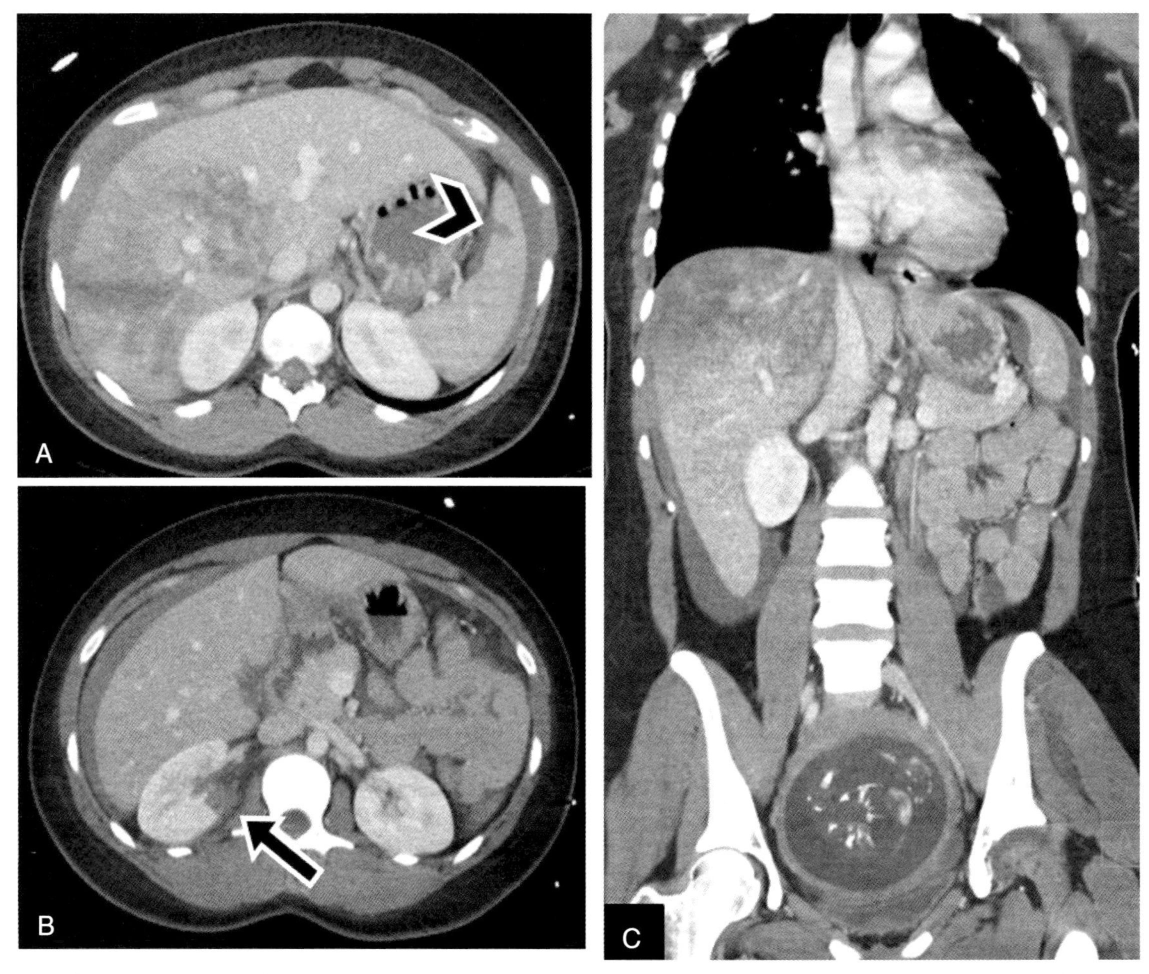


**Fig. 7.1** Computed tomography (CT) scan demonstrates multiple injuries in pregnant trauma patients. A 30-year-old woman, 19 weeks pregnant, who was involved in a motor vehicle collision. Axial (A, B) and coronal (C) CT with contrast demonstrate extensive liver lacerations (grade IV) with a perihepatic hematoma, a grade II splenic laceration (arrowhead) with subcapsular hematoma, and a posttraumatic segmental infarction in the right kidney (arrow).

trauma (FAST) examination in the trauma bay can be extremely useful for detecting intraabdominal bleeding or solid organ injury in a safe, rapid, and noninvasive manner.[20,24] The primary objective of FAST is to detect free fluid within the peritoneum or pericardium, which is generally taken to indicate hemoperitoneum and hemopericardium, respectively.[27] When compared with subsequent findings at CT or laparotomy, the combination of accumulated free fluid in the left and right upper quadrants of the abdomen plus free fluid in the pelvis is the most common pattern of FAST examination findings associated with intraabdominal injury in pregnant trauma victims with fetuses of all gestational ages.[28] Isolated free fluid in the pelvis is the second most common true-positive pattern of fluid accumulation on FAST examination in the setting of intraabdominal injury. However, this is also the most common false-positive finding, reflecting the limited ability of ultrasonography to differentiate free fluid secondary to injury and physiologic free fluid.[28]

Reported estimates of the sensitivity and specificity of FAST for detection of intraabdominal injuries in pregnant trauma patients range from 61% to 83% and 94% to 100%, respectively,[28–31] yet these values should be interpreted with a measure of caution, as they are largely based on small samples sizes. In the largest study on the topic to date, Richards and colleagues found that FAST was less sensitive for detection of intraabdominal injury in pregnant women compared with nonpregnant women following blunt abdominal trauma.[28] One potential explanation for this finding is that, in pregnant patients, small amounts of free fluid in the pelvis may be obscured by the enlarged gravid uterus.[32] In comparison to the transabdominal views obtained during the FAST exam, transvaginal ultrasonography is more sensitive for detection of free fluid in the cul-de-sac[33–36]; however, transvaginal ultrasonography is rarely practical to perform during active trauma resuscitation.

Although it has not been specifically studied in the pregnant patient population, contrast-enhanced ultrasonography (CEUS) has been proposed as a useful adjunctive imaging modality following trauma, given the potential benefit of minimizing exposure to ionizing radiation.[28, 37] CEUS allows visualization of parenchymal injuries of solid organs such as contusions, lacerations, and hematomas, which appear as nonenhancing lesions adjacent to hyperechoic and homogeneously enhancing normal tissue (Fig. 7.2).[38] Moreover, CEUS can detect findings that would be overlooked with conventional ultrasonography, including active bleeding, which will appear as a jet or pooling of hyperechoic material within the parenchyma of abdominal organs or within the peritoneal or retroperitoneal cavities.[37]

Despite its advantages, ultrasonography is best employed as a screening tool or for patients who are too clinically unstable to undergo CT imaging.

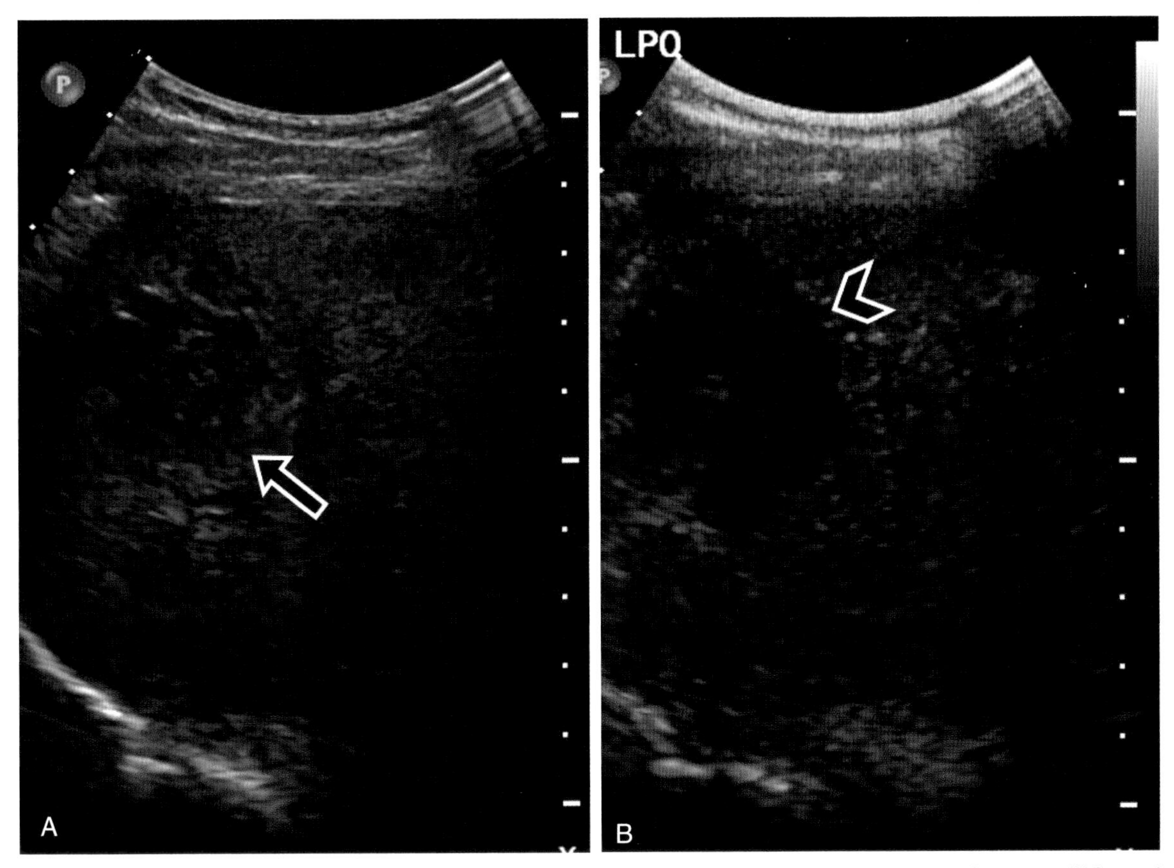


**Fig. 7.2** Contrast-enhanced ultrasound in imaging posttraumatic liver injury. An 18-year-old pregnant woman presented after trauma. (A) Greyscale ultrasound demonstrated a hypoechoic lesion in the right hepatic lobe (arrow). (B) Contrast-enhanced ultrasound demonstrates no internal enhancement (arrowhead) and no adjacent or internal pseudoaneurysm. Findings were consistent with an evolving hematoma.

Ultrasonography does not substitute a clinically necessary CT scan in the setting of major trauma and remains substantially inferior to CT in terms of detecting solid- and hollow-organ injuries in the abdomen.[20] In addition, it is insufficiently sensitive for detecting injuries in the chest, mediastinum, retroperitoneum, spine, and bony pelvis.[17] The detection of hemoperitoneum and visceral injuries based on ultrasound is also operator-dependent, requiring extensive training and sonographer proficiency.[20]

## CONVENTIONAL RADIOGRAPHY AND COMPUTED TOMOGRAPHY

Following major trauma, initial diagnostic imaging of a pregnant patient will typically include conventional radiographs of the chest, pelvis, and/or spine. If concerning findings are identified on conventional radiographs or ultrasonography, or if serious injuries are suspected clinically, further evaluation with CT is often necessary, provided that the patient remains hemodynamically stable.[17] A retrospective analysis of the clinical experiences at two level one trauma centers demonstrated that CT imaging was obtained for nearly 8% of pregnant trauma patients.[17] The advantages of CT include superior specificity and sensitivity compared with ultrasound, speed, widespread accessibility, cost-effectiveness, and relative technical ease.[17] The main disadvantages of CT include adverse effects due to the use of ionizing radiation and the risk of allergic reactions to the iodinated contrast media that are often employed.[28]

Exposure to ionizing radiation during pregnancy is associated with potential deleterious effects on the developing fetus, which has prompted concerns about use of ionizing radiation for diagnostic imaging during pregnancy. However, uncertainty regarding the safety of these modalities during pregnancy often prevents pregnant women from getting necessary diagnostic imaging.[39] Because conventional radiography and CT are often necessary for the evaluation of the pregnant trauma patient, radiologists and ordering providers should be familiar with the doses of ionizing radiation used for common imaging studies and how those doses compare to threshold levels for harmful effects to the fetus. According to the 2018 revision of the American College of Radiology (ACR) practice parameters for imaging pregnant or potentially pregnant patients and the 2017 American College of Obstetricians and Gynecologists (ACOG) guidelines for diagnostic imaging during pregnancy and lactation, radiation exposure of less than 50 mGy, regardless of the gestational age at the time of exposure, does not increase the risk of anomalies, growth restriction, or pregnancy loss for the fetus.[39,40] This statement has critical significance for the imaging evaluation of a pregnant trauma patient, because almost every diagnostic imaging that uses ionizing radiation will fall safely below this level (Table 7.1).[41] The rare exception to this principle could be a single prolonged fluoroscopic examination of the pelvis during which an intervention is performed.[20]

The risk of fetal harm due to ionizing radiation depends on both the gestational age and the radiation dose at the time of exposure[40] but should not be of concern if there is any risk to the mother's life.

Whenever necessary and possible, intravenous iodinated contrast should be used during body CT examinations of pregnant trauma patients.[20] The US Food and Drug Administration (FDA) classifies most intravenous contrast agents as category B medications, meaning that no adverse effects to the pregnancy have been demonstrated in animal or human studies.[42] Specifically, in response to prior theoretical concerns

**TABLE 7.1 Estimated Fetal Radiation Dose for Common Emergency Abdominal Imaging Studies**

| Procedure | Mean Fetal Dose (mGy) |
|---|---|
| Abdominal radiograph | 2.44 |
| Abdominopelvic radiograph | 3.60 |
| Lumbar radiograph | 4.92 |
| Contrast enhanced abdominal CT | 15.56 |
| Contrast enhanced abdominopelvic CT | 29.86 |
| Lumbar CT | 15.40 |

Based on values from Ozbayrak M, Cavdar I, Seven M, Uslu L, Yeyin N, Tanyildizi H, et al. Determining and managing fetal radiation dose from diagnostic radiology procedures in Turkey. Korean J Radiol. 2015;16(6):1276-1282.
*CT*, Computed tomography.

about potential effects of free iodide on fetal thyroid function, the ACR and ACOG guidelines both conclude that there is no evidence to date of neonatal hypothyroidism caused by maternal exposure to intravenous iodinated contrast material.[39,42] Nonetheless, given limited data on long-term effects, ACOG guidelines maintain that contrast should be reserved for situations where its administration will provide additional diagnostic information that may affect the management of a pregnant woman or the fetus. In the case of a pregnant trauma patient who needs CT imaging, the use of intravenous iodinated contrast media aids in detection of maternal and fetal injuries by demonstrating enhancement of soft tissues and opacification of vascular structures (including the placenta).[20,39] Because missing these injuries could be catastrophic for both the mother and the fetus, there should be a low threshold for using iodinated contrast when necessary. After all, a single diagnostic study performed with iodinated contrast is better than a potentially nondiagnostic study that must be repeated.

The administration of oral contrast material prior to imaging does not increase the sensitivity or specificity of CT for detection of injuries following blunt abdominal trauma and is not routinely recommended, as it may delay imaging and, consequently, diagnosis of injuries.[43] The use of oral or rectal contrast in cases of penetrating trauma, especially when penetrating trauma involves the pelvis, may help detect bowel injuries and should be used at the discretion of the radiologist and clinical team.[20] If they are needed, oral and rectal contrast agents can be administered safely to pregnant patients because the contrast is not absorbed into the maternal bloodstream.[39]

### MAGNETIC RESONANCE IMAGING

MRI plays a limited role in the initial imaging evaluation of pregnant trauma patients because a patient must be moved from the acute care setting for a relatively long time and may not be able to be adequately monitored during the exam.[20,24] Nonetheless, once the patient has been stabilized and the initial workup is complete, MRI can be extremely useful for evaluation of soft tissue, neurologic, and spinal injuries[20] (Fig. 7.3). Additionally, if follow-up imaging of injuries detected on CT is required, or if new symptoms arise, unenhanced MRI can be used in stable patients to minimize the cumulative dose of ionizing radiation that would be incurred by repeat CT examination.[10,20]

According to the 2020 ACR Manual for MR Safety, MRI can be safely performed at any time during a pregnancy when the risk-benefit ratio to the patient warrants doing so.[44] To date, there is no evidence of harmful fetal effects associated with MRI with magnetic field strength up to 3.0 T, although theoretical areas of concern include teratogenesis, acoustic damage, and heat deposition in tissue.[39,44,45] Reasonable steps to mitigate these potential risks include using the lowest magnetic field strength that will answer the clinical question (e.g., using a 1.5T scanner instead of a 3.0T scanner) and acquiring only the magnetic resonance (MR) sequences that are diagnostically relevant.[20] The FDA classifies gadolinium as a pregnancy category C drug based on evidence of teratogenic effects in animal models with insufficient data regarding the risks in humans. Given the potential risks, the ACR and ACOG recommend that MR contrast agents should not be routinely administered during pregnancy and should be reserved for rare situations where a gadolinium-based contrast is considered critical for diagnosis.[39,44] For the pregnant trauma patient, the most useful diagnostic information can be most often obtained with nonenhanced MRI.[20,39]

## Imaging of the Gravid Uterus and Placenta

By understanding the normal imaging appearance of the gravid uterus and placenta, the radiologist is better prepared to prospectively diagnose placental abruption and other pregnancy-specific traumatic injuries.[10,20] On ultrasound, the placenta initially appears at approximately 6 weeks of gestational age as an echogenic rind that surrounds the anechoic gestational sac.[46] A focal echogenic thickening of the echogenic rind develops by 10 weeks of gestation, and intervillous flow can be seen on color Doppler by the end of the first trimester.[46] By the beginning of the second trimester, the placenta will be well-formed and appear hyperechoic relative to the underlying myometrium (Fig. 7.4). The hypoechoic retroplacental zone (also known as the retroplacental complex) can also be seen around this time, located between the placenta and myometrium with linear horizontal echoes representing vascular channels.[46]

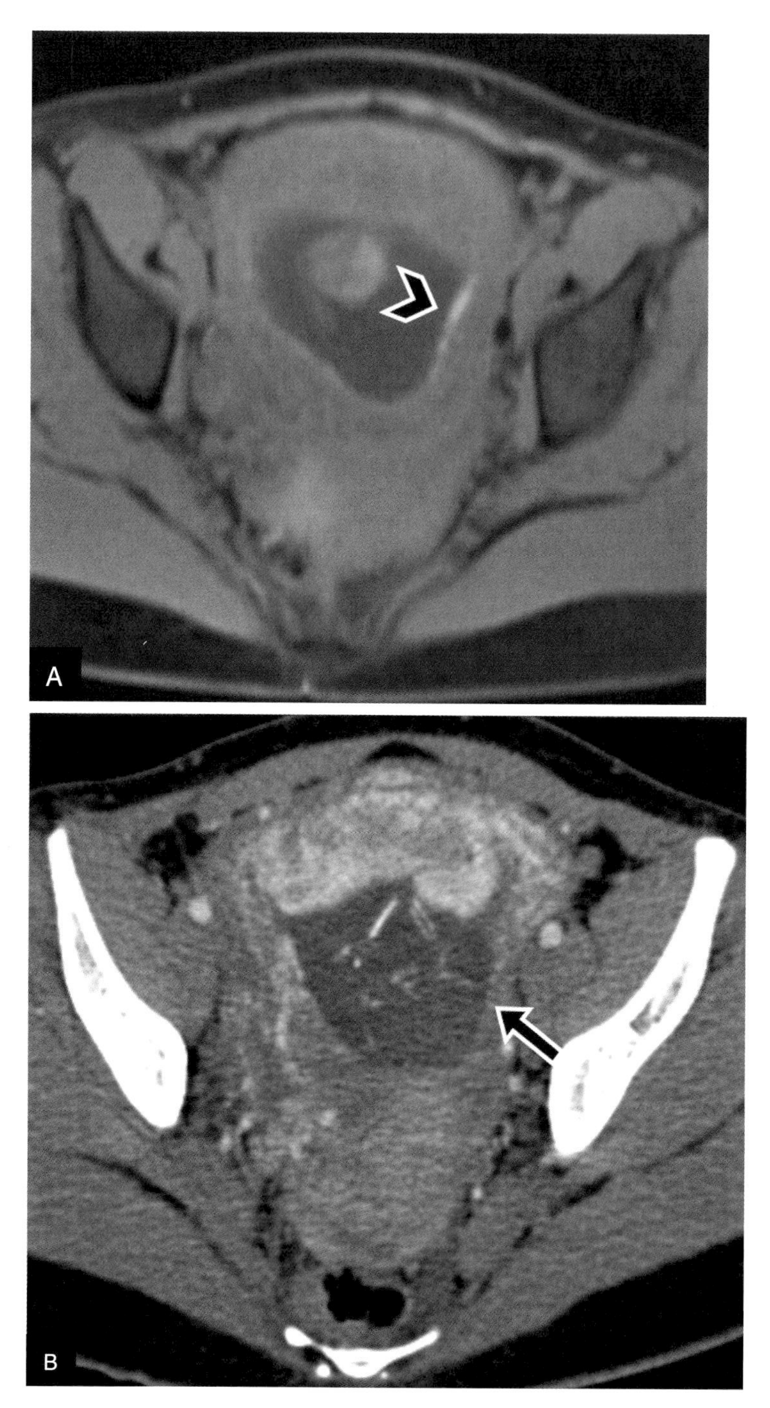


**Fig. 7.3** Complementary role of magnetic resonance imaging in imaging pregnant trauma patients. A 22-year-old woman, 14 weeks pregnant, presented after sustaining a fall with abdominal pain, low hematocrit, and a small amount of vaginal bleeding. (A) Axial noncontrast T1-weighted images demonstrate linear hyperintense signal (arrowhead) consistent with a small subchorionic hemorrhage. The patient developed peritoneal signs 2 days later, and contrast-enhanced computed tomography (CT) scan was performed. (B) The subchorionic hemorrhage is not appreciable in its known location (arrow) on this CT scan. There is no evidence of hematocrit level layering in the amniotic fluid.

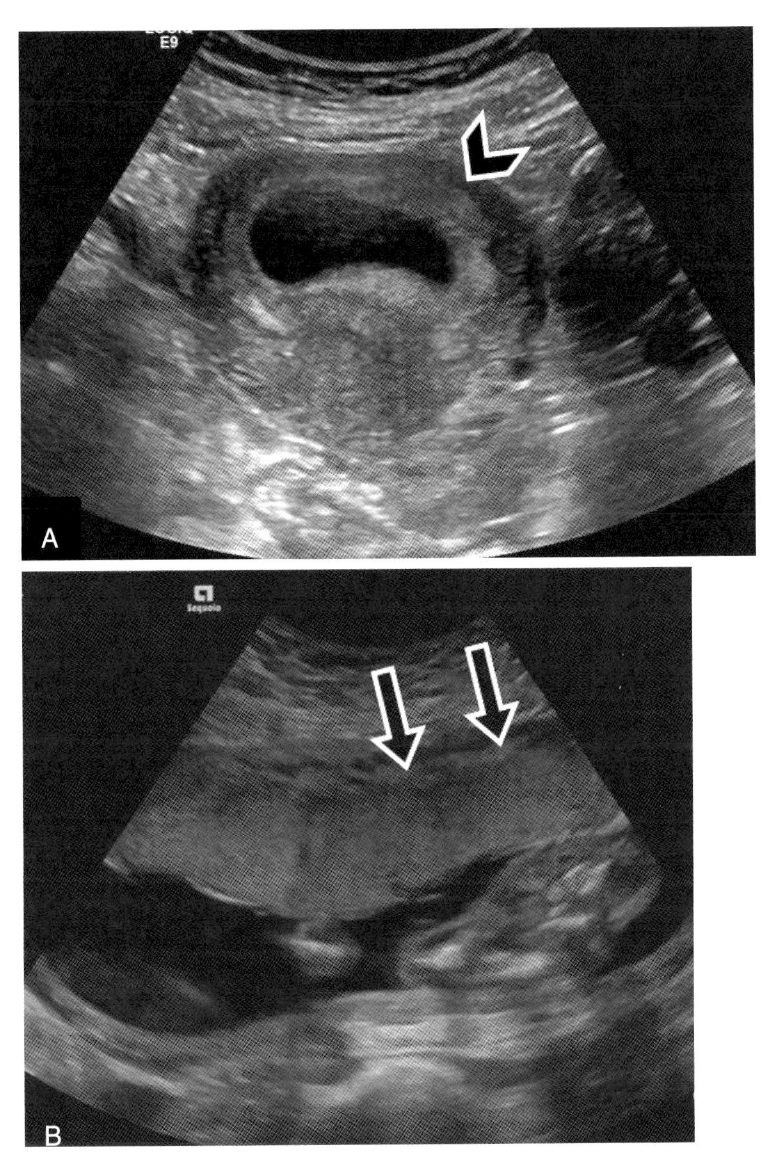

Fig. 7.4 Normal uteroplacental interface on ultrasound at different stages of pregnancy. (A) A 40-year-old woman, 8 weeks pregnant, with normal uteroplacental interface, demonstrating slightly hyperechoic placenta (arrowhead) relative to the myometrium. (B) A 22-year-old woman, 21 weeks pregnant, with normal uteroplacental interface (arrows).

Contrast-enhanced CT during the first trimester shows the gestational sac as a low-attenuation endometrial cystic structure and the placenta as a rind of homogenously enhancing tissue surrounding the gestational sac (Fig. 7.5). The placenta will typically be indistinguishable from the subjacent myometrium until late in the first trimester.[20,46] In the second trimester, the placenta becomes progressively more heterogeneous in appearance and more avidly enhances, allowing easily delineation of the placenta from the myometrium on contrast-enhanced CT.[20,46] The placental cotyledons, which are discoid subunits of the decidua basalis separated by placental septa, begin to form in the late second trimester.[46]

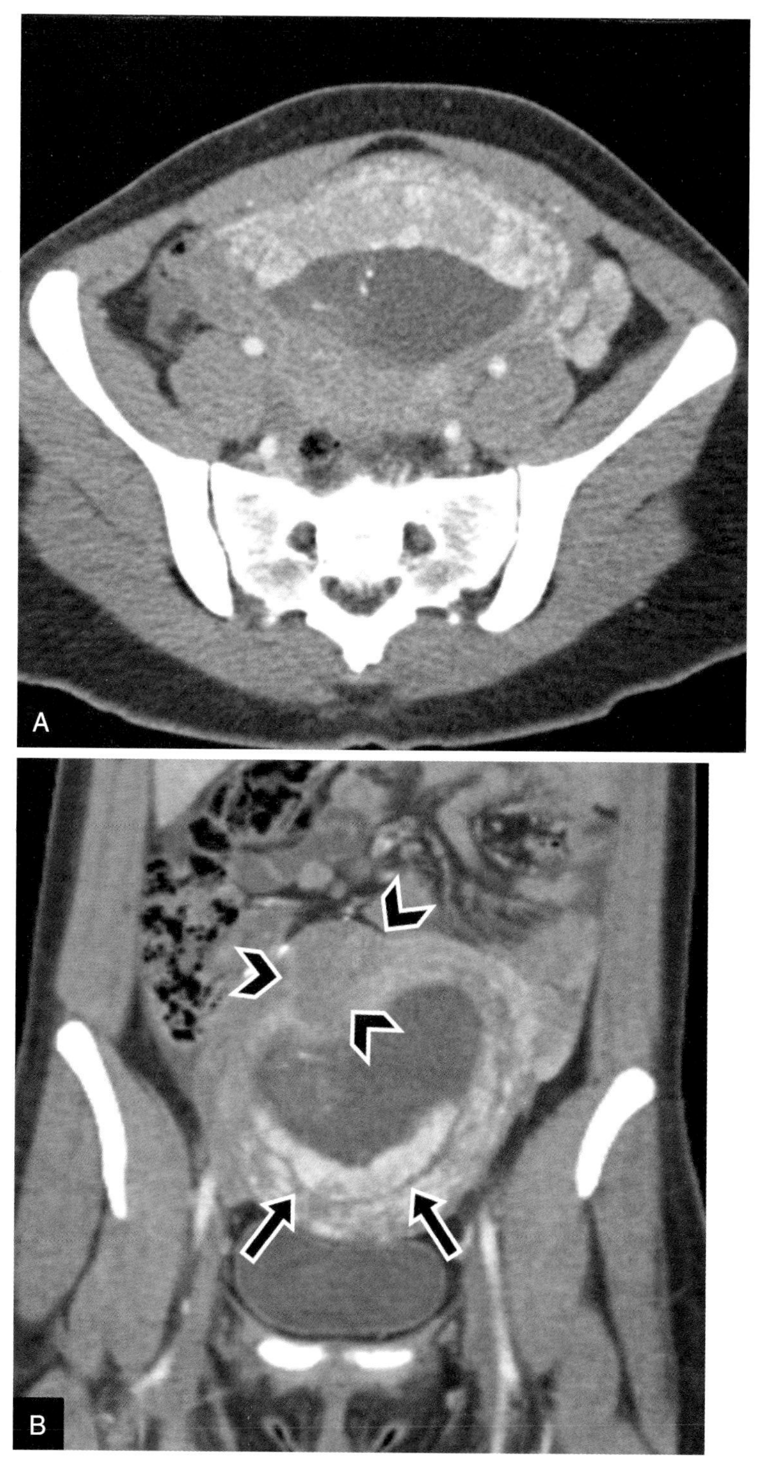


**Fig. 7.5** Normal uteroplacental interface on computed tomography (CT) scan. A 22-year-old woman, 14 weeks pregnant, with normal placenta. (A) Axial and (B) coronal contrast-enhanced CT images demonstrate normal uteroplacental interface (arrows). There is a hypoattenuating area in the cranial aspect of the placenta (arrowheads) with obtuse margins consistent with a myometrial contraction.

On contrast-enhanced CT, the cotyledons can be visualized as round, low-attenuation foci surrounded by enhancing placenta.[47] As the placenta matures through the third trimester, it becomes increasingly heterogeneous in appearance, with chorionic plate indentations becoming visible on the fetal side and venous lakes developing on the maternal side.[46,47]

On MRI in the second trimester, the normal placenta appears slightly hyperintense on T2-weighted images (T2WI) and slightly hypointense on T1-weighted images compared with the underlying myometrium. Like with CT, the imaging appearance of the placenta is initially homogenous, but becomes increasingly heterogeneous after 24 weeks' gestation as the placental cotyledons and placental septa form. Normal myometrium demonstrates a trilayered appearance on T2WI, with a thicker, heterogeneously hyperintense middle layer of vascular channels abutted by thinner, hypointense inner and outer layers.[48] As the pregnancy progresses, the myometrium becomes thinner and may appear as a single layer of uniform signal intensity at specific points of compression (e.g., adjacent to the aorta or spine).[48]

## Imaging of Pregnancy-Specific Injuries

### PLACENTAL ABRUPTION

Subchorionic placental abruption is the most common injury to the gravid uterus following blunt abdominal trauma, complicating 1% to 5% of minor traumas and 20% to 50% of major traumas. With a fetal mortality rate estimated at 67% to 75%, placental abruption is the most common cause of fetal death in cases of trauma where the mother survives.[7,49] If the fetus survives, placental abruption can lead to low birth weight and preterm delivery. Abruption is caused by shearing forces that separate the relatively rigid placenta from the more elastic uterus and can be classified based on the location of the separation between the placenta and the uterus into marginal and retroplacental (central).[26] Patients typically have uterine pain and irritability, with or without vaginal bleeding.

Imaging findings include retroplacental hemorrhage, bleeding into the amniotic fluid, and ingested fetal blood from the amniotic fluid.[10] On ultrasound, retroplacental hemorrhage appears hyperechoic to isoechoic relative to the overlying placenta in the acute phase, and gradually becomes hypoechoic then eventually sonolucent 2 weeks after the injury[50] (Fig. 7.6). The amniotic fluid might become echogenic or contain floating echogenic foci due to bleeding. Echogenic fetal bowel can also be seen due to the fetal swallowing of blood products in the amniotic fluid. Generally ultrasound is not accurate for the diagnosis of placental abruption, with relatively low sensitivity and a high false-negative rate of 50% to 80%.[10]

On CT, placental abruption appears as an area of decreased enhancement that forms acute angles with the myometrium and can be either full thickness or retroplacental[20] (Fig. 7.7). It might be difficult to identify a retroplacental hematoma, as it has similar attenuation to the subjacent myometrium. As such, it is important for the radiologist to examine the margins of the placenta and the adjacent myometrium. Blood products in the amniotic fluid are best identified in the dependent portions of the amniotic sac as areas of high attenuation. Based on retrospective evaluation, CT is reported to have a good sensitivity of 86% to 100% and a specificity of 80% to 98% for evaluation of placental abruption.[47,52] However, real-time performance is worse, with a sensitivity of only 43% and specificity 90% on analysis of original dictated reports.[47]

Causes of focal hypoattenuation that can be mistaken for placental abruption include focal myometrial contraction, venous lakes, placental infarcts, and subchorionic and preplacental hemorrhage. Myometrial contraction has bulging contours and can be differentiated from abruption by assessing the interface between the areas of high and low attenuation, as contractions will have obtuse margins, while abruption has acute angles[47] (Fig. 7.5). Placental infarcts manifest radiologically as small wedge-shaped hypoattenuating areas and become apparent as the pregnancy matures; they are often of no clinical significance.[20]

MRI performs better for evaluating retroplacental or marginal hematoma, which can be identified based on T1 and diffusion-weighted sequences. T2WI can help determine the age of the hematoma. In a small study, MRI accurately diagnosed placental abruption in 19/19 patients (compared with 10/19 patients diagnosed with ultrasound).[53]

### UTERINE RUPTURE AND PENETRATING INJURY

The incidence of uterine rupture and lacerations in pregnant trauma patients is less than 1%.[21] However, early diagnosis is crucial, as uterine rupture is associated with

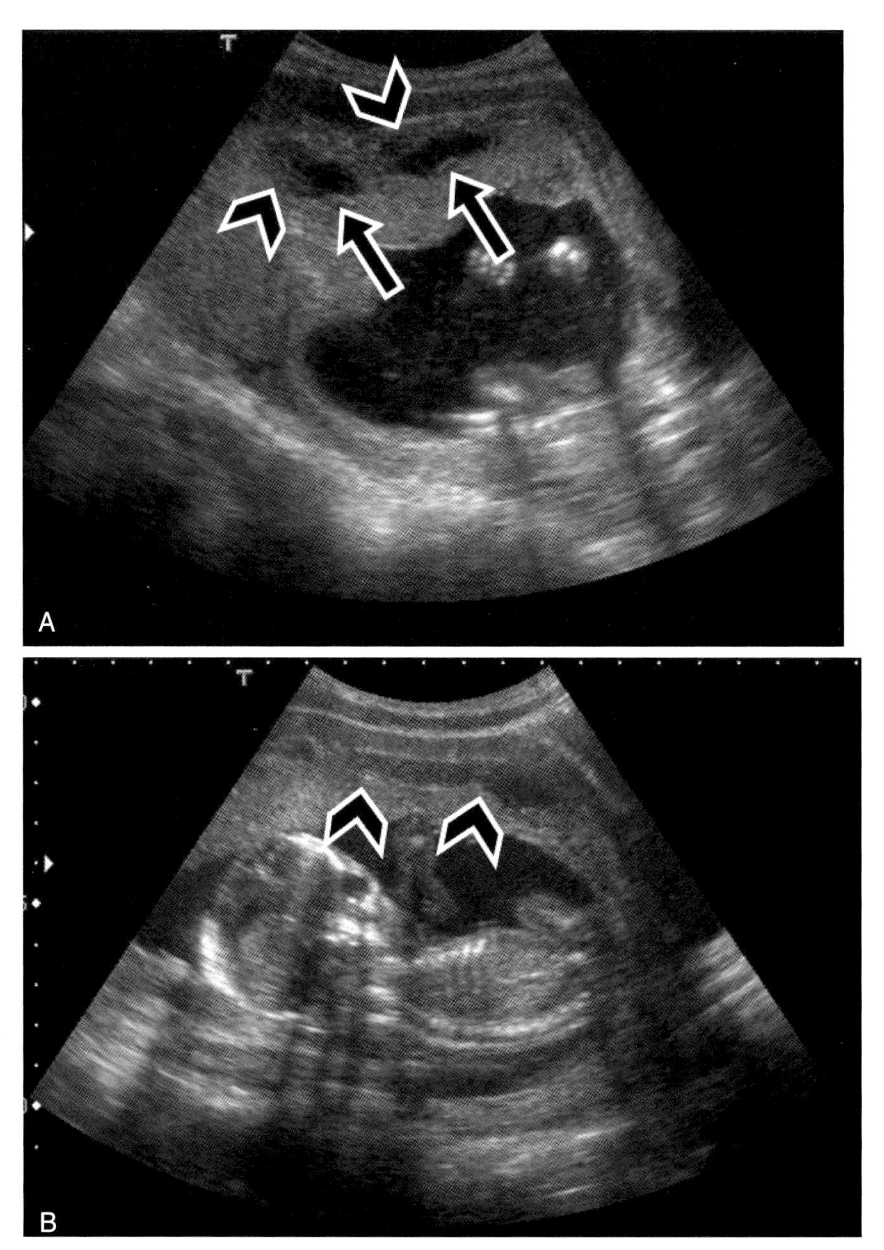


**Fig. 7.6** Ultrasound appearance of placental abruption in a 32-year-old woman, 17 weeks pregnant. Ultrasound demonstrates hypoechoic (arrowheads in A and B) and anechoic (arrows in A) areas between the placenta and the myometrium, consistent with retroplacental hemorrhage, underlying the majority of the placenta, in keeping with placental abruption. The patient had a miscarriage 7 days after this ultrasound.

nearly 100% fetal mortality and 10% maternal mortality (although typically due to other injuries). Penetrating abdominal trauma is generally associated with high fetal mortality; in a study of 321 pregnant patients with abdominal trauma, compared with overall fetal mortality of 16% and maternal morbidity of 10%, penetrating injuries result in significantly higher fetal mortality of 73% and maternal morbidity of 66%.[12] Patients present with pain, shock, and/or absent fetal heart tones.[21] Imaging features include hemoperitoneum and

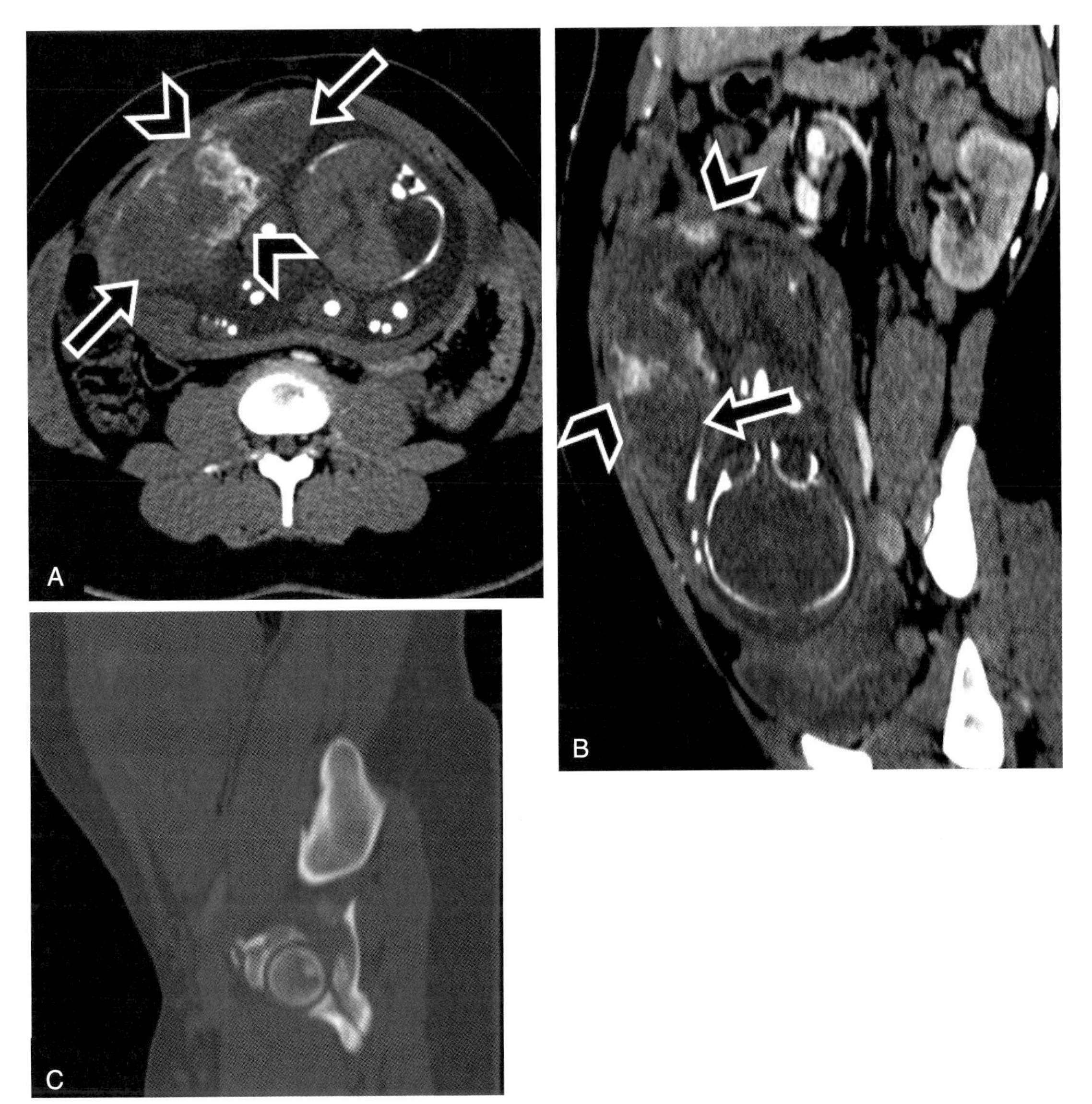


**Fig. 7.7** Computed tomography (CT) appearance of placental abruption. A 20-year-old woman, 29 weeks pregnant, presented after a motor vehicle collision. (A) Axial and (B) sagittal contrast-enhanced CT images demonstrate lack of enhancement of the placenta (arrows), with patchy areas of contrast extravasation (arrowheads). There was fetal demise at the accident scene. (C) Sagittal bone-window images also demonstrate a right acetabular fracture.

focal lacerations that appear as focal defects or areas of hypoattenuation in the uterine wall (Fig. 7.8). Gas or foreign bodies near the uterus can alert the radiologist to the path of the projectile.

## ADDITIONAL OBSTETRICAL INJURIES

Direct fetal injury is uncommon in abdominal trauma because the fetus is protected by the maternal body wall, uterus, and amniotic fluid. In the late third trimester, due to the decreased volume of amniotic fluid relative to fetal volume, there is less of a cushion effect. Most common direct fetal injuries include skull fracture and head injury, often seen in the late third trimester with cephalic presentation in the setting of a maternal pelvic fracture.[54] These are almost universally lethal to the fetus when they occur.[55]

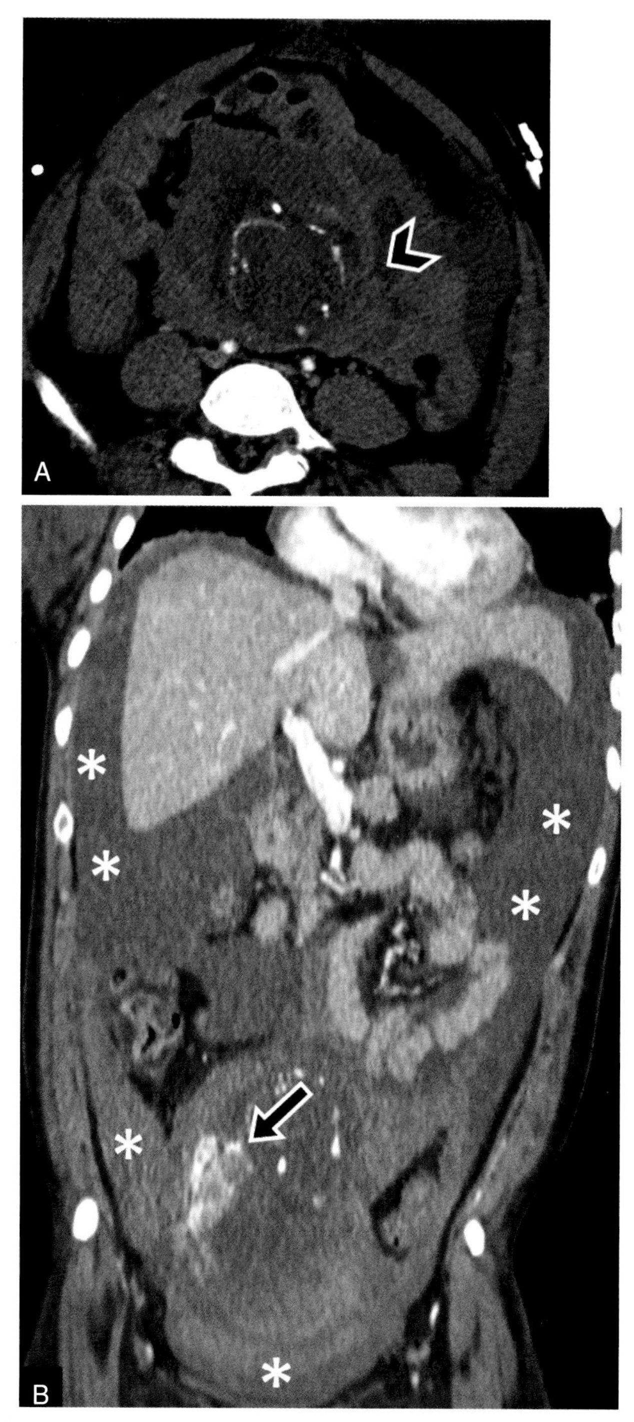


**Fig. 7.8** Computed tomography (CT) appearance of uterine rupture. A 22-year-old woman, 18 weeks pregnant, presented after a motor vehicle collision. (A) Axial contrast-enhanced CT images demonstrate lack of placental enhancement secondary to abruption, in addition to a focal area of myometrial discontinuity (arrowhead) consistent with uterine rupture, confirmed surgically. A large hematoma is seen anterior to the site of rupture. (B) Coronal images show large volume hemoperitoneum (asterisks) and areas of contrast extravasation in the placenta (arrow).

Premature rupture of membranes is another possible complication of abdominal trauma in the pregnant patient; the only imaging finding is decreased amniotic fluid volume. Spontaneous abortion, defined as noninduced loss of the pregnancy before 20 weeks of gestation, can also be encountered after abdominal trauma and can be seen on imaging as an empty uterus absent fetal components or products of conception, low-lying products of conception in the cervix, and/or blood in the cervix or vagina.

## Ectopic Pregnancy and Trauma

The incidence of ectopic pregnancy is 1% to 2%, and as such, it will complicate the presentation of some pregnant trauma patients.[56] As the majority of ectopic pregnancies manifest in the first trimester, it is expected that ectopic pregnancies in trauma patients are encountered early in the pregnancy. In one series, three of 328 pregnant patients with blunt abdominal trauma were found to have ruptured ectopic pregnancies on ultrasound examination, and all three were diagnosed in the first trimester.[28]

The only finding might be simple or hemorrhagic free fluid in the pelvis. Additional findings that might or might not be present include absent intrauterine products of conception in the setting of elevated human chorionic gonadotropin. An adnexal mass might be identified, with characteristic "ring of fire" appearance on color Doppler ultrasound.

## Imaging of Nonobstetric Injuries

In addition to obstetrical traumatic injuries, the pregnant patient is prone to various non–pregnancy-related injuries with abdominal trauma, including injury to solid organs, gastrointestinal tract, retroperitoneum, abdominal wall, diaphragm, and skeleton, less common injuries to the gallbladder, ureters, and adrenals, and hypoperfusion complex. There are a few key differences in the pattern of injury to the pregnant patient due to physiologic changes of pregnancy and anatomic displacement of organs by the gravid uterus.

Changes of pregnancy that can affect the patterns of injury with abdominal trauma in the pregnant patient include increased pelvic blood flow, which makes retroperitoneal hemorrhage more common, enlargement of the kidneys and spleen making them susceptible to injury, and displacement of the liver, spleen, and bladder causing an increased risk of injury[4,26,49,57,58] (Fig. 7.9). As mentioned earlier, with penetrating trauma the risk of bowel injury decreases in the third trimester due to cephalad displacement by the gravid uterus; nonetheless, stab wounds or gunshot wounds to the upper abdomen often result in complex bowel injuries for the same reason.[12]

Despite the slight change in patterns of abdominal injury to the pregnant patient, most cases of maternal mortality and morbidity are related to head injuries and hemorrhagic shock rather than injury to abdominal structures.

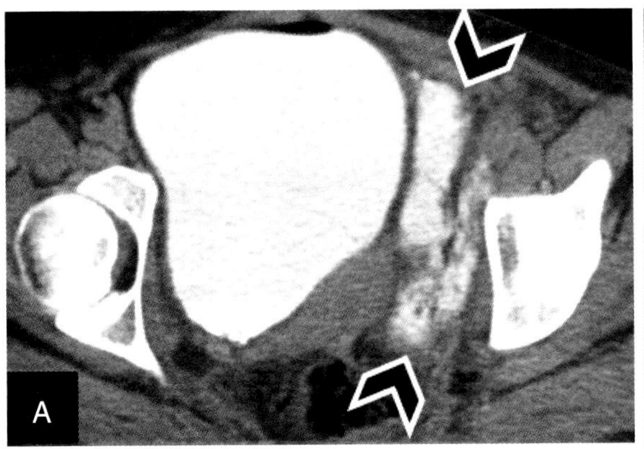


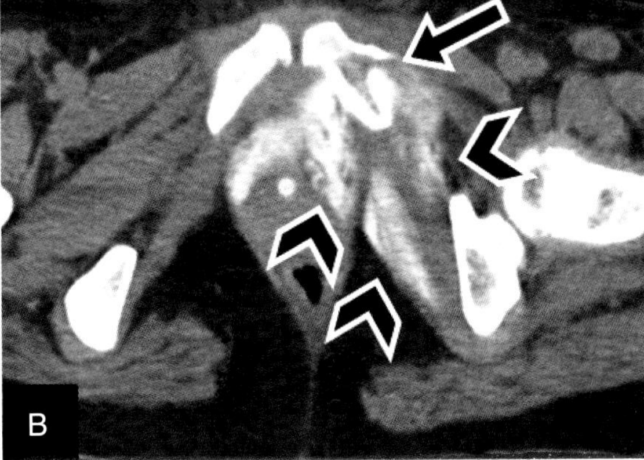


**Fig. 7.9** Bladder injury in a pregnant trauma patient. A 22-year-old woman, 28 weeks pregnant, presented after a motor vehicle collision. (A, B) Axial computed tomography cystogram images demonstrate extraperitoneal contrast leakage along the left bladder wall (arrowheads) and left pubic bone fracture (arrow).

In conclusion, radiologists play a vital role in management of the pregnant trauma patient by guiding the clinician to the most appropriate imaging modality, counseling the patient if required, and promptly and accurately evaluating for critical injuries with careful attention to the placenta and pelvic bones.

## Conclusion

Trauma is one of the leading causes of maternal nonobstetric mortality. Maternal stabilization is the primary goal of early management. If there is a risk to the life of the mother, potential fetal harm from radiation should not be a concern. Nonetheless, virtually all diagnostic imaging studies cause radiation exposure of less than 50 mGy and are not expected to significantly increase the risk of fetal damage. Radiologists are critical to managing the trauma of a pregnant patient. They can guide clinicians to the most appropriate imaging modality, advise the patient, and quickly and accurately assess critical injuries with particular attention to the placenta and pelvic bones.

### REFERENCES


1. Mattox KL, Goetzl L. Trauma in pregnancy. *Crit Care Med*. 2005;33(10 Suppl):S385–S389.
2. Towery R, English TP, Wisner D. Evaluation of pregnant women after blunt injury. *J Trauma*. 1993;35(5):731–735.
3. Connolly AM, Katz VL, Bash KL, McMahon MJ, Hansen WF. Trauma and pregnancy. *Am J Perinatol*. 1997;14(6):331–336.
4. Pearlman MD, Tintinalli JE, Lorenz RP. Blunt trauma during pregnancy. *N Engl J Med*. 1990;323(23):1609–1613.
5. Pearlman MD, Klinich KD, Schneider LW, Rupp J, Moss S, Ashton-Miller J. A comprehensive program to improve safety for pregnant women and fetuses in motor vehicle crashes: a preliminary report. *Am J Obstet Gynecol*. 2000;182(6):1554–1564.
6. Ikossi DG, Lazar AA, Morabito D, Fildes J, Knudson MM. Profile of mothers at risk: an analysis of injury and pregnancy loss in 1, 195 trauma patients. *J Am Coll Surg*. 2005;200(1):49–56.
7. Shah KH, Simons RK, Holbrook T, Fortlage D, Winchell RJ, Hoyt DB. Trauma in pregnancy: maternal and fetal outcomes. *J Trauma*. 1998;45(1):83–86.
8. Pape HC, Pohlemann T, Gansslen A, Simon R, Koch C, Tscherne H. Pelvic fractures in pregnant multiple trauma patients. *J Orthop Trauma*. 2000;14(4):238–244.
9. Mirza FG, Devine PC, Gaddipati S. Trauma in pregnancy: a systematic approach. *Am J Perinatol*. 2010;27(7):579–586.
10. Sadro C, Bernstein MP, Kanal KM. Imaging of trauma: Part 2, Abdominal trauma and pregnancy--a radiologist's guide to doing what is best for the mother and baby. *AJR Am J Roentgenol*. 2012;199(6):1207–1219.
11. Leggon RE, Wood GC, Indeck MC. Pelvic fractures in pregnancy: factors influencing maternal and fetal outcomes. *J Trauma*. 2002;53(4):796–804.
12. Petrone P, Talving P, Browder T, et al. Abdominal injuries in pregnancy: a 155-month study at two level 1 trauma centers. *Injury*. 2011;42(1):47–49.
13. Jain V, Chari R, Maslovitz S, et al. Guidelines for the management of a pregnant trauma patient. J Obstet Gynaecol Can. 2015;37(6):553–574.
14. Rothenberger D, Quattlebaum FW, Perry Jr. JF, Zabel J, Fischer RP. Blunt maternal trauma: a review of 103 cases. *J Trauma*. 1978;18(3):173–179.
15. Crosby WM, Costiloe JP. Safety of lap-belt restraint for pregnant victims of automobile collisions. *N Engl J Med*. 1971;284(12):632–636.
16. Rogers FB, Rozycki GS, Osler TM, et al. A multi-institutional study of factors associated with fetal death in injured pregnant patients. *Arch Surg*. 1999;134(11):1274–1277.
17. Lowdermilk C, Gavant ML, Qaisi W, West OC, Goldman SM. Screening helical CT for evaluation of blunt traumatic injury in the pregnant patient. *Radiographics*. 1999 19 Spec No:S243-S255; discussion S256-S248.
18. Weiss HB, Songer TJ, Fabio A. Fetal deaths related to maternal injury. *JAMA*. 2001;286(15):1863–1868.
19. Theodorou DA, Velmahos GC, Souter I, et al. Fetal death after trauma in pregnancy. *Am Surg*. 2000;66(9):809–812.
20. Raptis CA, Mellnick VM, Raptis DA, et al. Imaging of trauma in the pregnant patient. *Radiographics*. 2014;34(3):748–763.
21. Brown HL. Trauma in pregnancy. *Obstet Gynecol*. 2009; 114(1):147–160.
22. Milsom I, Forssman L. Factors influencing aortocaval compression in late pregnancy. *Am J Obstet Gynecol*. 1984;148(6):764–771.
23. Cohen WR. Hemorrhagic shock in obstetrics. *J Perinat Med*. 2006;34(4):263–271.
24. Greco PS, Day LJ, Pearlman MD. Guidance for evaluation and management of blunt abdominal trauma in pregnancy. *Obstet Gynecol*. 2019;134(6):1343–1357.
25. Murphy NJ, Quinlan JD. Trauma in pregnancy: assessment, management, and prevention. *Am Fam Physician*. 2014;90(10):717–722.
26. Sadro C, Bittle M, O'Connell K. Imaging the pregnant trauma patient. *Ultrasound Clin*. 2011;6(1):97–103.
27. McGahan JP, Rose J, Coates TL, Wisner DH, Newberry P. Use of ultrasonography in the patient with acute abdominal trauma. *J Ultrasound Med*. 1997;16(10):653–662. quiz 663-654.
28. Richards JR, Ormsby EL, Romo MV, Gillen MA, McGahan JP. Blunt abdominal injury in the pregnant patient: detection with US. *Radiology*. 2004;233(2):463–470.
29. Goodwin H, Holmes JF, Wisner DH. Abdominal ultrasound examination in pregnant blunt trauma patients. *J Trauma*. 2001;50(4):689–693. discussion 694.
30. Brown MA, Sirlin CB, Farahmand N, Hoyt DB, Casola G. Screening sonography in pregnant patients with blunt abdominal trauma. *J Ultrasound Med*. 2005;24(2):175–181; quiz 183-184.
31. Meisinger QC, Brown MA, Dehqanzada ZA, Doucet J, Coimbra R, Casola G. A 10-year restrospective evaluation of ultrasound in pregnant abdominal trauma patients. *Emerg Radiol*. 2016;23(2):105–109.
32. Nyberg DA, Laing FC, Jeffrey RB. Sonographic detection of subtle pelvic fluid collections. *AJR Am J Roentgenol*. 1984;143(2):261–263.
33. Nichols JE, Steinkampf MP. Detection of free peritoneal fluid by transvaginal sonography. *J Clin Ultrasound*. 1993;21(3):171–174.

34. Steinkampf MP, Blackwell RE, Younger JB. Visualization of free peritoneal fluid with transvaginal sonography: a preliminary study. *J Reprod Med*. 1991;36(10):729–730.
35. Rosen DJ, Ben-Nun I, Arbel Y, Altaras MM, Goldberger SB, Beyth Y. Transvaginal ultrasonographic quantitative assessment of accumulated cul-de-sac fluid. *Am J Obstet Gynecol*. 1992;166(2):542–544.
36. Mendelson EB, Bohm-Velez M, Joseph N, Neiman HL. Gynecologic imaging: comparison of transabdominal and transvaginal sonography. *Radiology*. 1988;166(2):321–324.
37. Miele V, Piccolo CL, Galluzzo M, Ianniello S, Sessa B, Trinci M. Contrast-enhanced ultrasound (CEUS) in blunt abdominal trauma. *Br J Radiol*. 2016;89(1061):20150823.
38. Cagini L, Gravante S, Malaspina CM, et al. Contrast enhanced ultrasound (CEUS) in blunt abdominal trauma. *Crit Ultrasound J*. 2013;5(Suppl 1):S9.
39. Committee Opinion No. 723 Guidelines for diagnostic imaging during pregnancy and lactation. *Obstet Gynecol*. 2017;130(4):e210–e216.
40. ACR-SPR practice parameter for imaging pregnant or potentially pregnant adolescents and women with ionizing radiation. Updated 2018. Accessed May 28, 2021. https://www.acr.org/-/media/acr/files/practice-parameters/pregnant-pts.pdf.
41. Ozbayrak M, Cavdar I, Seven M, et al. Determining and managing fetal radiation dose from diagnostic radiology procedures in Turkey. *Korean J Radiol*. 2015;16(6):1276–1282.
42. ACR Manual on Contrast Media. Updated 2021. Accessed May 28, 2021. https://www.acr.org/Clinical-Resources/Contrast-Manual.
43. Lee CH, Haaland B, Earnest A, Tan CH. Use of positive oral contrast agents in abdominopelvic computed tomography for blunt abdominal injury: meta-analysis and systematic review. *Eur Radiol*. 2013;23(9):2513–2521.
44. ACR Manual on MR Safety. Updated 2020. Accessed May 28, 2021. https://www.acr.org/-/media/ACR/Files/Radiology-Safety/MR-Safety/Manual-on-MR-Safety.pdf.
45. Ray JG, Vermeulen MJ, Bharatha A, Montanera WJ, Park AL. Association between MRI exposure during pregnancy and fetal and childhood outcomes. *JAMA*. 2016;316(9):952–961.
46. Fadl SA, Linnau KF, Dighe MK. Placental abruption and hemorrhage-review of imaging appearance. *Emerg Radiol*. 2019;26(1):87–97.
47. Wei SH, Helmy M, Cohen AJ. CT evaluation of placental abruption in pregnant trauma patients. *Emerg Radiol*. 2009;16(5):365–373.
48. Allen BC, Leyendecker JR. Placental evaluation with magnetic resonance. *Radiol Clin North Am*. 2013;51(6):955–966.
49. Puri A, Khadem P, Ahmed S, Yadav P, Al-Dulaimy K. Imaging of trauma in a pregnant patient. *Semin Ultrasound CT MR*. 2012;33(1):37–45.
50. Nyberg DA, Cyr DR, Mack LA, Wilson DA, Shuman WP. Sonographic spectrum of placental abruption. *AJR Am J Roentgenol*. 1987;148(1):161–164.
51. Glantz C, Purnell L. Clinical utility of sonography in the diagnosis and treatment of placental abruption. *J Ultrasound Med*. 2002;21(8):837–840.
52. Manriquez M, Srinivas G, Bollepalli S, Britt L, Drachman D. Is computed tomography a reliable diagnostic modality in detecting placental injuries in the setting of acute trauma? *Am J Obstet Gynecol*. 2010;202(6):e1–e5.
53. Masselli G, Brunelli R, Di Tola M, Anceschi M, Gualdi G. MR imaging in the evaluation of placental abruption: correlation with sonographic findings. *Radiology*. 2011;259(1):222–230.
54. Sadro CT, Zins AM, Debiec K, Robinson J. Case report: lethal fetal head injury and placental abruption in a pregnant trauma patient. *Emerg Radiol*. 2012;19(2):175–180.
55. Breysem L, Cossey V, Mussen E, Demaerel P, Van de Voorde W, Smet M. Fetal trauma: brain imaging in four neonates. *Eur Radiol*. 2004;14(9):1609–1614.
56. Mummert T, Gnugnoli DM. Ectopic pregnancy. Treasure Island (FL): StatPearls; 2021.
57. Goldman SM, Wagner LK. Radiologic ABCs of maternal and fetal survival after trauma: when minutes may count. *Radiographics*. 1999;19(5):1349–1357.
58. Brown S, Mozurkewich E. Trauma during pregnancy. *Obstet Gynecol Clin North Am*. 2013;40(1):47–57.

Chapter 8

# Abdominal Emergencies in Bariatric Patients

Omar Alwahbi, Abdullah Alabousi, Michael N. Patlas, Anahi Goransky, and Ehsan A. Haider

## Outline



## Key Points

- Bariatric surgical interventions require a multidisciplinary approach preoperatively and postoperatively.
- Fluoroscopy, abdominal ultrasound, and computed tomography are the most commonly utilized imaging modalities in assessing these patients.
- There are a number of common and uncommon complications (e.g., leaks, collections, bowel obstructions, internal hernias) associated with these procedures that the radiologist should be familiar with in order to help guide clinical and surgical management.
- A high index of suspicion and a low threshold for imaging are important for prompt detection of internal hernias.

## Introduction

Obesity is a disease of increasing global prevalence.[1] It has detrimental effects on individual health as well as on health care systems. In addition to lifestyle changes and medical management, several surgical procedures have been developed over the years to treat a subset of obese patients.[2,3] Some of the more well-known procedures are Roux-en-Y gastric bypass (RYGB) and laparoscopic adjustable gastric banding (LAGB). Other common surgical procedures include vertical banded gastroplasty (VBG), duodenal switch, and sleeve gastrectomy.[4–6] As with any surgical intervention, there is potential morbidity and mortality associated with these procedures. The radiologist plays an essential role in identifying and diagnosing the common and uncommon complications and can directly influence the management of these cases. Modalities such as fluoroscopy and computed tomography (CT) are most commonly used for investigating these suspected complications. This chapter will review and discuss the imaging findings of common and uncommon complications of some of the more widely utilized bariatric surgical procedures.[5]

## Presurgical Imaging and Workup

Bariatric operations require a multidisciplinary approach that includes surgical, medical, psychological, nursing, and radiology teams, both preoperatively and postoperatively. Comprehensive preoperative assessment and planning are required prior to any bariatric operation, including a psychological, social, medical, and anesthetic assessment. These are beyond the scope of this chapter. However, some centers also perform preoperative radiological assessment, which includes ultrasound of the abdomen to assess for, among other things, the presence of gallstones and kidney stones, as well as to measure the abdominal wall thickness. In some instances, surgeons may perform an elective cholecystectomy at the same time as certain bariatric procedures, namely RYGB, as these patients have a higher incidence of cholecystitis due to altered anatomy and therefore altered absorption.[7–12] Measurement of abdominal wall thickness is not a standard requirement but may assist the surgeons in choosing the appropriate laparoscopic equipment for each individual patient. This includes measuring the abdominal wall thickness from the skin surface to the ventral abdominal wall at the usual sites of laparoscopic ports, which are typically in the bilateral upper quadrants of the abdomen and in the supraumbilical region. Ultrasound could also be used to measure the left lobe of the liver, which could predict bariatric surgery difficulty.[13,14]

## Types of Commonly Performed Surgeries

The two main surgical approaches that have been adopted for achieving weight loss are restrictive procedures and bypass or malabsorptive procedures. The third category that has also gained popularity includes procedures with both restrictive and malabsorptive effects, such as the RYGB surgery. Many of these surgeries are now performed laparoscopically, which has been proven to decrease recovery time and reduce the complications associated with open surgical techniques.[15]

Some examples of restrictive procedures include LAGB, VBG, and sleeve gastrectomy. Each of these different techniques has been successful in achieving their goal, and each carries its own set of associated complications, some of which overlap. Examples of malabsorptive or bypass procedures include RYGB and biliopancreatic diversion gastric bypass (BPD). Interventions offering both restrictive and malabsorptive effects include RYGB, LAGB, and sleeve gastrectomy.[16]

## Imaging Modalities and Protocols

The evaluation of bariatric surgical complications depends on multiple factors. The modalities that may be used include abdominal radiographs, upper gastrointestinal (GI) fluoroscopic studies, and CT imaging.[5,17] Their utilization and applications are dictated by the clinical presentation. For instance, abdominal radiographs may be used for the initial evaluation of suspected bowel obstruction or to detect intraabdominal free air.

The fluoroscopic study is often a single-contrast study limited to evaluating for major complications. It can be helpful to assess for leaks or strictures, although the reliability and accuracy depend on the technique used and the radiologist's expertise.

CT is much more valuable, as it offers a detailed anatomic assessment, allows for characterization of any postprocedure complications, and allows for the detection of any alternative pathologies aside from bariatric surgery complications. The CT protocol should include both intravenous and oral contrast administration to accurately assess the anatomy and complications. The images are acquired in the portal venous phase (~70 seconds post–intravenous contrast administration). As well, administration of a small amount of positive oral contrast (~150 mL) is useful to evaluate for proximal leaks and to better delineate the anatomy. Images are then reconstructed in the coronal and sagittal planes, which is helpful in providing perspective on the anatomy as well as evaluating mesenteric and vascular distortion, especially in cases of RYGB.[17]

In the unique case of suspected bariatric surgery complications in pregnant patients, such as post-RYGB internal hernia, abdominal magnetic resonance imaging (MRI) has been shown to be a safe and a valuable imaging technique. MRI has specificity that is comparable to CT for diagnosing post-RYGB internal hernias, and its sensitivity approaches that of CT.[18]

Finally, the role of routine imaging following bariatric surgery is variable, and there are no consensus guidelines as to whether any routine imaging should be performed. For certain procedures, especially procedures with stapling or anastomosis, surgeons may elect to assess for any leak in the early postoperative period with an upper GI fluoroscopic study.[16,19]

## General Complications

As with all surgical procedures, some patients can experience one of a number of possible complications. Certain complications are similar to other surgical procedures, such as bleeding, infection, and wound-related complications, including dehiscence, delayed healing, hematoma, or fluid collections. Several complications have been noted to arise in relation to the different bariatric procedures commonly performed, some are common in every procedure, and a few complications are unusual or are seen more often in certain bariatric surgical procedures than others.[8,19,20]

### COLLECTIONS

These can be seen with any of the bariatric surgical interventions. They could be secondary to anastomotic leak with or without superimposed infection. CT is the modality of choice to assess for the presence of the different types of collections, including contained leaks and abscesses. Additionally, a hematoma is an important postoperative complication and may occur with RYGB, duodenal switch, or sleeve gastrectomy (Fig. 8.1). High-density fluid collections (60–80 HU) point to a hematoma.[5,17,21] A CT will also allow for the identification of active contrast extravasation in cases of ongoing active bleeding. Therefore, if there is a high index of suspicious for a hematoma and/or active hemorrhage, a multiphasic CT study could be performed to allow for the identification of active contrast extravasation.

### BOWEL OBSTRUCTION

Bowel obstruction is a common postsurgical complication and is most commonly seen secondary to

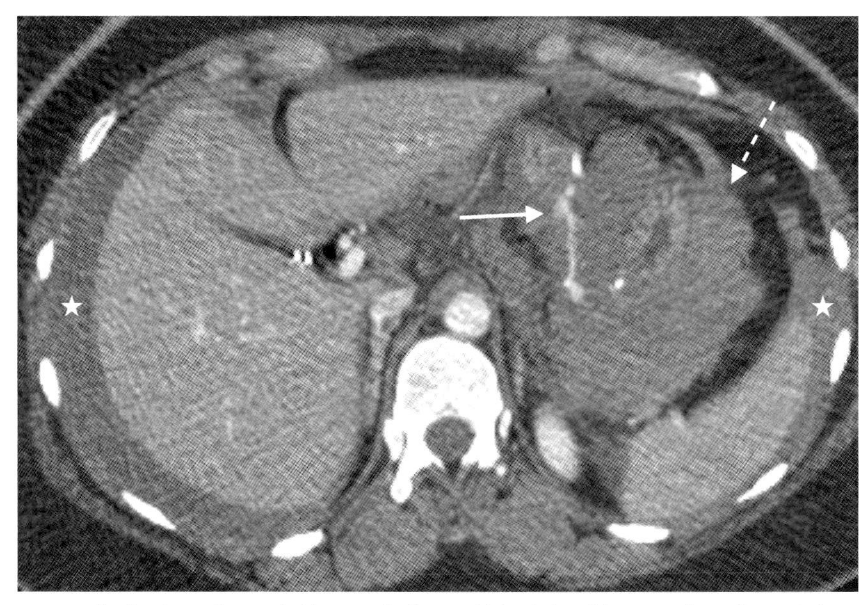

**Fig. 8.1** Axial intravenous contrast–enhanced computed tomography image obtained at portal venous phase demonstrates a contrast extravasation near the gastrojejunal anastomosis (arrow), in keeping with active bleeding. There is a large perigastric hematoma (dotted arrow), as well as perihepatic and perisplenic dense free fluid (white star), in keeping with hemoperitoneum.

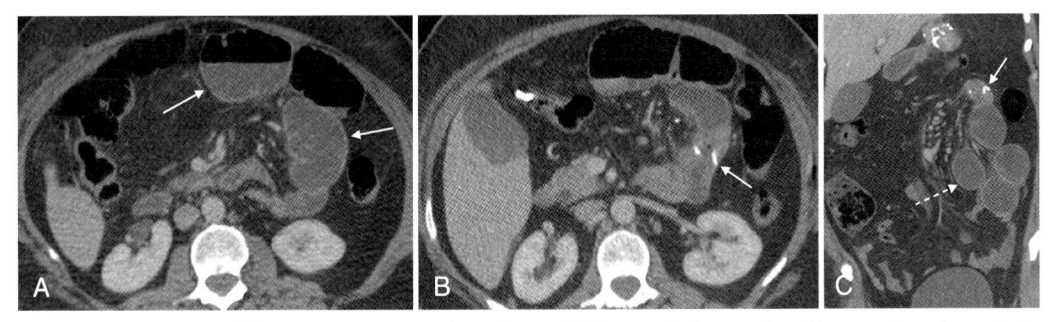


**Fig. 8.2** Axial (A and B) and coronal (C) intravenous contrast–enhanced computed tomography images at portal venous phase demonstrate evidence of a high-grade small bowel obstruction with transition point at the jejunojejunal anastomosis. This is secondary to adhesions. (A) Dilated roux limb (arrows). (B) Change in bowel caliber with a transition point at the jejunojejunal anastomosis (arrow). (C) Multiple dilated loops of proximal small bowel (dotted arrow) with transition point at the jejunojejunal anastomosis (arrow).

adhesions (Fig. 8.2). This may be detected after any of the aforementioned bariatric surgical procedures. In patients who have undergone RYGB or duodenal switch, care must be taken to exclude an internal hernia as the cause of obstruction, as it may have important consequences and unique management. Internal hernias will be further discussed below. Strictures are also a common cause of obstruction and should be considered. CT examination is the modality of choice to evaluate for suspected obstruction.[17,21,22]

### SUTURE DEHISCENCE OR LEAK

These usually occur along the suture lines, such as in sleeve gastrectomy, or at the sites of anastomosis, particularly in procedures such as duodenal switch and RYGB. Suture dehiscence appears as focal interruption of the staple line and is readily evaluated by CT with or without oral contrast.[17] Anastomotic leaks are best assessed with oral contrast, whether through an upper GI fluoroscopic assessment or CT (Fig. 8.3). The latter is helpful in identifying further complications that may or may not be related directly to leaks such as hematomas and abscesses.[5,17,21]

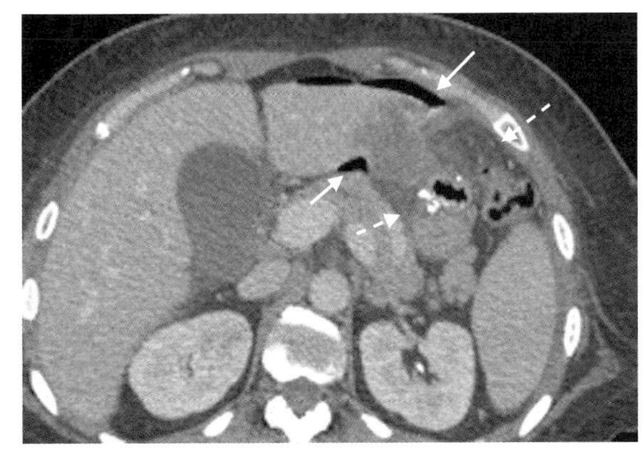

**Fig. 8.3** Axial intravenous contrast–enhanced computed tomography image demonstrates fatty stranding in the region of the gastrojejunal anastomosis (dotted arrows), with free air seen in the upper abdomen (arrows), in keeping with dehiscence.

## Surgical Procedures and Associated Complications

### LAPAROSCOPIC ADJUSTABLE GASTRIC BAND

#### Anatomy and Technique

The LAGB procedure is a restrictive bariatric technique, the goal of which is to induce the sensation of early satiety. This is achieved by placing a gastric band, usually made of silicone, at the proximal stomach, creating a small gastric pouch that is separated from the remaining stomach by a narrow stoma. A reservoir is connected via plastic tubing and placed within the anterior abdominal wall to permit an adjustable volume balloon within the band to be altered, allowing variation in band tightness. The band position is maintained by suturing it into the gastroesophageal junction, with care taken not to penetrate the lesser sac, as this was noted to be associated with higher incidence of complications, namely band slippage.[23,24]

#### Imaging Follow-Up and Evaluation

Abdominal radiographs and upper GI fluoroscopic studies are the modalities commonly used to evaluate the anatomy and complications that are specific to LAGB procedures. The normal appearance of an appropriately positioned gastric band on an abdominal radiograph is a "rectangular" appearance. Upper GI series are used to evaluate for leaks or strictures. Immediate postoperative evaluation is not usually recommended unless there is a concern for perforation or early leakage. However, these have become exceedingly rare with new surgical techniques. The normal upper GI contrast examination should reveal a small upper gastric pouch with passage of contrast through the narrow stoma into the remainder of the stomach. CT evaluation for complications related specifically to LAGB are not usually performed but may be useful to assess for other associated complications, such as abscesses, ascites, and/or hemoperitoneum.[25–27]

### Complications

Some complications that are associated with this procedure include a tight band, gastric band slippage, band erosion, and band opening. Perforation may further complicate any of the previously mentioned complications or, rarely, may occur as an early postoperative complication.[25,28]

As with all devices with reservoirs and tubing, complications related to these should always be considered, and include port infection, tube fracture, catheter disconnection, and failure to access the subcutaneous port site.[23]

## Band Slippage

Band slippage occurs when the gastric band is dislocated or has migrated from its original position. This results in herniation of parts of the stomach through the gastric band, causing eccentric dilatation of the pouch and band malposition. The two observed types that can occur are anterior and posterior band slippage. Anterior band slippage occurs due to instability of the fixation sutures and result in herniation of the superior and anterior portions of the stomach and a clockwise rotation of the gastric band. Posterior slippage is usually seen in patients with retrogastric band placement, a technique that is no longer performed. This results in herniation of the inferior and posterior portions of the stomach and counterclockwise rotation of the gastric band.[23,25]

An abdominal radiograph can confirm the diagnosis if there is evidence of an abnormal configuration of the gastric band, usually resulting in an abnormal "O-shaped" configuration (the "O" sign), as opposed to its normal rectangular appearance (Fig. 8.4). An

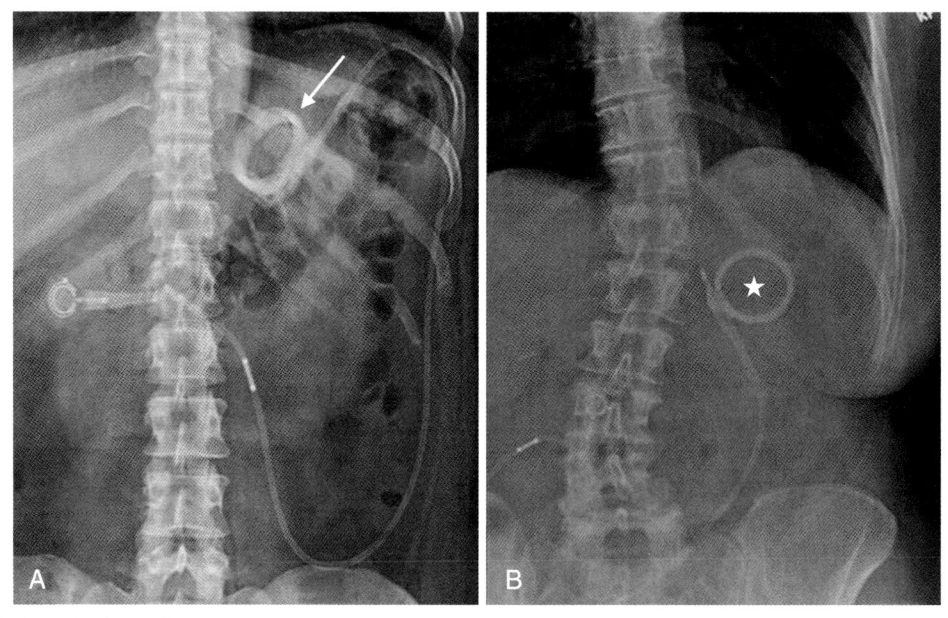


**Fig. 8.4** (A) Supine abdominal radiograph demonstrates the normal oblique orientation of a gastric band on a frontal radiograph (arrow). (B) Supine abdominal radiograph shows gastric band slippage, with an O-shaped configuration seen (star).

upper GI study can support the diagnosis with minimal or decreased passage of contrast through the gastric band, as well as eccentric dilation of the gastric pouch.[29] Complications that can result from band slippage include ischemia and necrosis of the gastric pouch.

## Band Migration

This is a rare and underreported long-term complication. The estimated prevalence is between 2% and 10%.[30–32] This has become exceedingly rare with the experience and skill of bariatric surgeons and new surgical techniques.

In band migration, the gastric band gradually erodes into the gastric wall, resulting in a local tear through the gastric wall that gradually expands, and the band may enter the gastric lumen.[28] This is thought to be secondary to multiple factors, including intraoperative damage to the outer gastric wall, chronic irritation and subsequent inflammation of the gastric wall by the band, excessive vomiting and retching, infection, or use of nonsteroidal antiinflammatory drugs. The spectrum of clinical presentations ranges from nonspecific abdominal pain to peritonitis secondary to perforation and/or gastrointestinal hemorrhage.

Upper GI fluoroscopic studies demonstrate a gastric intraluminal filling defect representing the band that has migrated into the lumen. Other findings on abdominal radiographs or on CT include pneumoperitoneum, ascites, and/or hemoperitoneum. Abscess near the site of the access port may also be seen. Urgent surgical removal of the band and repair of the stomach is required. If the defect is small, or if there has been only partial migration of the band, endoscopic removal of the band may be performed.

## Concentric Pouch Dilatation

Dilatation of the gastric pouch has been one of the major long-term complications of LAGB, occurring in around 25% of patients.[23,25] However, with increasing surgical experience and modifications of the surgical technique, this has decreased in incidence. Gastric pouch dilatation is not necessarily related to the width of the stoma; while significant narrowing of the stoma might be a cause, dilatation may also be seen with a normal or a widened stoma or may be secondary to gastric band slippage.

## Concentric Dilatation Secondary to Stomal Stenosis

A narrow stoma may be a result of overinflation of the gastric band. This results in acute prestenotic dilatation of the gastric pouch, leading to symptoms such as vomiting, dysphagia, pseudoachalasia, or obstruction. Upper GI examinations demonstrate a narrow stoma with upstream concentric dilatation of the gastric pouch. When this abnormality is seen, immediate deflation of the band must be performed, as pouch dilatation may recur if not treated promptly. A repeat upper GI study postadjustment is also important to perform, because as many as half of these patients may have recurrent or irreversible pouch dilatation.[30,32]

## Concentric Dilatation Without Stomal Stenosis

Gastric pouch dilatation may be seen with a normal or even a widened stoma with chronic concentric gastric pouch dilatation. This is often seen due to overfilling rather than the outflow obstruction described previously and is likely due to dietary noncompliance. On upper GI series, the stoma is usually widened or normal caliber; however, the gastric pouch is concentrically dilated. The larger gastric pouch results in a cycle of overeating due to the increased capacity, resulting in further pouch dilatation.[25,30]

# SLEEVE GASTRECTOMY

### Anatomy and Technique

Sleeve gastrectomy, first performed in 1999, is one of the most common bariatric surgeries and has achieved good results.[16] It is a restrictive surgery performed laparoscopically by creating a vertical transection along the greater curvature of the stomach, removing the fundus, a large portion of the body, and the antrum (Fig. 8.5). This results in a long tubular remnant consisting of the remaining body, cardia, and pylorus, effectively decreasing the capacity of the stomach by reducing the stomach size by approximately 75%. Additionally, removing the stomach fundus results in a decrease in circulating levels of the hormone ghrelin,

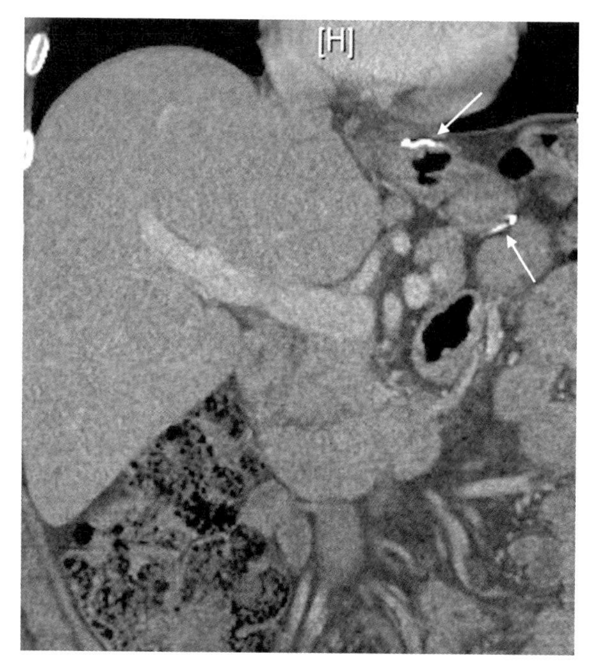


**Fig. 8.5** Coronal intravenous contrast–enhanced computed tomography image in a patient post–sleeve gastrectomy showing the surgical staple line (arrows) in an otherwise collapsed stomach.

which is responsible for increasing appetite and driving satiety, further increasing the effectiveness of this procedure in promoting and maintaining weight loss.[6,33]

### Imaging Appearance and Complications

The normal imaging appearance of a sleeve gastrectomy upper GI series is a tubular or a banana-shaped gastric pouch or residual stomach, with a surgical staple line across the greater curvature. The oral contrast should pass freely into the stomach, and there may be slight dilatation or transient holdup at the antrum, especially in the early postoperative period. Upper GI fluoroscopy is considered the first-line study to detect leaks. Complications of this procedure include both functional and postsurgical entities, as described below.[5,17,27,34]

## Gastric Dilatation

Presents as inadequate weight loss or as weight gain due to an increase in the capacity of the gastric pouch. This often leads to reoperation and is one of the drawbacks of this procedure. Imaging findings on fluoroscopy include an increased stomach diameter and loss of the normal tubular or banana-shaped configuration.

## Stricture or Gastric Outlet Obstruction

May develop secondary to scarring along the staple line, which results in luminal narrowing. Upper GI fluoroscopy may reveal focal areas of luminal narrowing with delayed passage of contrast material and delayed gastric emptying of the ingested contrast. CT may also demonstrate a similar appearance. The added advantage of fluoroscopy is that it is a dynamic examination, and the operator may choose to wait a few additional minutes to differentiate complete gastric outlet obstruction due to stricture from delayed gastric emptying. A delayed single-view abdominal radiograph may also be obtained after fluoroscopic assessment to assess for contrast extending beyond the stomach. Cases of short segment narrowing may be treated endoscopically by dilation. However, longer segments may require further surgical intervention and revision.

## Suture Dehiscence

May occur anywhere along the staple line, but most commonly occurs at the proximal portion of the staple line at the gastroesophageal junction. This appears as a focal interruption of the staple line on CT. The addition of oral contrast is helpful to delineate the presence of a leak. Therefore, most centers utilize a specific bariatric CT protocol to evaluate postoperative bariatric complications. Complications of suture line dehiscence include leak and perforation, and subsequently may result in collections or abscesses, or even peritonitis.[35]

## Gastric Leak

Results from a disruption in the vertical staple line. This is a major concern postoperatively due to the significant gastric resection and long staple line. The clinical presentation includes abdominal pain, fever, and leukocytosis. The most common site of leak is along the proximal portion of the staple line at the gastroesophageal junction. Leaks may be evaluated with upper GI fluoroscopy and manifest by extravasation of contrast material from the gastric lumen. CT examination with oral contrast may also demonstrate not only the presence of the leak, but also the site and associated complications, such as the resulting fluid collection or abscess.[35]

## ROUX-EN-Y GASTRIC BYPASS SURGERY

### Preoperative Workup

In some centers, there may be standard preoperative imaging workup prior to RYGB. This may include ultrasound examination of the abdomen assessing for the presence of gallstones, as surgeons may opt to perform a concomitant cholecystectomy during the bariatric procedure if gallstones are present. There has been mixed literature on this topic, with some studies citing an increased incidence of cholecystitis with rapid weight loss and some citing cost-benefit as a factor. This remains center-specific and not the standard of care at this time.[9,36–38] Ultrasound evaluation of abdominal wall thickness may also be performed to assist the surgeons in surgical planning and choosing the appropriate devices for laparoscopic surgery.

### Surgical Technique and Anatomy

RYGB is now the most commonly performed bariatric procedure owing to its good results and association with sustained weight loss and long-term successful outcomes. It is both a restrictive and malabsorptive procedure. It involves the creation of a gastric pouch by isolating the fundal component of the stomach, which excludes the remainder of it. The jejunum is then divided approximately 25 to 50 cm from the ligament of Treitz, creating an efferent limb from distal limb of the divided jejunal loops that is brought up and anastomosed to the small gastric pouch, either as an end-side anastomosis, which is more common, or as an end-to-end anastomosis (Fig. 8.6). This creates the alimentary tract, or the "Roux" limb, and represents the restrictive portion of the procedure, as the tract from the gastric pouch through the Roux limb may be as small as 8 to 12 cm in diameter. The Roux limb may be brought up to anastomose to the stomach either anterior or posterior to the transverse colon. The latter necessitates the creation of a window through the posterior aspect of the transverse mesocolon. The gastrojejunal anastomosis may also be antegastric or retrogastric in location. The afferent limb, or the "Y" limb, is then created by anastomosing the proximal limb of the jejunal loop to the small bowel, usually 100 to 150 cm distal to the gastrojejunal anastomosis; this is usually a side-side anastomosis. This creates the biliopancreatic limb that diverts the digestive enzymes and biliary secretions. At this point, the small bowel becomes a common channel throughout its length to the terminal ileum. The creation of this diversion represents the malabsorptive component of this procedure, where digestion occurs in a different location than the stomach. This also has physiological effects, as it may alter the levels of peptides and hormones, such as glucagon-like peptide-1, as well as bile acids, which further contributes to weight loss. Adjusting the degree of malabsorption is achieved by altering the distance of the anastomosis from the terminal ileum: the more distal the anastomosis, the greater the malabsorptive effect.[4,27,39,40]

### Imaging Evaluation and Complications

As with other bariatric procedures, patients post-RYGB may be assessed with upper GI series or CT. Knowledge

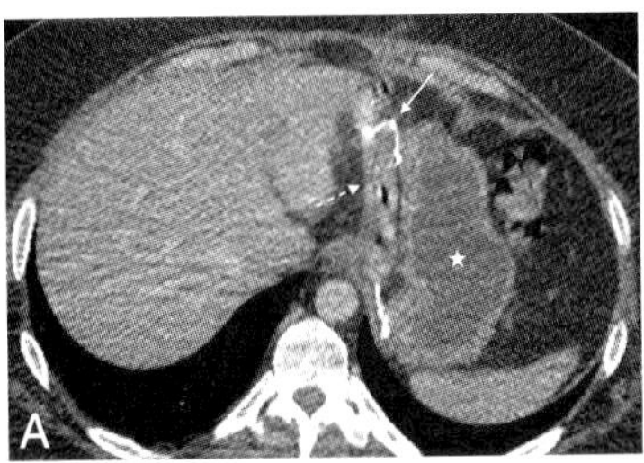


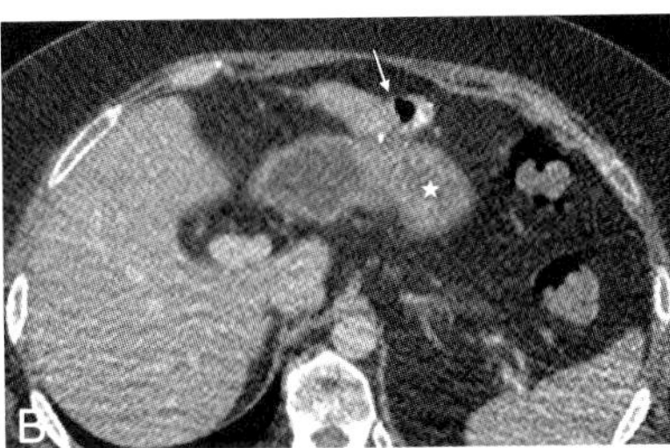


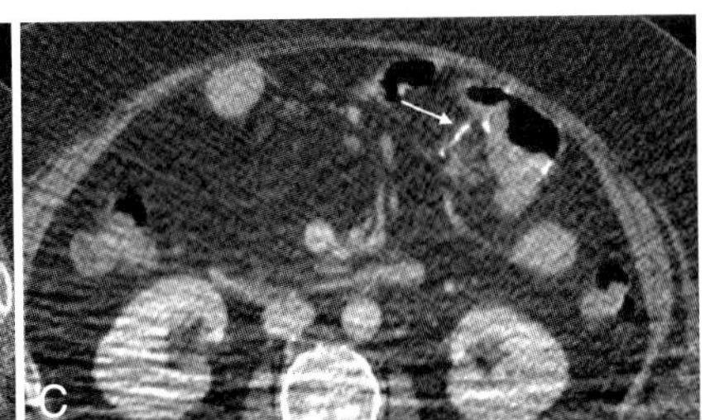


**Fig. 8.6** Axial intravenous contrast–enhanced computed tomography images demonstrating the expected anatomy post–Roux-en-Y gastric bypass. (A) Gastric pouch (dashed arrow), gastrojejunal anastomosis (arrow), and excluded stomach (star). (B) Roux limb (arrow) and excluded stomach (star). (C) Jejunojejunal anastomosis (arrow).

of the altered anatomy is key for proper evaluation in both modalities. Complications that occur post-RYGB include complications that are common among many other bariatric surgeries. In addition, there are some complications that are more commonly seen or only seen post-RYGB.[8,27]

## Leaks

Extraluminal leaks usually occur at the sites of anastomosis. Anastomotic leaks from RYGB are the most serious early complication, occurring in around 2% to 5% of cases[16] and usually occurring within 7 to 10 days of the procedure. Classic clinical presentation is usually abdominal pain with or without peritoneal signs, fever, tachycardia, and leukocytosis. In many cases, tachycardia was found to be the most common, and sometimes the only, symptom. Most leaks occur at the gastrojejunal anastomosis, in up to 75% of cases.[5] Leaks may also occur due to perforation, such as at the gastric pouch or at the level of the jejunojejunostomy. Initial abdominal radiographs may or may not demonstrate free intraabdominal air and may be helpful to assess for the site of the suture line so as not to mistake the anastomotic line for contrast leak. Evaluation with upper GI series may be difficult, as abnormalities can be challenging to delineate depending on the site of leakage and on the patient's position. Evaluation with CT requires ingestion of oral contrast material prior to scanning, as well as aiming to opacify the Roux limb to the level of distal jejunojejunal anastomosis. In both modalities, contrast should not be administered through a nasogastric tube, as a contrast leak from the proximal gastrojejunal limb may be missed. As mentioned earlier, CT has the added advantage of assessing for other complications that may or may not be related to a leak, such as the presence of fluid collections, abscesses, hematoma, or other complications, such as bowel obstruction or internal hernia.

## Suture Breakdown or Dehiscence

Suture dehiscence may lead to extraluminal leaks, as discussed above, and are best evaluated with CT, ideally with oral contrast. Breakdown of the gastric staple line may also occur and may result in an intraluminal leak into the excluded stomach; most of these cases have an associated incidence of extraluminal leaks. If occurring early, these intraluminal leaks are not always treated surgically because they have a chance of spontaneous healing. However, late intraluminal leaks are less likely to heal spontaneously and result in failure of the surgery and recurrent weight gain, necessitating surgical revision.[5]

## Small Bowel Obstruction

Small bowel obstruction (SBO) is a common postsurgical complication and is most often seen secondary to adhesions (Fig. 8.2). SBO may be seen following any of the aforementioned bariatric surgical procedures. However, in patients who have undergone RYGB (or biliopancreatic diversion, which is discussed subsequently in the chapter), care must be taken to exclude internal hernia as a cause of obstruction, as it may have important consequences and unique management. Strictures are also a common cause of obstruction and should be considered. A CT examination is the modality of choice to evaluate for suspected obstruction.[17,21,22]

An ABC classification system has been devised to classify the three different patterns of SBO that can occur in patients post RYGB. This is based on the location of anatomic alteration in relation to the distal (jejunojejunal) anastomosis.[5,41,42] The types are described below:

- Type A. In this type, the Roux limb is dilated, and the excluded stomach and biliopancreatic limb are decompressed above the distal jejunojejunal anastomosis. This type of obstruction may be difficult to assess on CT examination.
- Type B. Type B is a closed-loop obstruction causing significant distention of the biliopancreatic limb and excluded stomach at or above the level of the distal jejunojejunal anastomosis. These patients are at high risk for perforation, and therefore prompt intervention is required. This diagnosis is readily apparent on CT with a dilated and fluid-filled biliopancreatic limb, as well as a dilated excluded stomach with a collapsed alimentary or Roux limb.
- Type C. This is due to obstruction at the level of the common channel, distal to the jejunojejunal anastomosis, and manifests as dilation of both the Roux and biliopancreatic limbs above the distal anastomosis.

## Internal Hernia

Laparoscopic RYGB is performed by creating surgical defects in the mesentery, whether it is to create the jejunojejunostomy or with a retrocolic Roux limb (creating a defect in the transverse mesocolon). Rapid weight loss also decreases the amount of visceral fat, and as a result the bowel loops are usually mobile and may herniate through the acquired mesenteric defects. Internal hernia is a feared complication of RYGB, as it can lead to small bowel incarceration and ischemia and even perforation, which could be fatal. What is also worrisome is that the clinical presentation is often nonspecific. A high index of suspicion and a low threshold for imaging are important. Knowledge of the postsurgical anatomy, as well as an appropriate imaging protocol, will aid in the identification of the internal hernia and any associated complications. A CT examination with intravenous and oral contrast is important to identify internal hernias and any secondary bowel obstruction. Interestingly, not all internal hernias are symptomatic, and many hernias may be seen with no associated bowel obstruction.[21,22]

An internal hernia may be suspected when there is an abnormal cluster of bowel loops in an unusual location. This may be seen with or without concomitant obstruction. An internal hernia may also be suspected if there is an abnormal right-sided location of the distal jejunojejunal anastomosis, which is usually in the left hemiabdomen. Another feature that supports this diagnosis is the presence of mesenteric swirling. A sign that has been described and found to be highly specific for internal hernia is the superior mesenteric vein (SMV) cutoff sign, where there is an abrupt cutoff or beaking of the SMV at the site of mesenteric swirling.[18, 43] Mesenteric and small bowel swirling may also result in small bowel loops coursing posterior to the superior mesenteric vascular root, a finding that is considered highly specific for internal hernia.

Table 8.1 breaks down the sensitive and specific CT signs of internal hernias. There are multiple types of internal hernias, which include transmesenteric hernias (Figs. 8.7 and 8.8) and Petersen hernias (Fig. 8.9).[43] Petersen hernias can occur if bowel herniates through a defect in the mesentery posterior to the Roux limb and inferior to the transverse mesocolon into what is referred to as Petersen's space. This can occur with both types of RYGB surgeries, although it is more common with the retrocolic version. This is often seen 6 to 18 months post-RYGB following significant weight loss. Patients can present with chronic intermittent abdominal pain. On CT, the "mushroom" sign can be seen, which is related to the shape of the hernia sac as the bowel loops pass through an opening between the superior mesenteric artery and the root of the mesentery.[43] In pregnant patients, MRI could be used instead of CT to assess for internal hernia and could depict the same findings that could be seen on CT (Fig. 8.10).[18]

**TABLE 8.1 Signs of Internal Hernia**

| High Sensitivity | High Specificity |
|---|---|
| Swirled mesentery | Small bowel passing behind superior mesenteric artery |
| Mushroom shape of the herniated noesenteric root with crowding and stretching of the mesenteric vessels | Tubular or round shape of distal mesenteric fat closely surrounded by bowel loops |
| Small bowel obstruction | Right-sided location of distal jejunal anastomosis |
| Clustered loops | |

## Intussusception

A less common complication that can be seen in patients post-RYGB is intussusception. This can be detected when one segment of bowel is displaced into an adjacent segment or into itself. In the case of patients post-RYGB, this can be seen in relation to the jejunojejunal anastomosis (Fig. 8.11).

## Marginal/Perianastomotic Ulcer

These have been reported in up to 13% of patients following RYGB surgery. Ulcers usually occur at or near the gastrojejunal anastomosis and develop secondary to tension and ischemia at the anastomosis. It has been thought that these ulcers occur due to chronic irritation by the stomach acid entering the Roux limb.

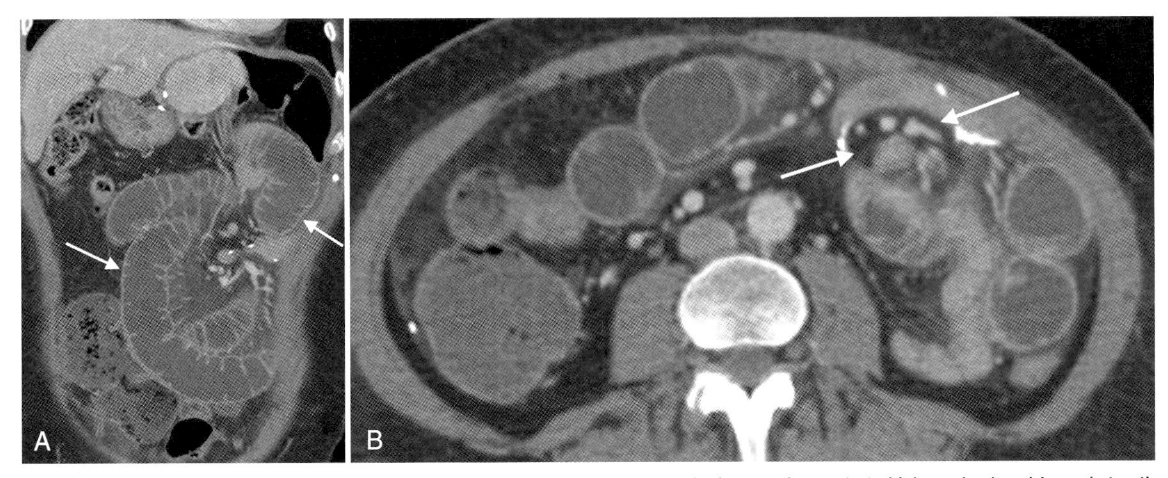


Fig. 8.7 Coronal (A) and axial (B) intravenous contrast–enhanced computed tomography images demonstrate high-grade closed-loop obstruction secondary to an internal hernia. (A) Multiple dilated loops of proximal small bowel (arrows). (B) Swirling of the mesentery focally in the left midabdomen with round shape of mesenteric fat closely surrounded by bowel loops (arrows). At the time of surgery, this was found to be a transmesenteric internal hernia.

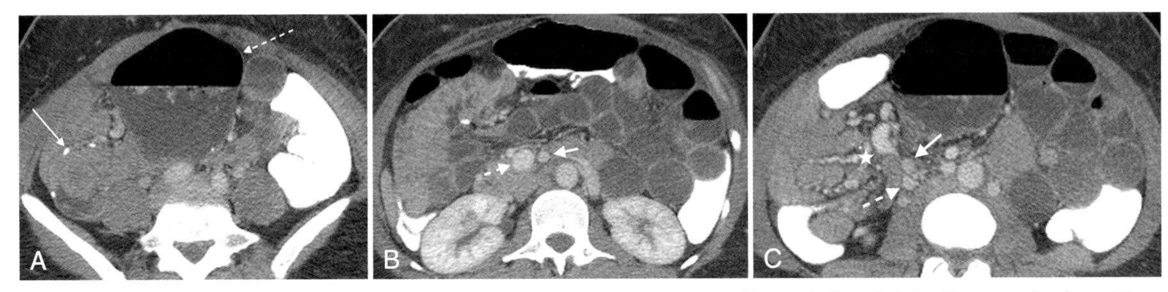


Fig. 8.8 Axial intravenous contrast–enhanced computed tomography images demonstrate evidence of a bowel obstruction secondary to an internal hernia. (A) Dilated cecum, which is displaced toward the midline (dotted arrow), with an abnormal location of the jejunojejunal anastomosis in the right lower quadrant (arrow). (B) Normal superior mesenteric vein (SMV; dotted arrow) and superior mesenteric artery (SMA; arrow) relationship proximally. (C) Evidence of abnormal twisting and abnormal orientation of the SMV (dotted arrow) with respect to the SMA (arrow) secondary to an internal hernia. Multiple engorged veins are noted in the right lower quadrant secondary to the internal hernia (star). At the time of surgery, the patient was found to have a transmesenteric internal hernia along with an associated cecal volvulus.

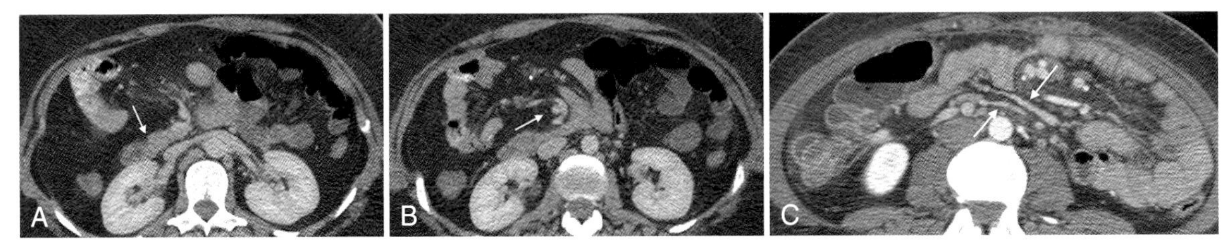


Fig. 8.9 Axial intravenous contrast–enhanced computed tomography images demonstrate evidence of a Petersen internal hernia without evidence of obstruction. (A) The duodenojejunal anastomosis is abnormally located to the right of midline (arrow). (B) There is some twisting of the mesenteric vessels (arrow). (C) A different case with a Petersen hernia showing abnormal parallel orientation of the mesenteric veins side by side (arrows).

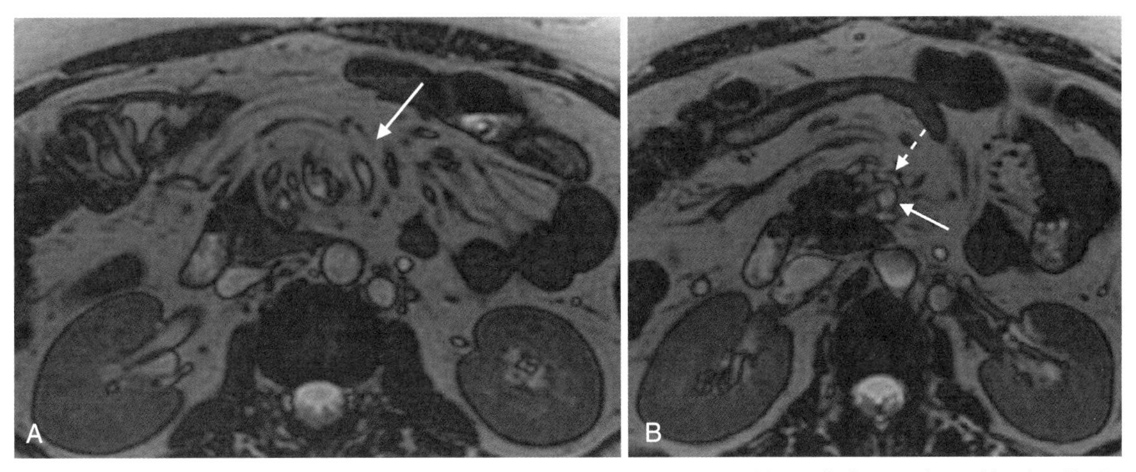

Fig. 8.10 Axial T2-weighted magnetic resonance images in a pregnant patient demonstrate evidence of a Petersen internal hernia without secondary obstruction. (A) Swirling of the mesenteric vessels is seen in the midabdomen (arrow). (B) The superior mesenteric vein (dotted arrow) is compressed and abnormally located anterior to the superior mesenteric artery (arrow).

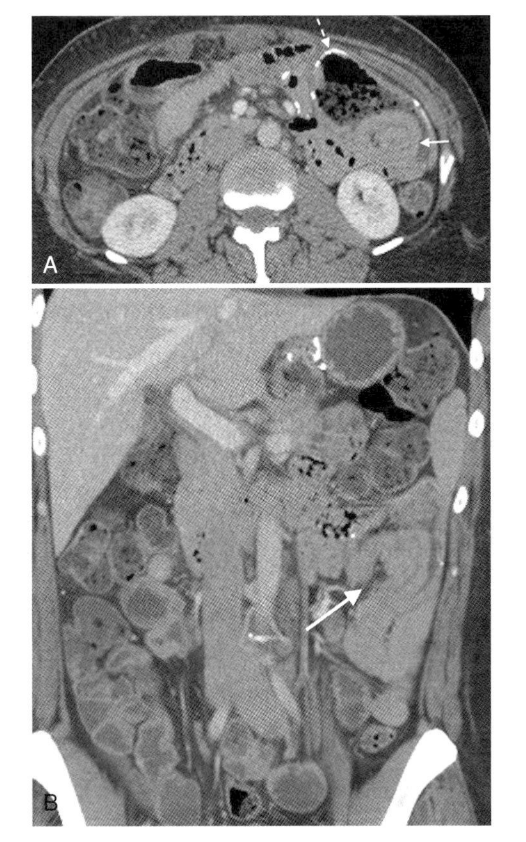

Fig. 8.11 Axial (A) and coronal (B) intravenous contrast–enhanced computed tomography images demonstrate evidence of small bowel intussusception near the jejunojejunal anastomosis, without evidence of secondary obstruction. (A) Intussusception (arrow) and jejunojejunal anastomosis (dotted arrow). (B) Intussusception (arrow).

Clinical presentation is usually vague epigastric pain, and some patients may even present with upper GI bleeding. Ulcers are difficult to assess radiologically and usually require direct visualization through endoscopy. Upper GI fluoroscopy may demonstrate discrete ulceration at the proximal gastrojejunal anastomosis or along the proximal aspect of the Roux limb. Focal bowel wall thickening and edema can occasionally be seen on CT studies. These findings, however, need to be confirmed with direct visualization. Possible complications of marginal ulcers include perforation and/or fistula formation (Fig. 8.12).[5,44]

## Candy Cane Syndrome

This entity is specific to RYGB and occurs due to an excessive length of the afferent nonfunctional blind-end Roux (alimentary) limb proximal to the gastrojejunostomy site (Fig. 8.13). This leads to nonspecific upper GI symptoms, including progressive nausea and vomiting, as well as reflux. It requires a high index of suspicion and may be suggested on upper GI series or CT.[45] The length of the candy cane could range from 3 to 22 cm (mean 7.6 cm). The syndrome resolves after resection of the blind-end limb.

## DUODENAL SWITCH/BILIOPANCREATIC DIVERSION

### Anatomy and Technique

The duodenal switch procedure is also known as BPD with duodenal switch. It is a procedure that combines

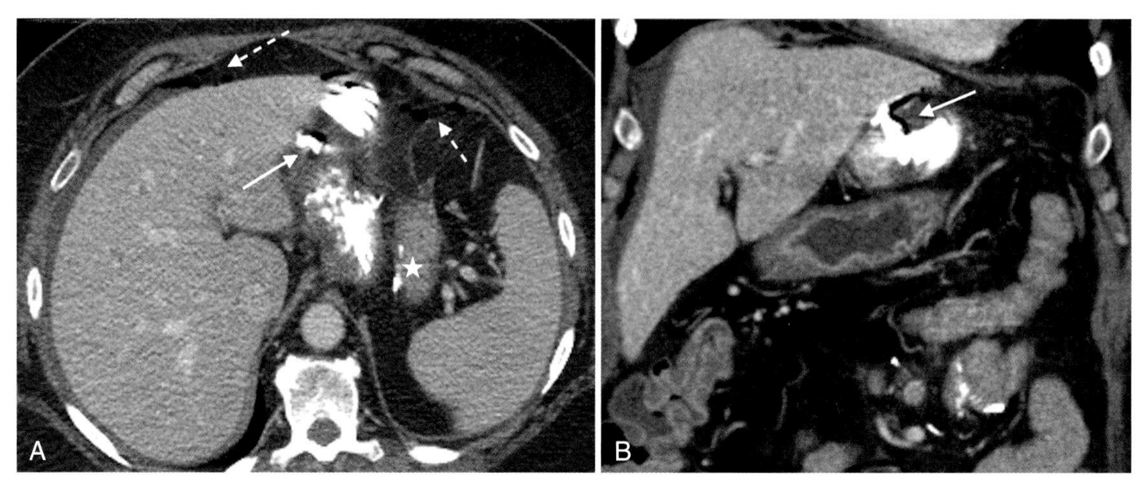

**Fig. 8.12** Axial and coronal intravenous contrast– and oral contrast–enhanced computed tomography images demonstrate evidence of a perforated marginal ulcer with oral contrast extravasation and free air. (A) Perforated marginal ulcer with oral contrast extravasation (arrow) located proximal to the gastrojejunal anastomosis (star). Free air and free fluid are also seen in the perihepatic region and epigastric region (dotted arrows). (B) Perforated marginal ulcer with oral contrast extravasation (arrow).

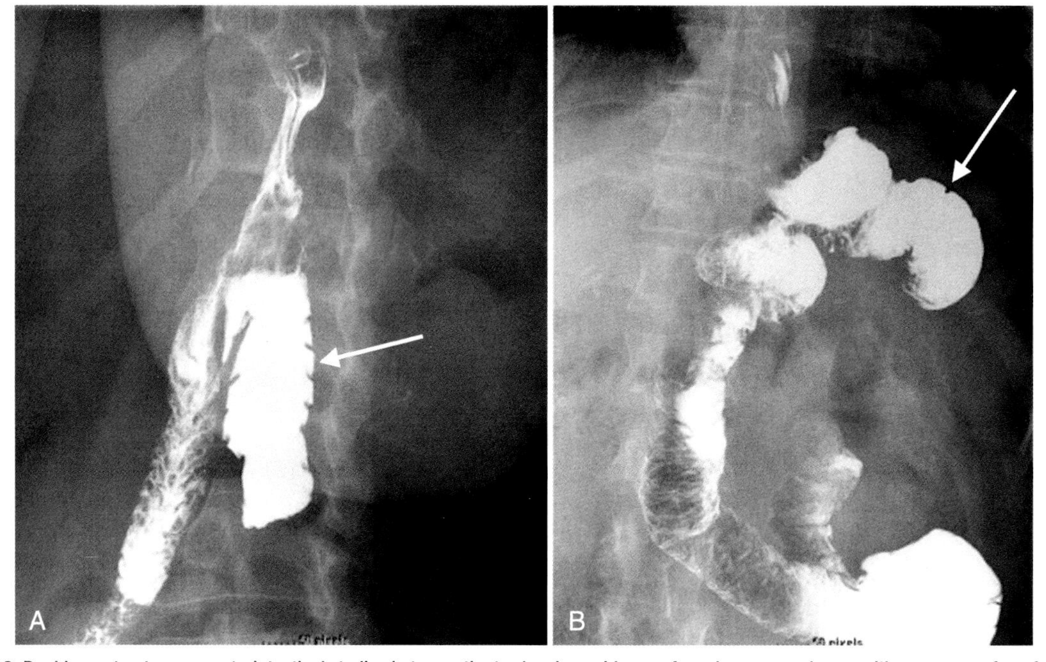

**Fig. 8.13** Double-contrast upper gastrointestinal studies in two patients showing evidence of candy cane syndrome with an excess of nonfunctioning Roux limb (arrows A and B).

restriction and malabsorption. Duodenal switch consists of a pylorus-sparing sleeve gastrectomy at the greater curvature, which is the restrictive component. The duodenum, jejunum, and proximal ileum are then excluded from the stomach and from the biliary limb. Subsequently, the ileum is transected approximately 350 cm from the ileocecal valve and used to create a 250 cm alimentary limb. The alimentary limb is then anastomosed to the pylorus in an antecolic fashion. Approximately 75 to 100 cm from the ileocecal valve, the distal biliary limb is anastomosed to the alimentary limb, and that segment of ileum is called the common limb. Hence, in this procedure, the malabsorptive component is the main element determining weight loss, as only a small portion of small bowel is available for absorption.[21]

### Imaging Evaluation and Complications

Immediate postoperative imaging is not usually performed unless a concern or an indication arises. Imaging modalities used to evaluate patients post-BPD are similar to the aforementioned procedures and include upper GI fluoroscopy and/or CT. The imaging appearance is that of a narrowed gastric pouch to the level of the pylorus, which is preserved, with a proximal gastroenteric anastomosis seen in the right upper quadrant. This is in contrast with RYGB, where the anastomosis is in the left hemiabdomen. The alimentary limb, which consists of distal ileal loops, has the characteristic ileal fold pattern on fluoroscopy. The biliary limb, consisting of excluded duodenum, jejunum, and proximal ileum, can be seen on CT but is nonopacified on fluoroscopy.[21]

### Bowel Obstruction

As described earlier, bowel obstruction may complicate any of the bariatric procedures. Obstruction may happen at the level of the proximal anastomosis, usually involving the gastric pouch or the distal anastomosis. Early obstruction occasionally occurs within the first week after the operation and is usually secondary to postoperative edema at the anastomosis. Most patients presenting with obstructions, however, develop it after 1 month to 4 years postsurgery, in which case adhesions are the most likely etiology.

### Anastomotic Leak

Leaks post-BPD may occur at any of the staple or suture lines, including the gastric staple line or the anastomotic sites proximally and distally. Leaks commonly occur in the early postoperative period but may also occur a few years later. Complications include abscess or fistula formation, especially if left untreated (Fig. 8.14).

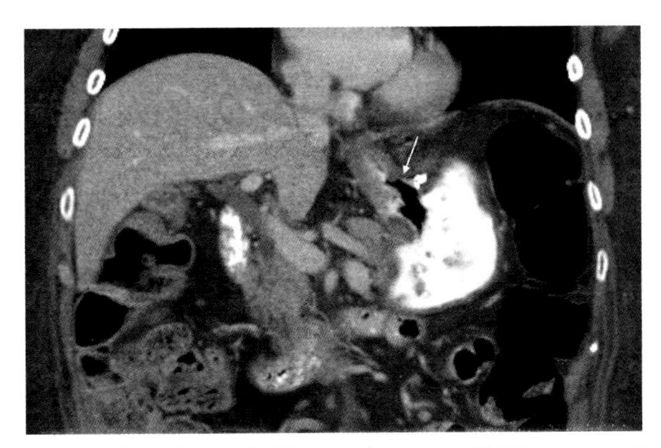

**Fig. 8.14** Coronal computed tomography image with intravenous and oral contrast in a patient post–Roux-en-Y gastric bypass demonstrates a widely patent gastrogastric fistula between the gastric pouch and excluded stomach (arrow). There is passage of oral contrast from the gastric pouch through the fistula to the excluded stomach.

### Hernia

Ventral abdominal wall hernias may complicate any abdominal surgery. These usually occur at the incision sites (incisional hernias) and as a late complication secondary to laxity of the abdominal wall musculature after healing. Another hernia that may occur post-BPD is symptomatic hiatal hernia. These may present with symptoms of reflux or even chest or phrenic pain.

### Unintentional Ligature of the Bile Duct

Although extremely rare, complete bile duct obstruction could occur due to unintentional application of surgical clips and ligatures. In such cases, significant bile duct dilatation with abrupt change in caliber at the ligation site could be seen on CT and magnetic resonance cholangiopancreatography studies (Fig. 8.15).

## Conclusion

This chapter has provided an overview of multiple bariatric surgical procedures, with a review of the radiologic anatomy and imaging techniques, as well as a discussion of common and uncommon associated complications. It is essential for the radiologist to be familiar with these procedures and their associated complications in order to be able to best assist the clinical and surgical teams in making a timely diagnosis and to guide appropriate management.

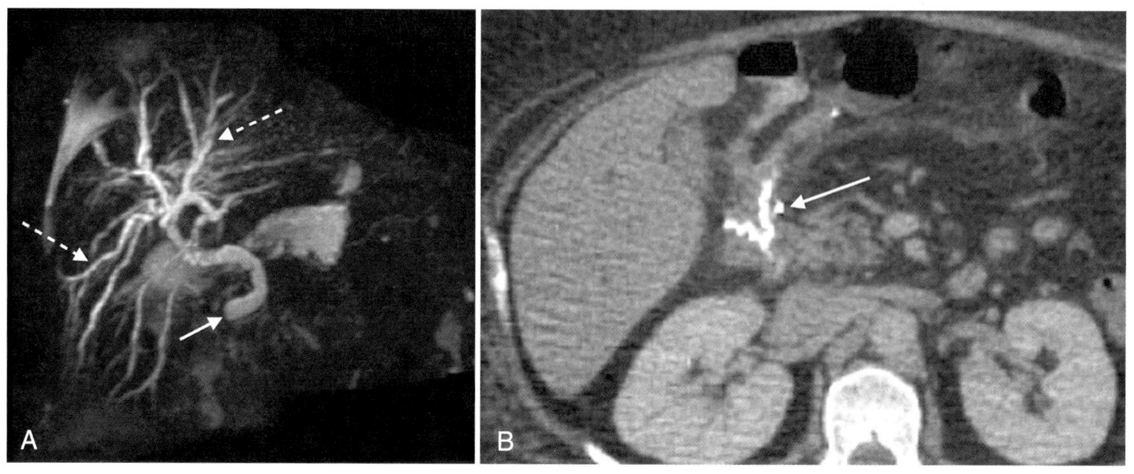


**Fig. 8.15** Coronal magnetic resonance cholangiopancreatography image (A) and axial intravenous contrast–enhanced computed tomography image (B) show evidence of intrahepatic biliary duct dilatation (dotted arrows) with abrupt termination of the common bile duct at the level of the ampulla (arrow in A) secondary to surgical sutures at the level of the ampulla (arrow in B). In this case, the ampulla was inadvertently sutured at the time of the duodenal switch.

## REFERENCES


1. Hurt Ryan T., Kulisek Christopher, Buchanan Laura A., McClave Stephen A., et al. The obesity epidemic: challenges, health initiatives, and implications for gastroenterologists.. Gastroenterology & Hepatology. Millenium Medical Publishing; 2010:6(12):780–792.
2. Cawley John, Meyerhoefer Chad. The medical care costs of obesity: An instrumental variables approach. *J Health Econ*. 2012:31(1):219–230.
3. Biertho Laurent, Marceau Simon, Biron Simon. A Canadian and historical perspective on bariatric surgery. *Can J Diabetes*. 2017:41(4):341–343.
4. Yu Jinxing, Turner Mary Ann, Shao-Ro Cho, Fulcher Ann S, DeMaria Eric J, Kellum John M, et al. Normal anatomy and complications after gastric bypass surgery: Helical CT findings. *Radiology*. 2004:231(3):753–760.
5. Levine Marc S., Carucci Laura R. Imaging of Bariatric Surgery: Normal Anatomy and Postoperative Complications. *Radiology*. 2014:270(2):327–341.
6. Buchwald H. The evolution of metabolic/bariatric surgery. *Obes Surg*. 2014;24(8):1126-1135.
7. Doulamis Ilias P., Michalopoulos George, Boikou Vasileios, Schizas Dimitrios, Spartalis Eleftherios, Menenakos Evangelos, et al. Concomitant cholecystectomy during bariatric surgery: The jury is still out. *Am J Surg*. 2019:218(2): 401–410.
8. Lewis Kyle D., Takenaka Katris Y., Luber Samuel D. Acute abdominal pain in the bariatric surgery patient. *Emerg Med Clin North Am*. 2016;34(2):387–407.
9. Swartz Daniel E., Felix Edward L. Elective cholecystectomy after Roux-en-Y gastric bypass: why should asymptomatic gallstones be treated differently in morbidly obese patients? *Surg Obes Relat Dis*. 2005:1(6):555–560.
10. Liem Robert K., Niloff Paul H. Prophylactic cholecystectomy with open gastric bypass operation. *Obes Surg*. 2004:14(6):763–765.
11. Sioka Eleni, Zacharoulis Dimitris, Zachari Eleni, Papamargaritis Dimitris, Pinaka Ourania, Katsogridaki Georgia, et al. Complicated gallstones after laparoscopic sleeve gastrectomy. *J Obes*. 2014;Epub.
12. Manatsathit Wuttiporn, Leelasinjaroen Pornchai, Al-Hamid Hussein, Szpunar Susanna, Hawasli Abdelkader. The incidence of cholelithiasis after sleeve gastrectomy and its association with weight loss: A two-centre retrospective cohort study. *Int J Surg*. 2016:30:13–18.
13. Escalona Alex, Boza Camilo, Munoz Rodrigo, Perez Gustavo, Rayo Sabina, Crovari Fernando, et al. Routine preoperative ultrasonography and selective cholecystectomy in laparoscopic roux-en-Y gastric bypass. why not? *Obes Surg*. 2008:18(1):47–51.
14. Passos Teivelis Marcelo, Faintuch Joel, Ishida Robson, Sakai Paulo, Bresser Adriano, Gama-Rodrigues Joaquim Endoscopic and ultrasonographic evaluation before and after Roux-en-Y gastric bypass for morbid obesity. Arquivos de Gastroenterologia. 2007;44(1):8–13.
15. Needleman Bradley J., Happel Lynn C. Bariatric surgery: choosing the optimal procedure. *Surgical Clin North Am*. 2008:88(5):991–1007.
16. Shah S., Shah V., Ahmed A.R., Blunt D.M. Imaging in bariatric surgery: service set-up, post-operative anatomy and complications. *Br J Radiology*. 2011:84(998):101–111.
17. Riaz Rehan M., Myers Daniel T., Williams Todd R. Multidetector CT imaging of bariatric surgical complications: a pictorial review. *Abdom Radiology*. 2016:41(1):174–188.
18. Krishna Satheesh, McInnes Matthew D.F., Schieda Nicola, Narayanasamy Sabarish, Sheikh Adnan, Kielar Ania Diagnostic accuracy of MRI for diagnosis of internal hernia in pregnant women with prior Roux-en-Y gastric bypass. *Am J Roentgenology*. 2018;211(4):755–759.
19. Byrne T. K. Complications of surgery for obesity. *Surgical Clin North Am*. 2001:81(5):1181–1193. vii-viii.
20. Kassir Radwan, Debs Tarek, Blanc Pierre, Gugenheim Jean, Ben Amor Imed, Boutet Claire, et al. Complications of

bariatric surgery: Presentation and emergency management. *International Journal of Surgery*. 2016:27:77–81.
21. Mitchell Myrosia. T., Carabetta Joseph M., Shah Rajshri N., O'Riordan Moira A., Gasparaitis Arunas E., Alverdy John C. Duodenal switch gastric bypass surgery for morbid obesity: imaging of postsurgical anatomy and postoperative gastrointestinal complications. *Am J Roentgenol*. 2009:193(6):1576–1580.
22. Lockhart Mark E., Tessler Franklin N., Canon Cheri L., Smith J. Kevin, Larrison Matthew C., Fineberg Naomi S., et al. Internal hernia after gastric bypass: Sensitivity and specificity of seven CT signs with surgical correlation and controls. *Am J Roentgenol*. 2007:188(3):745–750.
23. Prosch H., Tscherney R., Kriwanek S., Tscholakoff D. Radiographical imaging of the normal anatomy and complications after gastric banding. *Br J Radiol*. 2008:81(969):753–757.
24. Beitner M, Kurian MS Laparoscopic adjustable gastric banding. Abdom Imaging. 2012;37(5):687–689
25. Carucci Laura R., Turner Mary Ann, Szucs Richard A. Adjustable laparoscopic gastric banding for morbid obesity: imaging assessment and complications. *Radiol Clin North Am*. 2007:45(2):261–274.
26. Blachar Arye, Blank Annat, Gavert Nancy, Metzer Ur, Fluser Gideon, Abu-Abeid Subhi Laparoscopic adjustable gastric banding surgery for morbid obesity: imaging of normal anatomic features and postoperative gastrointestinal complications. *Am J Roentgenol*. 2007:188(2):472–479.
27. Clayton Ryan D., Carucci Laura R. Imaging following bariatric surgery: Roux-en-Y gastric bypass, laparoscopic adjustable gastric banding and sleeve gastrectomy. *Br J Radiol*. 2018;91(1089):Epub.
28. Hainaux Bernard, Agneessens Emmanuel, Rubesova Erika, Muls Vinciane, Gaudissart Quentin, Moschopoulos Constantin, et al. ntragastric band erosion after laparoscopic adjustable gastric banding for morbid obesity: imaging characteristics of an underreported complication. *Am J Roentgenol*. 2005:184(1):109–112.
29. Pieroni Sabrina, Sommer Eric A., Hito Rania, Burch Miguel, Tkacz Jaroslaw N. The "O" sign, a simple and helpful tool in the diagnosis of laparoscopic adjustable gastric band slippage. *Am J Roentgenol*. 2010;195(1):137–141.
30. Mehanna Mayssoun J., Birjawi Ghina, Moukaddam Hicham A., Khoury Ghattas, Hussein Maher, Al-Koutoubi Aghiad Complications of adjustable gastric banding, a radiological pictorial review. *Am J Roentgenol*. 2006;186(2):522–534.
31. Nocca D, et al. Migration of adjustable gastric banding from a cohort study of 4,236 patients. Surg Endosc. 2005;19(7):947–950.
32. Hainaux B, et al. Laparoscopic adjustable silicone gastric banding: radiological appearances of a new surgical treatment for morbid obesity. Abdom Imaging. 1999;24(6):533–537.
33. Gumbs Andrew A., Gagner Michel, Dakin Gregory, Pomp Alfons Sleeve gastrectomy for morbid obesity. *Obes Surg*. 2007;17(7):962–969.
34. Quigley S., Colledge J., Mukherjee S. Patel K. Bariatric surgery: A review of normal postoperative anatomy and complications. *Clin Radiology*. 2011:66(10):903–914.
35. Burgos Ana Maria, Braghetto Italo, Csendes Attila, Maluenda Fernando, Korn Owen, Yarmuch Julio, et al. Gastric leak after laparoscopic-sleeve gastrectomy for obesity. *Obes Surg*. 2009:19(12):1672–1677.
36. Benarroch-Gampel Jaime, Lairson David R., Boyd Casey A., Sheffield Kristin M., Ho Vivian, Riall Taylor S. Cost-effectiveness analysis of cholecystectomy during Roux-en-Y gastric bypass for morbid obesity. *Surgery*. 2012:152(3):363–375.
37. Moon Rena C., Teixeira Andre F., DuCoin Christopher, Varnadore Sheila, Jawad Muhammad A. Comparison of cholecystectomy cases after Roux-en-Y gastric bypass, sleeve gastrectomy, and gastric banding. *Surg Obes Relat Dis*. 2014:10(1):64–68.
38. Weiss Anna C., Inui Tazo, Parina Ralitza, Coker Alisa M., Jacobsen Garth, Horgan Santiago, et al. Concomitant cholecystectomy should be routinely performed with laparoscopic Roux-en-Y gastric bypass. *Surgical Endoscopy*. 2015:29(11):3106–3111.
39. Lutz Thomas A., Bueter Marco. The physiology underlying Roux-en-Y gastric bypass: A status report. *Am J Physiol - Regulatory Integr Comp Physiol*. 2014:307(11):R1275–R1291.
40. Damian JM, Tolan-Keith M, Deepak H, Mehta P-SP. The Stomach and Duodenum. In Brittenden J and Tolan DJM (eds) Radiology of the Post Surgical pp. 71–126, 2012. Springer-Verlag: London.
41. Carucci Laura R. Role of imaging in bariatric procedures: Roux-en-Y gastric bypass and laparoscopic adjustable gastric banding. *Imaging in Medicine*. 2011;3(1):81–92.
42. Tucker Olga N., Escalante-Tattersfield Tomas, Szomstein Samuel, Rosenthal Raul J. The ABC System: a simplified classification system for small bowel obstruction after laparoscopic Roux-en-Y gastric bypass. *Obes Surg*. 2007;17(12):1549–1554.
43. Miao Timothy L., Kielar Ania Z., Patlas Michael N., iordon Michele, Chong Suzanne T., Robins Jason, et al. Cross-sectional imaging, with surgical correlation, of patients presenting with complications after remote bariatric surgery without bowel obstruction. *Abdom Imaging*. 2015;40(8):2945–2965.
44. Lemanowiczabef A, Serafinabef Z Imaging of patients treated with bariatric surgery. Pol J Radiol. 2014;79:12–19.
45. Dallal Ramsey M., Cottam Daniel. "Candy cane" Roux syndrome--a possible complication after gastric bypass surgery. *Surg Obes Relat Dis*. 2007:3(3):408–410.

Chapter 9

# Abdominal Emergencies in Geriatric Patients

Iain D.C. Kirkpatrick

## Outline



## Key Points

- Acute abdominal diseases frequently have atypical presentations in geriatric patients. Patients with intraabdominal sepsis may not have a fever or elevated white cell count, and conditions usually associated with abdominal pain (e.g., cholecystitis, pyelonephritis) may present as generalized sepsis without localizing signs.
- When performing emergency computed tomography (CT) on geriatric patients, scanning with the highest pitch available can be desirable, and weight-based contrast dosing is recommended.
- Gallstone ileus, colonic volvulus, stercoral colitis, and Ogilvie syndrome are rarely seen causes of bowel dilatation in younger patients but are not uncommon in this age group.
- Geriatric patients are at increased risk of acute mesenteric ischemia, and if there is any clinical suspicion of ischemia, a biphasic CT protocol is recommended. Many of the earliest signs of ischemia (embolus, thrombosis, or vascular signs of nonocclusive ischemia) are only well seen on CT mesenteric angiography.

## Introduction

The investigation of acute illnesses in geriatric patients (those aged ≥65 years) poses a number of unique challenges. These patients more frequently present with atypical symptoms for a given condition, can delay seeking medical care (which allows for more advanced or multisystem disease upon presentation), and often have other medical conditions and multiple prescription medications, which can confound diagnosis or compound the impact of an illness.[1–3] Geriatric patients are less likely to manifest fever and leukocytosis.[4] A number of normal anatomic variants that occur with age can mimic disease processes on diagnostic imaging. These factors combine to result in reduced diagnostic accuracy for geriatric emergency patients, increased morbidity and mortality, and increased time in the emergency department (ED) until a diagnosis is made.[3,5]

While radiography, ultrasound (US), computed tomography (CT), and magnetic resonance imaging (MRI) all play roles in evaluating the emergency patient, there is evidence that the early use of CT in particular leads to a significant alteration in patient diagnosis and management, as well as time to patient disposition.[6,7] Conventional radiography still has a role to play in the rapid identification of free intraperitoneal air, exclusion of a pulmonary process as the cause of upper abdominal pain, and evaluation for bowel obstruction, but CT is increasingly recognized as the primary diagnostic modality for geriatric patients with an acute abdomen. The assessment of right upper quadrant pain may still begin with US to assess for gallbladder pathology or biliary dilatation, and US can also exclude obstructive uropathy in the elderly patient presenting with acute kidney injury. MRI plays a much more limited role in these patients, primarily when biliary dilatation has been identified and choledocholithiasis is to be excluded.

This chapter will begin by discussing special considerations in the acquisition of CT and MRI abdominal studies unique to geriatric patients, as well as the use of iodinated contrast material in this population. Following this, anatomic variations and unique pathologies that develop with age will be addressed on a system-by-system basis.

## Technical Considerations

### COMPUTED TOMOGRAPHY

CT is ideally suited for imaging elderly patients who may have limited breath-holding capacity, or who may have difficulty lying supine and still. The use of standard CT protocols may not be ideal for this group of patients, however, and it is worth developing a specialized approach for them.

The key parameter to consider in this group is scan time, in order to obtain images that preserve spatial resolution and are free of artifacts. It is thus desirable to scan with a higher pitch than one might use for a routine outpatient exam, recognizing that the reduction in motion artifact will usually far outweigh any theoretical reduction in image quality due to less redundant data sampling. In fact, it is rare to appreciate a significant difference in quality with modern scanners until above a pitch of 1.5.[8] Many standard preinstalled vendor protocols will have the pitch set to a value of less than 1 in order to maximize image quality, whereas a pitch of 1 or more would be more appropriate for older emergency patients. The maximum pitch that could be deemed acceptable will be scanner dependent. While higher-pitch scans can be associated with a lower signal-to-noise ratio (for a static tube output, fewer photons will be able to penetrate the patient at each slice level as the patient moves more rapidly through the gantry), geriatric patients typically have a lower body mass index, and this is rarely a problem in practice. A higher-pitch technique also has the advantage of an overall lower radiation dose. A recent study evaluating the use of a pitch of 1.5 for emergency thoracoabdominal CT found a reduction in overall motion artifacts with no significant effect on image quality otherwise when scanning unconscious patients using single-source CT.[9] A much higher pitch still can be utilized with dual-source CT, because each tube-and-detector combination can acquire 90 degrees of data simultaneously. A study of second-generation dual-source CT using pitch values of 2.1 to 2.5 allowed for the diagnostic assessment of the diaphragm free of motion artifact in more than 99% of blunt trauma patients, and third-generation scanners can reach a pitch of 3.2.[10] Image noise will eventually become a limiting factor when the maximum pitch is approached, and additionally, if using both tubes simultaneously in a dual-tube system to achieve an ultrafast pitch, one must be aware of potential limitations on the field of view of the scan depending on the generation (33–35.6 cm for second- and third-generation systems). For both single- and dual-tube systems, the use of most dual-energy techniques across vendors is generally associated with a reduction in the maximum allowable pitch, and unless there is a specific use case in mind for a dual energy acquisition, this downside is often enough to avoid dual-energy scans in geriatric patients.

If using software that automatically selects an appropriate kVp based on the CT topogram, radiologists should be aware that levels of 80 to 100 kVp may be selected with smaller geriatric patients. While increased tube output will attempt to compensate for the lower photon energy level with increased photon flux (mA) and largely maintain signal-to-noise, the lower mean energy level of the photons will be closer to the k-edge of iodine and result in increased beam attenuation by iodinated contrast (Fig. 9.1). This has definite advantages, in that the vasculature will be brighter and easier to assess (particularly smaller vessels), but also the disadvantage that at standard window/level (W/L) settings many solid organs will be too bright to optimally assess for parenchymal abnormalities without manual W/L adjustment.[11] Beam

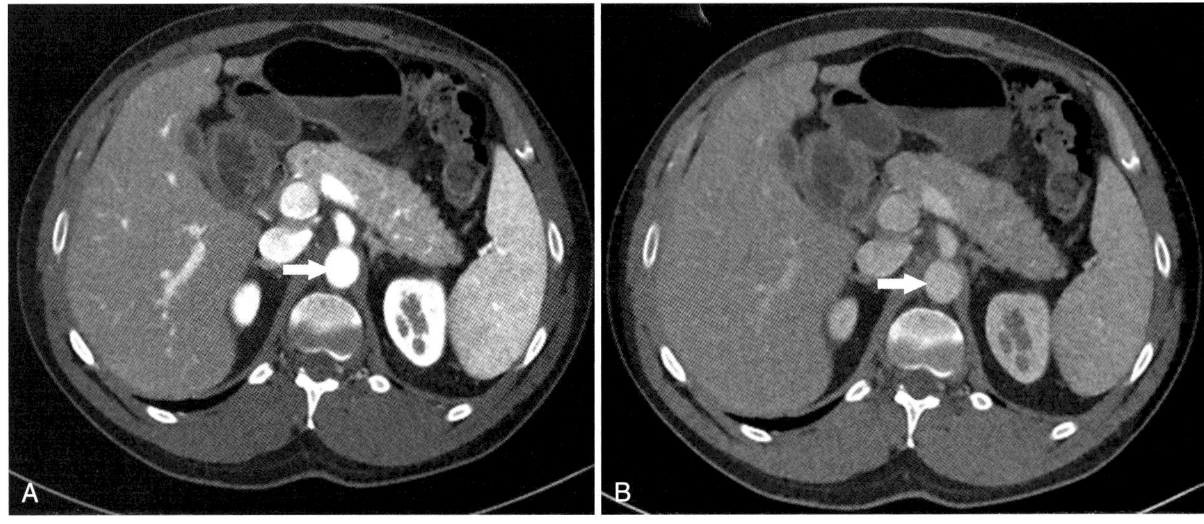


**Fig. 9.1** Transverse contrast-enhanced computed tomography image of the same patient at 80 kVp (A) and 120 kVp (B). As long as the scanner tube capacity is capable of increasing mA to accommodate a lower kV and keep image noise similar, the primary impact will be an increase in attenuation of iodine at the lower kV, manifested here as an increased brightness of the aorta (arrows), other vessels, and solid organs.

hardening artifacts will also be more pronounced, and it may be advantageous to manually select a higher kVp if surgical hardware is identified on the topogram.

### MAGNETIC RESONANCE IMAGING

While MRI can be a valuable modality in scanning patients with a contraindication to iodinated contrast, in the elderly it may be still preferable to perform a noncontrast CT due to the challenges posed by motion artifact. One area where MRI is often unavoidable is in the exclusion of choledocholithiasis. Single-shot fast-spin echo techniques are extremely valuable in this case, as they are performed in single-slice acquisitions, and image quality is often satisfactory even when a patient is free breathing. Following thick (7–8 mm) and thin (3–4 mm) stack acquisitions in the axial and coronal planes, three-dimensional (3D) magnetic resonance cholangiopancreatography (MRCP) is acquired. Breath-holding 3D fast/turbo spin echo techniques usually require longer breath holds than an elderly patient can maintain, unless newer compressed sensing methods are used to heavily accelerate the acquisition, and respiratory triggering using a navigator echo on the diaphragm is generally advised for the 3D MRCP acquisition.[12] In the event postcontrast imaging is felt to be necessary, scan time can be reduced to accommodate for breath-holding capacity by reducing the acquisition matrix or by increasing the parallel imaging factor. Newer scanners also offer novel T1-weighted 3D spoiled gradient echo sequences that utilize compressed sensing for acceleration to the point where a diagnostic free-breathing acquisition is possible, or radial stack-of-stars k-space acquisition, either of which would be preferable for challenging patients.[13,14]

## Contrast Considerations

The degree of enhancement achieved on CT with iodinated contrast depends on many factors, but a few are particularly important when assessing geriatric patients. Cardiac output and circulation are critical in determining enhancement, with a reduction in cardiac output associated with delayed arrival of the intravascular contrast bolus and delayed but stronger enhancement of the solid organs. If empiric scan timing is used, the abdominal CT of a patient with heart failure may have the appearance of an arterial phase exam as a result. It is thus strongly recommended that either a test bolus or automated bolus tracking technique be used to optimize scan timing (Fig. 9.2).[15,16] The greater a patient's blood volume, the more a

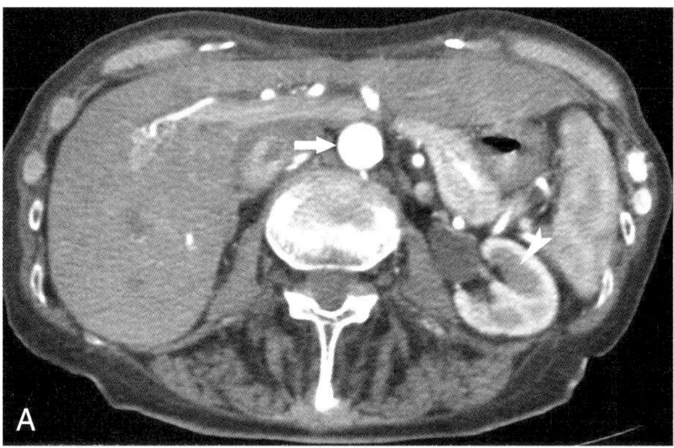


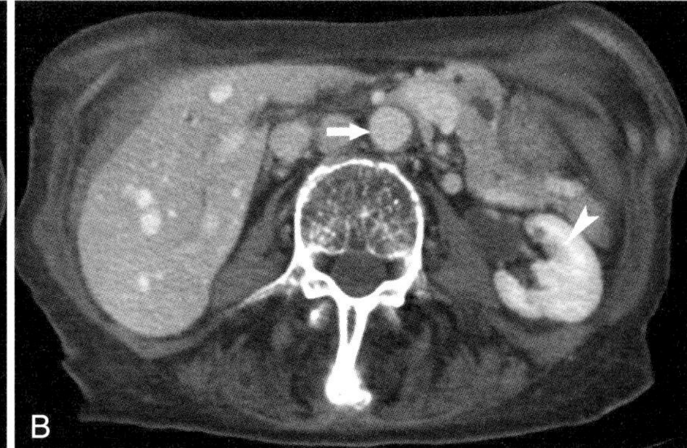


**Fig. 9.2** Transverse contrast-enhanced computed tomography examinations performed on the same patient on two occasions using empiric scan timing (A) and timing with bolus tracking (B). Geriatric patients will often have reduced cardiac output, which can result in an earlier phase of enhancement than expected with empiric timing. In this case, the aortic enhancement (arrows) is brighter, and renal enhancement (arrowheads) is corticomedullary with empiric timing (A), but enhancement is more typical of a portal venous phase as intended when bolus tracking is used (B).

contrast bolus will be diluted. Blood volume generally correlates well with body weight, although it can be overestimated in obese patients, and for these reason adjustments based on lean body weight or body surface area are sometimes used. In the geriatric population, morbid obesity is less common, and the relationship of blood volume to body weight is mostly linear. Because many elderly patients are of low body weight, one can expect greater vascular and parenchymal enhancement for the same injected contrast volume on average compared with larger and younger patients.[15]

In recent years, the existence of contrast-induced acute kidney injury (AKI) has become controversial, after a number of papers concluded that the incidence of AKI in patients receiving iodinated contrast was similar to that of matched patients who did not receive contrast.[17–19] It is likely that historical literature has overstated the risk of contrast-induced AKI due to the lack of proper control groups and the presence of other confounding factors, including dehydration. At this time, it is the position of the American College of Radiology that contrast-induced AKI is a real phenomenon, but a rare one.[20,21]

Geriatric patients undergoing emergent CT imaging should be considered at risk due to age, but there are a number of other factors that may compound this risk, including the presence of cardiovascular disease, dehydration, diuretic use, diabetes, and hypertension. Unless there are well-documented laboratory records, the baseline creatinine and estimated glomerular filtration rate (eGFR) obtained in the ED cannot be assumed to be that patient's steady state. Nevertheless, an eGFR of less than 30 mL/min/1.73 $m^2$ is considered the strongest risk factor for AKI, and for these patients the use of either noncontrast CT or alternative imaging (US or MRI) should be entertained. That said, the risk-benefit proposition for each patient must be considered separately, and there will be scenarios where contrast-enhanced CT will still be the best test for these patients, regardless of renal risk. Volume expansion is recommended for patients who are felt to require contrast-enhanced CT and have an eGFR of less than 30 mL/min/1.73 $m^2$, and should be strongly considered for those with an eGFR of 30 to 44 mL/min/1.73 $m^2$, but in consultation with the referring service or ED, given that many geriatric patients may have preexisting congestive heart failure. Although prolonged infusion of 0.9% normal saline (100 cc/hour) for 6 to 12 hours prior to the study and 4 to 12 hours afterwards is ideal, this is not usually practical for emergency patients, and a normal saline bolus is a reasonable alternative in this setting if felt safe. The use of specific contrast agents, N-acetylcysteine or sodium bicarbonate is not currently recommended.[20,21]

Adjusting contrast volume is another potential intervention that may affect renal risk, although a direct dose-to-toxicity relationship for intravenous iodinated contrast has not been clearly established as it has for intraarterial injection.[20] Studies of isoosmolar contrast dosing for coronary angiography patients have shown a consistent decrease in the risk of contrast-associated AKI with lower volumes, particularly when the volume of contrast is limited to double the eGFR (for example, significantly lower risk if a patient with an eGFR of 35 mL/min/1.73 $m^2$ receives no more than 70 cc of contrast).[22,23] On one hand, some argue that *ad hoc* manipulation of contrast protocols is dangerous, as it may result in a nondiagnostic study if insufficient contrast has been administered.[21] At the same time, as previously noted, the mean lower body weight and cardiac output of geriatric patients provide more opportunity to reduce contrast volume because these factors increase vascular and parenchymal enhancement independent of the contrast bolus.[15] The best compromise may be for a department to adopt weight-based contrast dosing protocols, so that every patient may benefit from a reduction in contrast volume but the emergency radiologist is not at risk of making a time-sensitive decision on dosing that could compromise a scan. Several examples of these protocols have been published, and weight-based dosing has consistently been shown to decrease overall contrast volume while maintaining overall image quality.[16,24–27]

The routine administration of positive oral contrast for CT is not advised in geriatric patients, as it is associated with increased time to scanning, can result in vomiting or aspiration, could potentially mask important diagnoses such as mesenteric ischemia or intestinal hemorrhage (intraluminal or mural), and does not significantly improve the diagnosis of most emergent conditions.[28,29]

## Clinical Considerations by Organ System

### LOWER CHEST

An incidental malignancy or pneumonia at the lung bases could present as upper abdominal pain. The left atrium is usually largely outside the field of view of an abdominal CT, but care should be taken to assess the left ventricle for evidence of hypoenhancement that may indicate myocardial ischemia/infarction, or the presence of fat or calcium within the myocardium or papillary muscles that can indicate a remote infarct (Fig. 9.3).[30] Cardiac ischemia can manifest as upper abdominal discomfort, and left ventricular thrombus can be a source of embolism to the abdomen, resulting in mesenteric ischemia or solid organ infarction as a cause of pain.

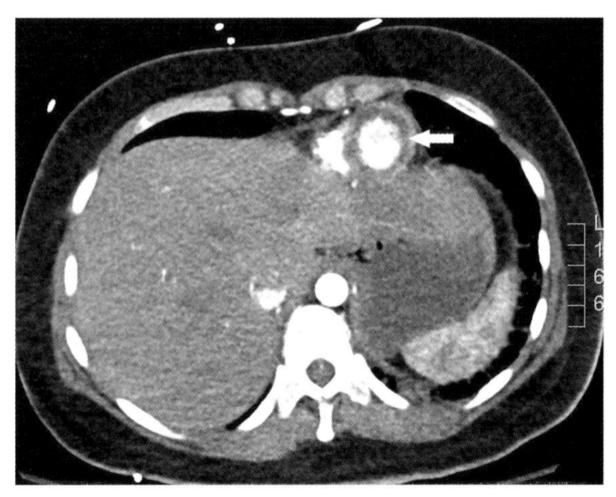

**Fig. 9.3** Transverse contrast-enhanced computed tomography through the upper abdomen in a patient with epigastric pain ultimately found to be secondary to myocardial infarction. There is prominent subendocardial hypoenhancement at the left ventricular apex (arrow), which prompted investigation for cardiac source of the pain.

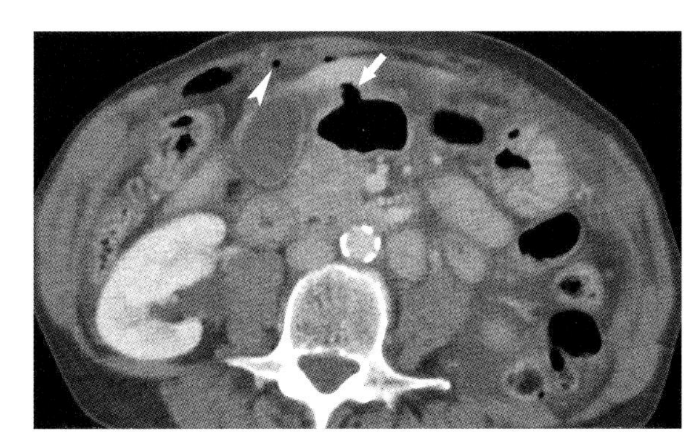

**Fig. 9.4** Transverse contrast-enhanced computed tomography of a perforated duodenal ulcer seen as an eccentric outpouching of gas arising from the duodenal bulb (arrow) and associated with a small amount of adjacent fluid and bubbles of free air (arrowhead).

### GASTROINTESTINAL

Gastrointestinal pathology accounts for more geriatric emergency visits for abdominal pain than any other organ system.[2,6] Peptic ulcer disease and bowel obstructions account for most of these cases. Peptic ulcer disease may show thickening of the gastric or duodenal wall with associated fat stranding and free air if a perforation has occurred. In some cases, the ulceration itself may be visible (Fig. 9.4).[31]

Most small bowel obstructions (SBOs) in the elderly are secondary to either adhesions or hernias, particularly through the abdominal wall or inguinal canals.[32] Large bowel obstructions are usually due to diverticulitis or carcinoma, although volvulus can occur in this age group.[1,3,5,33] When diverticulitis presents with a clearly inflamed diverticulum, the diagnosis is straightforward, but chronic diverticulitis may result in segmental colonic thickening without focal inflammation around any particular diverticulum, and these cases can be difficult to differentiate from colonic carcinoma. Both conditions can perforate, form abscesses, and be associated with pericolonic edema and pericolonic lymph nodes. The degree of wall thickening is usually not a helpful discriminator. Particularly large, necrotic, or distant nodes (or metastatic disease) will favor carcinoma. Chronic diverticulitis is associated with more diverticula and is more likely to extend over more than 10 cm. Carcinoma is more likely to demonstrate shouldering.[34–37]

Colonic volvulus can occur at sites of mesenteric laxity, usually at the level of the cecum or sigmoid colon (most common). To make this diagnosis, one must identify a mechanical transition point and visualize a beak at that point followed by a swirl ("whirl sign") consisting of the twisted bowel and associated mesenteric vessels, after which decompressed bowel follows. The mesenteric vessels may be engorged from the volvulus and easier to follow into the twist. Identification of the twist is mandatory to avoid diagnosing colonic spasm as a volvulus (Fig. 9.5).[36,38]

Acute colonic pseudo-obstruction (Ogilvie syndrome) is related to altered colonic motility in the absence of mechanical obstruction and usually occurs in the hospitalized or institutionalized elderly with underlying risk factors such as neurologic disease, significant systemic illness, recent major trauma or surgery, or motility-inhibiting drugs such as opioids.[39] A transition point may be visible, most frequently near the splenic flexure, but no mass or thickening should be present, and often the entire colon is dilated. The small bowel is nondistended. This is generally a diagnosis of exclusion when no obstructing lesion can be identified.[36,39]

Geriatric patients are prone to constipation, and fecal impaction may increase intraluminal pressure and cause stercoral colitis. On CT this appears as a fecal-filled and usually dilated (often >6 cm) segment of distal (usually rectosigmoid) colon with wall thickening and pericolonic edema (Fig. 9.6). Wall ulceration and perforation can occur in advanced cases.[40]

Acute mesenteric ischemia (AMI) can occur as a result of mesenteric artery embolism, primary mesenteric arterial thrombosis, mesenteric venous thrombosis, or a low-flow state (termed nonocclusive mesenteric ischemia [NOMI]). Geriatric patients are at particular risk given the incidence of underlying atherosclerotic disease, higher rates of atrial fibrillation and cardiac thrombus, reduced cardiovascular reserve, and increased likelihood of conditions leading to NOMI (e.g., sepsis, cardiogenic shock, major surgery). Any patient suspected of AMI should be scanned with a biphasic protocol consisting of either an arterial or combined arterial/enteric phase followed by a venous phase. In AMI due to mesenteric embolus or thrombus, the CT angiogram may show the arterial occlusion as the earliest sign of disease, and in NOMI, the CT findings include a small superior mesenteric artery (<4 mm), impaired filling of mesenteric branches, spasm of branch origins, and diffuse spasm or beading of the mesenteric vascular arcade. An ischemic ileus and bowel wall hypoenhancement are the next signs to appear, and as the ischemia progresses and becomes transmural, CT findings of mesenteric edema, ascites, pneumatosis intestinalis (due to mucosal breakdown), mesenteric/portal venous gas, and eventually free air from perforation can be seen. If the patient is reperfused (a common occurrence for patients with NOMI who are resuscitated prior to being scanned), the bowel may be thickened and hyperenhancing because of the ischemic insult and associated inflammation. Other signs of reperfusion include hyperenhancing adrenals, gallbladder wall thickening, heterogeneous solid organ perfusion or frank infarction, and rarely ischemic pancreatitis (Fig. 9.7). Mesenteric venous thrombosis and prominent bowel wall thickening are common in the venous form of ischemia.[41–43]

## HEPATOBILIARY

Measurements of the extrahepatic biliary tree increase with age, and 6 mm plus 1 mm for every decade after the age of 60 years is considered the upper limit of normal. Following cholecystectomy, the common bile duct can measure up to 10 mm and still be considered normal-caliber, and mild intrahepatic dilatation can be

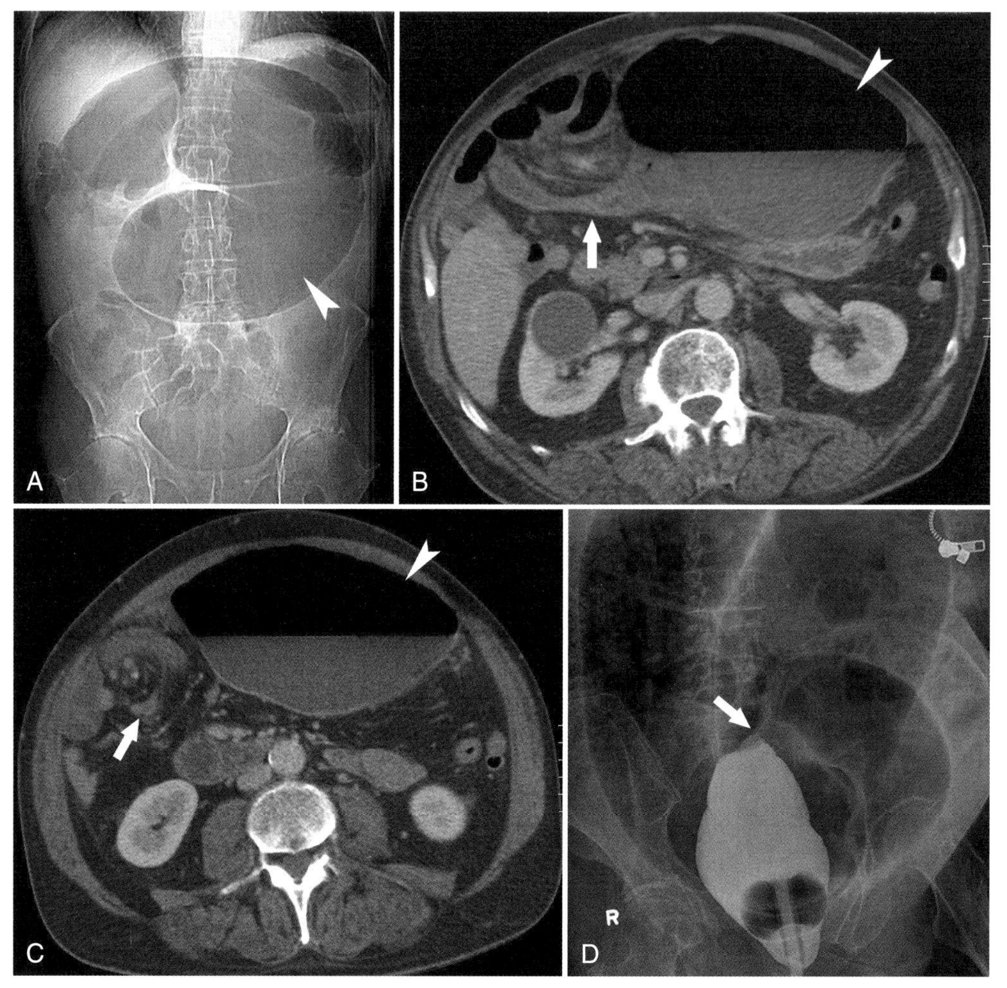


**Fig. 9.5** Imaging of colonic volvulus. (A) A computed tomography (CT) topogram shows a grossly dilated cecum and ascending colon extending into the left abdomen (arrowhead), with minimal distal colonic gas. (B and C) Transverse contrast-enhanced CT images show the dilated cecum (arrowheads) and ascending colon twisted along with its mesentery (arrows). The swirling of the mesenteric vessels and bowel is vital to identify before making this diagnosis. (D) An abdominal radiograph performed on a different patient with large bowel obstruction following instillation of water-soluble contrast via a rectal tube shows a "beak" (arrow) at the distal margin of a sigmoid volvulus.

seen as an incidental finding. Even if the extrahepatic tree measures 7 mm or more (or >10 mm in patients postcholecystectomy), if a patient is asymptomatic with a normal alkaline phosphatase and bilirubin, the finding is unlikely to be significant.[44] Age-related biliary ectasia may result in overinvestigation or distract from the real underlying illness if care is not taken to correlate the finding to the hepatobiliary enzyme profile.

With age, the likelihood of a patient having a condition that may result in benign gallbladder wall thickening increases. Hepatitis, cirrhosis, congestive heart failure, volume overload, renal failure, and hypoalbuminemia can all cause wall thickening that may raise concern for cholecystitis. The possibility of benign wall thickening should be strongly considered whenever the gallbladder is nondistended, or in the absence of calculi. The wall contacting the liver may be more significantly affected, particularly when the thickening is related to adjacent hepatocellular disease. These conditions would not be expected to result in mass-like thickening.[45]

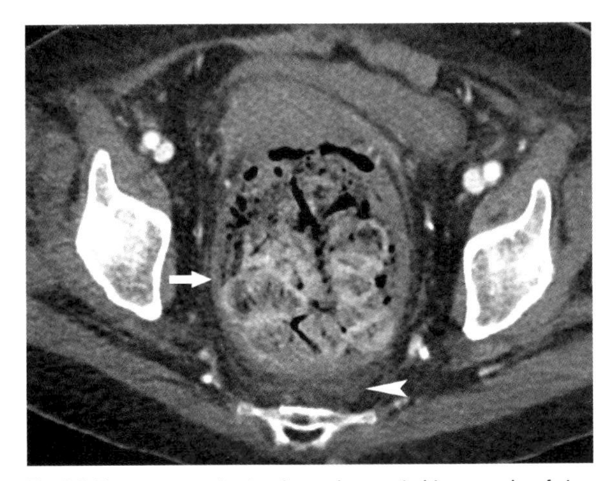

**Fig. 9.6** Transverse contrast-enhanced computed tomography of stercoral colitis. The rectum is grossly distended with fecal material, the rectal wall is thickened (arrow), and there is mild perirectal and presacral edema (arrowhead).

Congestive hepatopathy can be mistaken for heterogeneous enhancement due to contrast timing but is an important potential cause of right upper quadrant pain and elevated liver enzymes in older patients, who are more likely to have increased central venous pressure (secondary to right heart failure or constrictive pericarditis). The liver is often enlarged and may be fatty, and hepatic enhancement is patchy and heterogeneous (Fig. 9.8). The hepatic veins and suprahepatic inferior vena cava may be distended, possibly with evidence of iodinated contrast reflux from the right atrium. Signs of cirrhosis may be present if the condition is chronic.[46]

Cholecystitis and choledocholithiasis are common causes of right upper quadrant pain in older patients, but atypical manifestations are more common in the elderly.[7] Gallbladder wall gangrene and

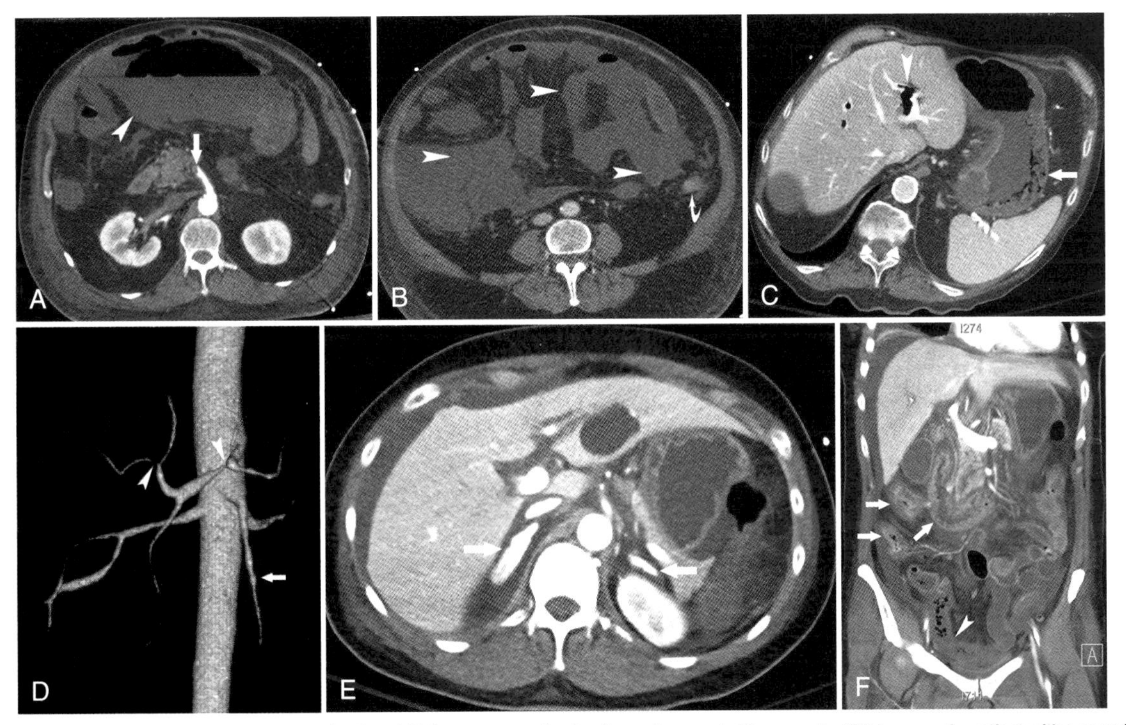


**Fig. 9.7** Imaging of acute mesenteric ischemia. (A and B) Transverse contrast-enhanced computed tomography (CT) images of a patient with a superior mesenteric artery (SMA) embolus show complete occlusion of the vessel (arrow) and complete nonenhancement of bowel in the SMA distribution (arrowheads). The descending colon, supplied by the inferior mesenteric artery, continues to enhance (curved arrow). (C) Another patient with severe ischemia shows gastric pneumatosis (arrow) and air within the portal venous system (arrowhead). (D–F) Nonocclusive mesenteric ischemia. Volume rendered image of a CT angiogram (D) shows a small and spasmed/beaded SMA with impaired filling of its branches (arrow) as well as spasm of celiac branch origins (arrowhead) in a resuscitated intensive care unit patient on vasopressors. Transverse contrast-enhanced CT through the upper abdomen (E) demonstrates hyperenhancing adrenals (arrows), and a coronal image (F) displays thickened small bowel loops with mucosal hyperenhancement (arrows) commonly seen in reperfusion after ischemia. One bowel loop in the pelvis did not reperfuse and remains hypoenhancing and ischemic (arrowhead).

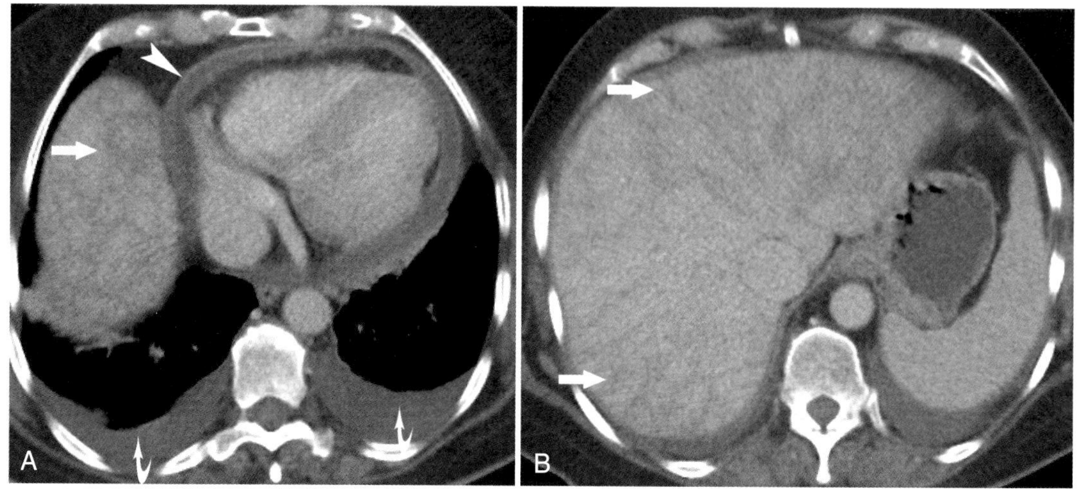


**Fig. 9.8** (A and B) Transverse contrast-enhanced computed tomography images of congestive hepatopathy. The pericardium is mildly thickened and hyperenhancing (arrowhead) in this patient with adhesive constrictive pericarditis, and the elevated right sided cardiac pressure is resulting in hepatic congestion with a mottled hepatic enhancement pattern (arrows). Bilateral pleural effusions are also present (curved arrows). The patient presented with jaundice and right upper quadrant pain rather than cardiac symptoms.

perforation are more common in geriatric patients and appear on imaging as regions of wall irregularity, decreased or absent Doppler flow on US, intraluminal membranes, or frank wall discontinuity upon perforation.[47] Emphysematous cholecystitis is more common in older men, particularly those with underlying diabetes and peripheral vascular disease. It is much more likely than conventional cholecystitis to have an atypical clinical presentation, including sepsis in the absence of abdominal pain or generalized abdominal pain without a Murphy's sign. Fever and leukocytosis may be absent.[47–49] Vascular compromise of the cystic artery and bacterial infection (commonly *Escherichia coli* and *Clostridium welchii*) result in the presence of air that can be found in the gallbladder lumen, wall, or pericholecystic tissues (Fig. 9.9).[47, 49] Acalculous cholecystitis is the result of biliary stasis and gallbladder ischemia and usually occurs in already critically ill patients. As geriatric patients are more likely to undergo procedures that place them at risk (e.g., coronary artery bypass, surgical aortic repair) and are more prone to blood pressure lability when acutely ill, this places them at increased risk for the condition. On imaging, findings are similar to acute cholecystitis (gallbladder distension, wall thickening, wall hyperenhancement), but without the presence of stones.[50,51]

Gallbladder carcinoma can present with right upper quadrant pain, and the imaging appearance may overlap with that of complicated cholecystitis. Polypoid intraluminal tumor could potentially be mistaken for a calculus or intraluminal hemorrhage, and diffuse malignant wall thickening may overlap with the appearance of acute cholecystitis, particularly if the gallbladder is distended, as 70% to 100% of cases of gallbladder carcinoma are associated with cholelithiasis. The most challenging scenario is when a necrotic gallbladder carcinoma invades the adjacent liver because this may mimic perforated cholecystitis with adjacent abscess formation. Key differentiating factors that favor carcinoma include the absence of clinical sepsis, a density of the lesion greater than expected for fluid, the presence of periportal adenopathy or hepatic metastases, or biliary obstruction at the porta hepatis (Fig. 9.10). In challenging cases, percutaneous aspiration may be necessary.[47,52]

Gallbladder torsion is rare but mostly occurs in elderly women and clinically can mimic acute cholecystitis. Complete torsion can result in vascular compromise and perforation. On imaging, the gallbladder is distended, may be edematous, and is often in an unusual position, with twisting of the neck or cystic duct possibly visible on CT.[51]

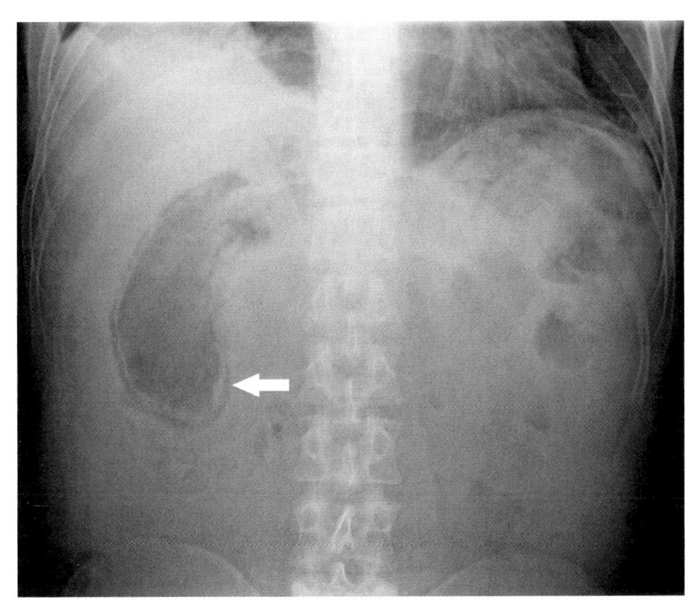

**Fig. 9.9** Abdominal radiograph demonstrating air in the wall (arrow) and lumen of the gallbladder in a patient with emphysematous cholecystitis.

Gallstone ileus is a relatively rare cause of SBO overall (1%–5% of cases), but in the elderly has been reported to be the cause of SBO in up to 25% of cases, and is more common in women.[2,53] This occurs when an impacted stone results in recurrent or chronic cholecystitis with adhesions and inflammation sufficient to extend to a nearby loop of bowel, causing a biliary-enteric fistula. The calculus subsequently erodes into the enteric lumen, where it can be prone to becoming lodged at areas of physiologic narrowing (for example, at the ligament of Trietz or ileocecal valve) or in regions where the lumen may already be partially compromised by adhesions. Erosion into the proximal duodenum can result in obstruction at that level and a clinical presentation of gastric outlet obstruction, termed Bouveret syndrome (Fig. 9.11). The obstruction in gallstone ileus rarely resolves spontaneously. On imaging, the gallbladder is typically thick-walled and hyperenhancing. It may be collapsed due to decompression from the fistula, and air within the gallbladder or biliary tree is characteristic (Fig. 9.12). If these findings are present with an associated SBO, great care should be taken to assess the transition point for evidence of a calculus. These are often non-calcified and may be nearly isodense to enteric lumen. The combination of air within the biliary system, evidence of a SBO, and an ectopic gallstone is termed Rigler's triad and can sometimes be visible on abdominal radiography.[47,53]

## PANCREAS

Mean pancreatic ductal diameter increases with age, and ductal diameter may gradually increase from the tail through the head.[54–56] Ductal dilatation should only be diagnosed if the maximum diameter is greater than 3.5 mm or if the upstream duct is dilated relative to the downstream duct.[54–57] The increased incidence of pancreatic carcinoma in older patients should prompt further assessment with multiphasic pancreatic CT or MRI if a ductal stricture is suspected.

Pancreatic calcifications can be seen in older patients, and their presence is not necessarily diagnostic of chronic pancreatitis. Punctate (<3 mm) parenchymal calcifications can occur, usually secondary to remote pancreatitis, in the absence of chronic pancreatitis. The diagnosis of chronic pancreatitis should be reserved for cases where there are multiple calcifications (especially coarse calcifications ≥3 mm), ductal calcifications (particularly when combined with parenchymal calcifications), or calcifications combined with other evidence of chronic pancreatitis such as glandular atrophy, cysts, or ductal dilatation.[57–59]

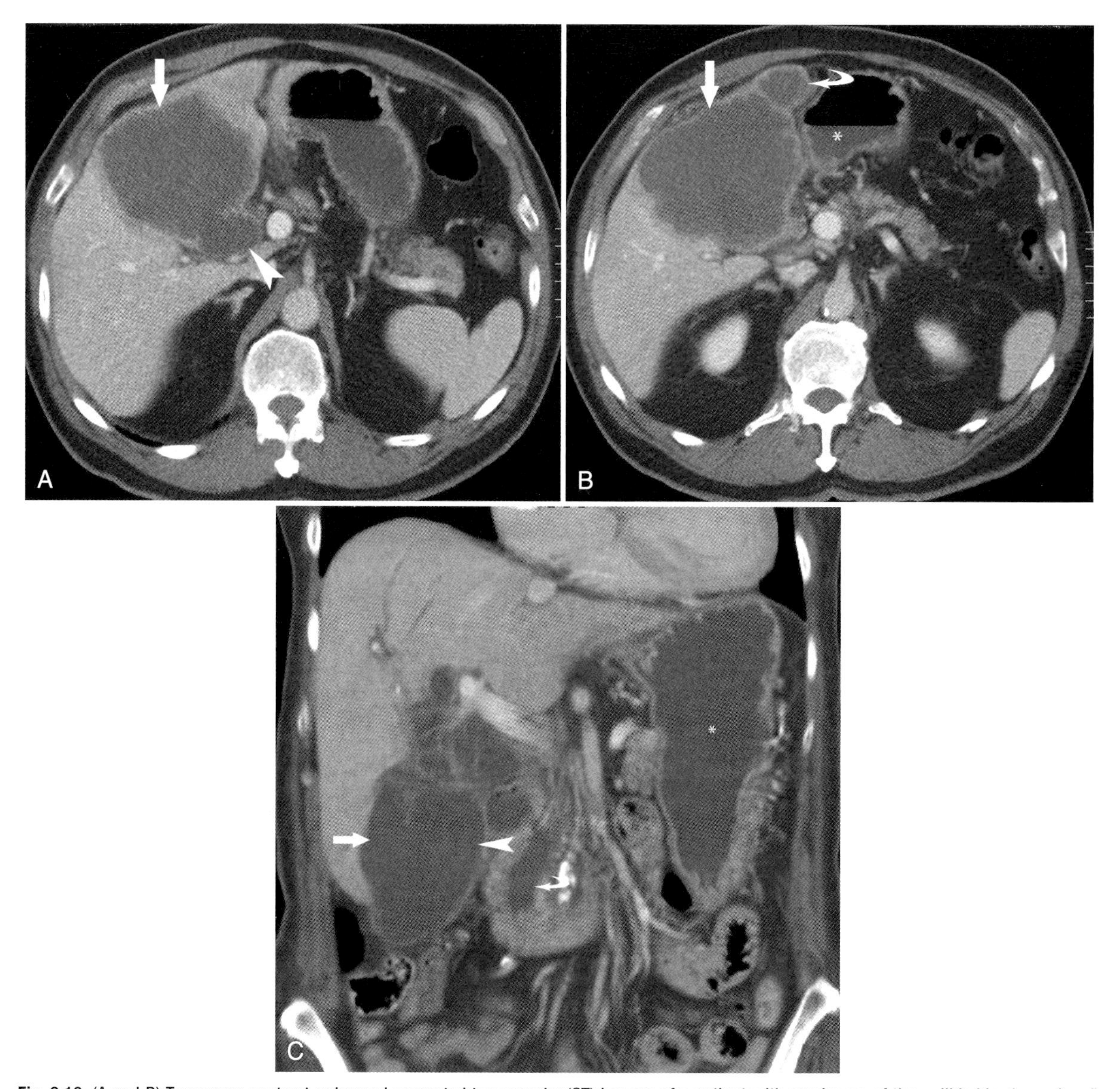


**Fig. 9.10** (A and B) Transverse contrast-enhanced computed tomography (CT) images of a patient with carcinoma of the gallbladder (arrowhead) invading the liver. The hepatic component of the tumor (arrows) and a smaller satellite mass (curved arrow) are both more dense than the water in the stomach (*), raising concern for malignancy rather than perforated cholecystitis. (C) In contrast, coronal contrast-enhanced CT in another patient with perforated cholecystitis shows that the collection (arrow) beside the gallbladder (arrowhead) is the same density as the water in the stomach (*), and there is also biliary dilatation present as a result of choledocholithiasis (curved arrow), all findings that favor a benign process.

Pancreatic fatty replacement/lipomatosis is common in older patients, and while it can be seen in association with chronic pancreatitis, its presence alone is not indicative of exocrine insufficiency. It is more commonly seen in obese patients, diabetics, and patients with atherosclerotic disease.[60,61] Pancreatic bulk also naturally decreases with age, and parenchymal thickness normally decreases by 0.5 to 0.7 cm from the second through eighth decades, with volume loss accelerating after 80 years of age.[55]

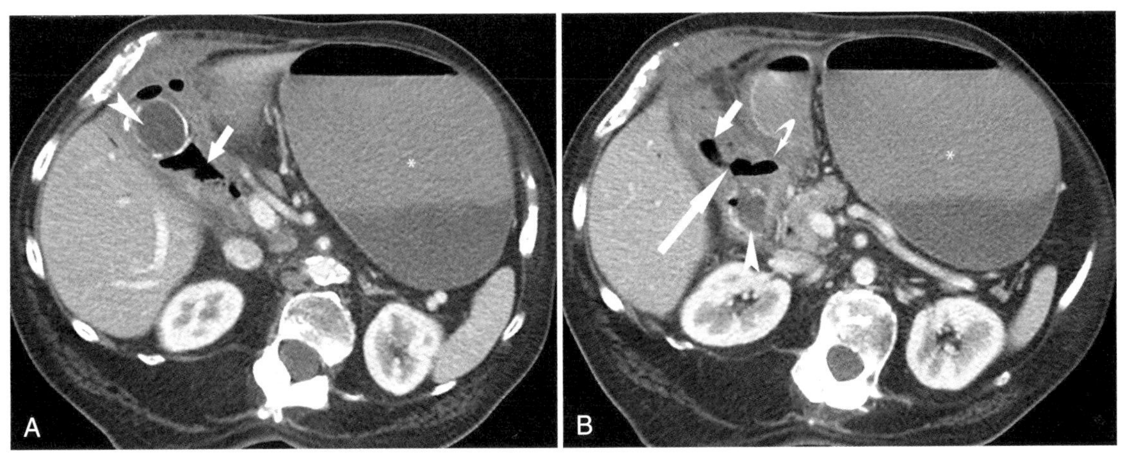


**Fig. 9.11** (A and B) Transverse contrast-enhanced computed tomography images in an elderly patient presenting with nausea and vomiting. Gallstones are present in the gallbladder and duodenum (arrowheads), with the latter resulting in gastric distension (*) from obstruction, termed Bouveret syndrome. Air is seen tracking from the duodenum (curved arrow) into the thick-walled gallbladder lumen (arrows) via a cholecystoduodenal fistula (long arrow).

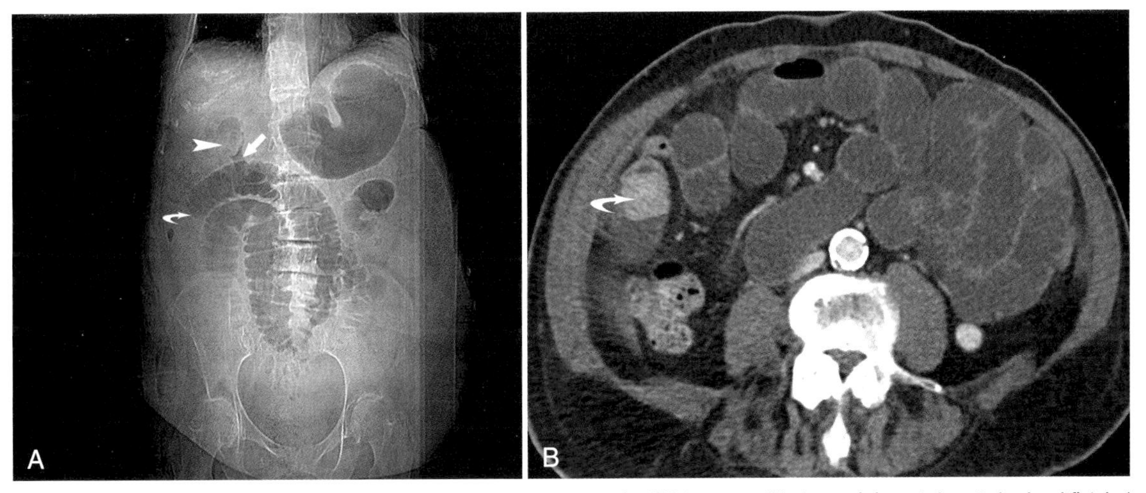


**Fig. 9.12** (A and B) In this patient with gallstone ileus, the computed tomography (CT) topogram (A) shows air in a cholecystoduodenal fistula (arrow) and outlining a gallstone in the gallbladder (arrowhead). Distended air-filled loops of small bowel come to an abrupt end in the right abdomen (curved arrow). Transverse contrast-enhanced CT shows another gallstone (arrowhead) in the small bowel lumen as the cause of the obstruction.

Acute pancreatitis does not seem to occur significantly more frequently in the elderly, but as the incidence of pancreatic carcinoma increases with age, radiologists should look closely for any evidence of an underlying mass that may have resulted in obstructive pancreatitis and have a low threshold for follow-up imaging with multiphasic pancreatic CT or MRI, particularly if there is associated ductal dilatation or atrophy (Fig. 9.13).[3,6,7]

## GENITOURINARY

Renal cortical volume and overall renal size naturally decrease with age, and the incidence of renal cysts increases.[62] Urinary tract infection (UTI) is a very common cause of hospital visits in the elderly, and they are less likely than younger individuals to present with classic features such as dysuria or flank pain, sometimes manifesting only confusion or sepsis. When abdominal pain occurs, it may be without

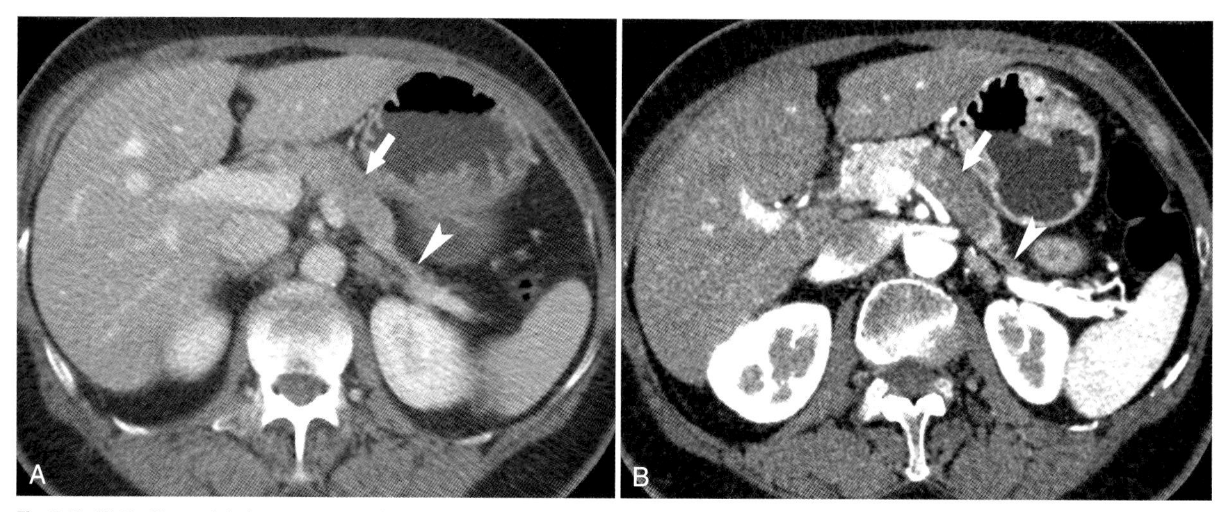


**Fig. 9.13** (A) Routine portal phase contrast-enhanced abdominal computed tomography (CT) was performed for a patient with abdominal pain and elevated lipase. Subtle hypoattenuation in the pancreatic body was suspected (arrow), and pancreatitis was initially questioned, but because the pancreatic tail appeared atrophic (arrowhead), follow-up with a dual-energy pancreatic protocol CT was recommended. (B) A 70keV transverse reconstruction of a subsequent thin-section pancreatic phase dual energy CT markedly increases the conspicuity of a pancreatic body carcinoma (arrow) as well as ductal ectasia in the atrophic tail (arrowhead), subsequently biopsied under endoscopic ultrasound.

localizing signs.[2, 7] Imaging findings of infection may be subtle or absent, but pyelonephritis may manifest as patchy, streaky, or wedge-shaped regions of hypoenhancement on CT. If the abnormalities become rounder, more confluent, and lower in density, renal abscess development must be suspected (Fig. 9.14).[63] Associated ureteritis may be present and demonstrate diffuse urothelial enhancement. Cystitis may appear as bladder wall thickening, wall hyperenhancement, and perivesical edema, and can sometimes be difficult to differentiate from wall redundancy if the bladder is not adequately distended. An indwelling Foley catheter places patients at increased risk of cystitis.[64] The risk of acute bacterial prostatitis increases over the age of 50 years, especially in those with indwelling Foley catheters or diabetes, and while it may be occult on imaging, findings of prostatomegaly, periprostatic edema, or cystic changes that may indicate abscess formation can indicate the diagnosis. The clinical presentation can be quite variable.[64]

Older patients are additionally at risk of complicated UTIs, such as emphysematous pyelonephritis, a severe necrotizing gram-negative bacterial infection with a propensity for poorly controlled diabetics.[63] In addition to the previously described findings of pyelonephritis, gas is present: in class 1, also known as emphysematous pyelitis, gas is limited to within the renal collecting system, and this form has the best prognosis (and is the most responsive to antibiotic treatment); in class 2, gas is within the renal parenchyma; in class 3, there is gas or abscess in the perinephric (3A) or pararenal (3B) space; and class 4 is bilateral emphysematous changes, or emphysematous pyelonephritis in a solitary kidney (Fig. 9.15). Increasing classes are associated with increasing morbidity and mortality, as well as an increasing need for percutaneous drainage or nephrectomy to achieve cure.[65,66] Emphysematous cystitis occurs in older patients with diabetes, neurogenic bladder, immunosuppression, or indwelling catheters and can be life-threatening. Air is present within the bladder lumen or wall, but bear in mind that recent instrumentation, vesicoenteric fistulization, or an indwelling catheter can also explain air in the bladder lumen, and thus a small amount of luminal air alone should not be used solely to make the diagnosis (Fig. 9.16).[64,65]

Urinary retention can present as nonspecific abdominal pain, is more common in this patient group due to the increased frequency of neurogenic bladder and medications that can contribute to retention (antihistamines and anticholinergics), and should be considered if an otherwise normal bladder appears particularly distended on imaging.[2]

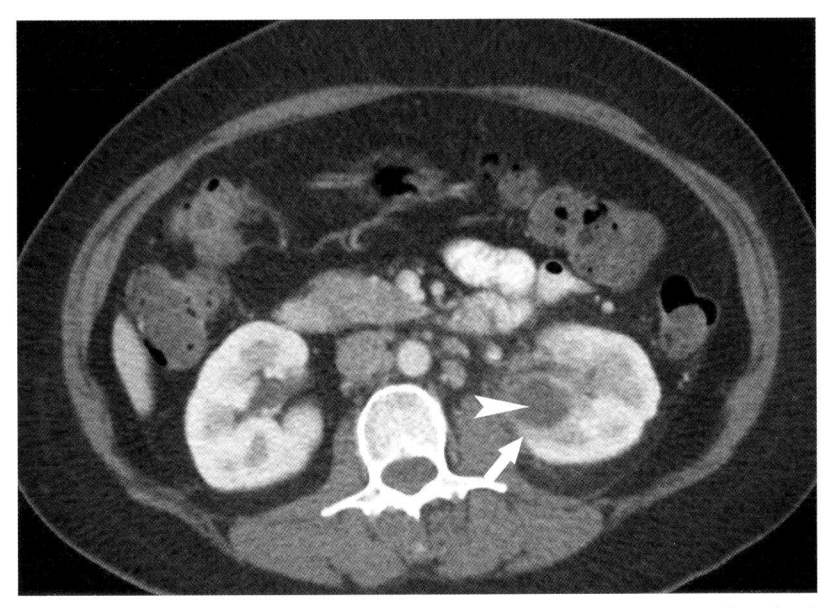

**Fig. 9.14** Transverse contrast-enhanced computed tomography showing left renal cortical hypoenhancement (arrow) and cystic change (arrowhead) in a patient with pyelonephritis and renal abscess formation. The patient presented with fever and chills but no pain or urinary symptoms. Urine cultures grew *Escherichia coli*.

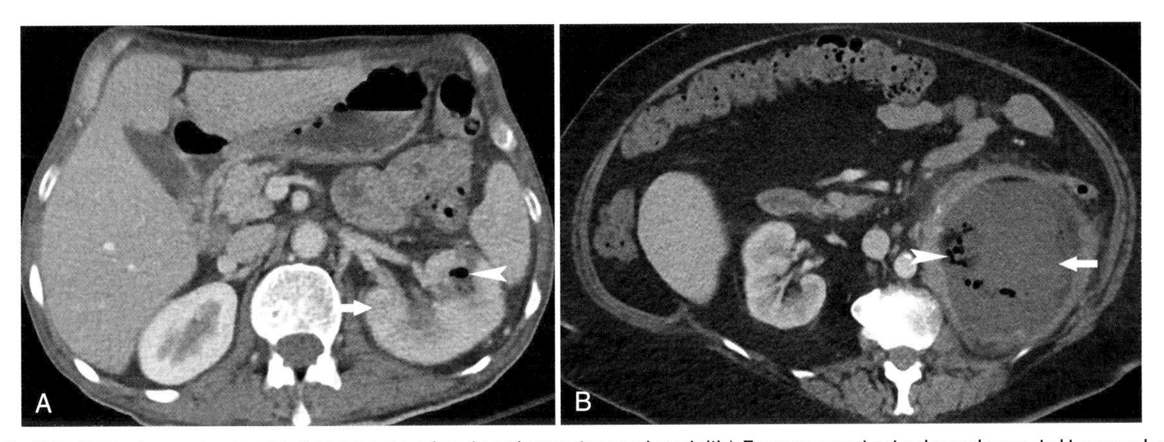


**Fig. 9.15** (A) Emphysematous pyelitis (also known as class 1 emphysematous pyelonephritis). Transverse contrast-enhanced computed tomography shows left renal cortical hypoenhancement consistent with pyelonephritis (arrow) and air in the left renal collecting system (arrowhead). (B) class 3 emphysematous pyelonephritis. The left kidney is necrotic, and the renal bed is filled with gas (arrowhead) and complex fluid (arrow). The patient was unstable and drained percutaneously immediately after the scan, extracting pus, gas, and flecks of necrotic tissue.

Adrenal insufficiency/crisis can present in very nonspecific fashion, including as fever and abdominal pain, as a flu-like illness, or with confusion and hypotension. It should be considered as a potential cause of symptoms when there is evidence of bilateral adrenal hemorrhage, atrophy, calcification, or adrenalitis (enlargement and edema) on CT (Fig. 9.17).[67]

## VASCULAR

The likelihood of rupture of an abdominal aortic aneurysm increases with size, and while there is a 1% annual risk of rupture for an aneurysm 4.5 to 4.9 cm in size, this risk increases to 11% at 5.0 to 5.5 cm and up to 50% for aneurysms of 8.0 cm or more.[68,69] While a frankly ruptured aortic aneurysm is rarely a

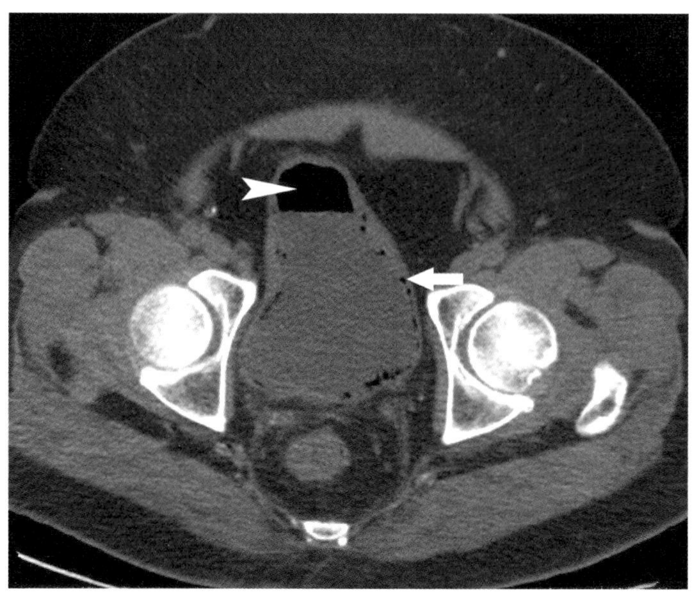

**Fig. 9.16** Transverse contrast-enhanced computed tomography showing air in the bladder wall (arrow) and lumen (arrowhead) in a patient with emphysematous cystitis. Similar to the patient in Fig. 9.14, there was a history of fever but no pain or dysuria, and cultures grew *Escherichia coli*.

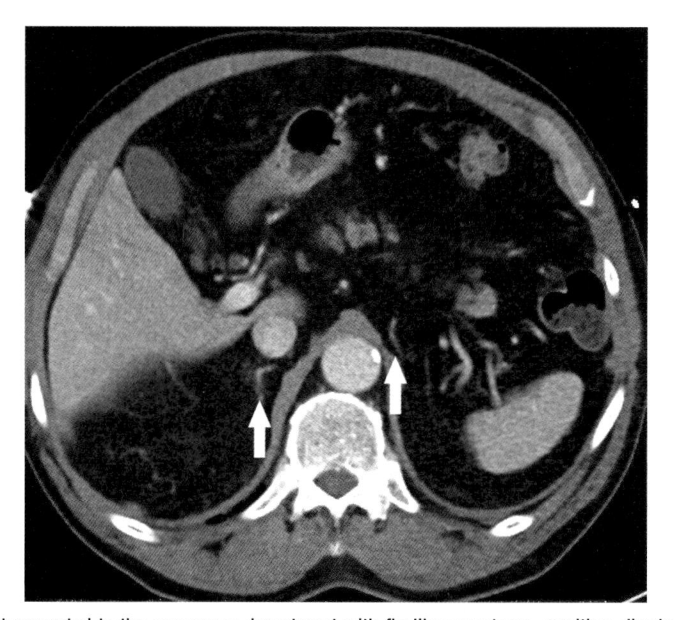

**Fig. 9.17** A 68-year-old patient presented to the emergency department with flu-like symptoms, vomiting, diarrhea, and hypotension. Contrast-enhanced computed tomography was performed and showed no explanation aside from markedly atrophic adrenal glands (arrows), raising concern for adrenal insufficiency. Upon further questioning, it was discovered that the patient had recently run out of a prescription for prednisone that was being given chronically for chronic obstructive pulmonary disease.

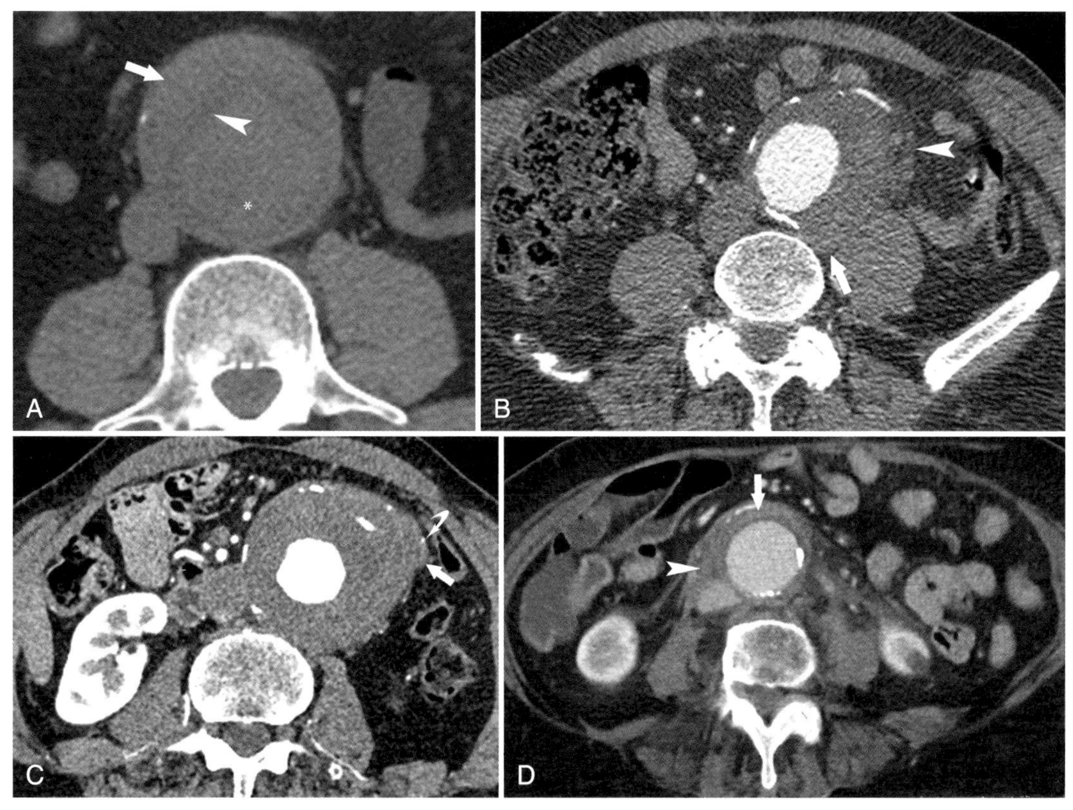


**Fig. 9.18** Findings of impending abdominal aortic aneurysm rupture. (A) Noncontrast computed tomography (CT) shows the subtle density differences between blood in the aortic lumen (*), chronic thrombus in the aneurysm (arrowhead), and the hyperdense "crescent sign" (arrow) that can be indicative of more recent bleeding into the thrombus and aneurysm instability. As a symptomatic aneurysm could present with flank pain, this sign may be identified on a noncontrast renal colic CT. (B) CT angiogram demonstrating the "draped aorta" sign (arrow), which is a pseudoaneurysm conforming to the margin of the adjacent lumbar vertebral body, along with perianeurysmal fat stranding (arrowhead), which in this case was a small amount of blood around the aneurysm found in the operating room. (C) Another CT angiogram showing focal aneurysm convexity consistent with pseudoaneurysm formation (arrow) and outward displacement of the calcium ring (curved arrow), both of which are signs of impending rupture. (D) Transverse contrast-enhanced CT of a patient with abdominal pain and an unexpected aortic aneurysm rupture. A hyperdense crescent is seen in the aneurysm (arrow) along with retroperitoneal hemorrhage (arrowhead).

diagnostic dilemma, due to the retroperitoneal hemorrhage surrounding the aneurysm, a symptomatic aneurysm with impending rupture is a significant clinical challenge to diagnose. It is important to report any abdominal aortic aneurysm and provide double oblique measurements of size axial to the lumen. If the patient has symptoms felt to be attributable to an aneurysm or a tender aneurysm, these are independent risk factors for rupture and may prompt treatment.[69] Aside from size, several CT signs have been described as portents of impending rupture, including growth of 5 mm or more in 6 months, a focal break in or outward displacement of intimal calcifications, focal aneurysm convexity (indicative of pseudoaneurysm formation), penetrating ulceration, the "draped aorta" sign (a pseudoaneurysm draped over the adjacent vertebral body), the "hyperdense crescent" sign (indicating acute intramural hematoma), perianeurysmal fat stranding, and lysis of thrombus in the aneurysm relative to prior scans (Fig. 9.18).[68,70–75]

## MULTISYSTEM

Geriatric patients have a significantly increased risk of major hemorrhage from pelvic fractures, and also have lower cardiovascular reserve. A low threshold for performance of abdominal CT following blunt trauma is advised.[76] Radiologists should note that, in this age range, patients are more likely to have trace amounts of benign free fluid (4% of men and 17% of postmenopausal women), and should be careful about attributing this to trauma if the scan is otherwise normal. This fluid is almost always less than 10 cc, watery in attenuation, and limited to the pelvis.[77] Other underlying conditions such as congestive heart failure, cirrhosis, and volume overload may result in larger amounts of ascites unrelated to trauma as well.

Several medications that radiologists should be familiar with, as well as their complications (Fig. 9.19) that may be visible on CT, are shown in Table 9.1.[78]

# Conclusion

Geriatric patients presenting for emergent abdominal imaging are more likely to manifest atypical symptoms of common intraabdominal diseases or suffer from pathologies that are uncommon in younger patients. CT is generally the imaging modality of choice in this patient population, and every effort should be made to minimize scan time (using as high a pitch as feasible) and optimize contrast dosing and timing (using weight-based contrast dosing and contrast timing tied either to a test bolus or a bolus triggering method). Care must be taken to recognize normal anatomic variants in this age group that can mimic disease. The diseases outlined above are of particular importance to recognize in elderly patients.

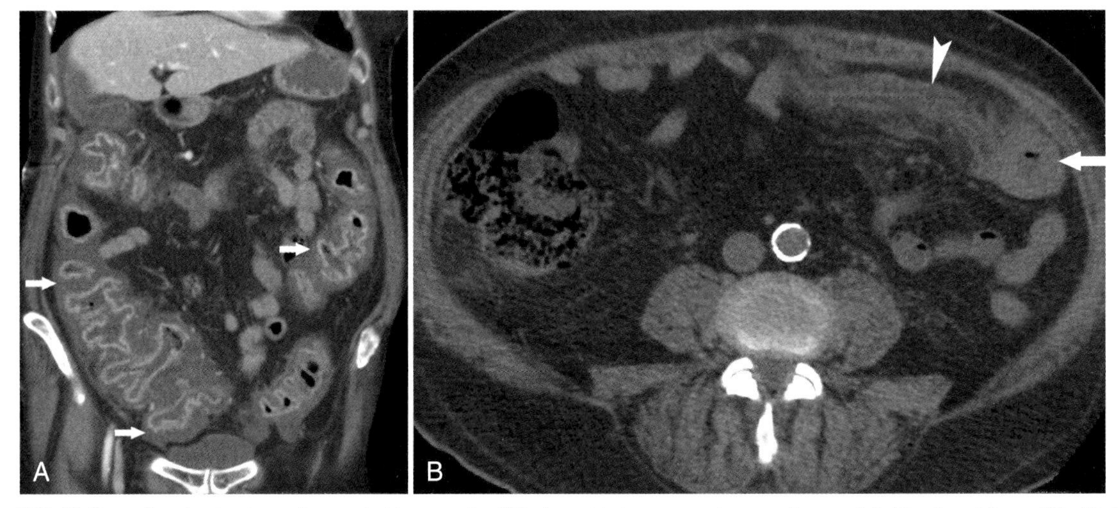


**Fig. 9.19** (A) Coronal contrast-enhanced computed tomography (CT) of an elderly woman who recently completed treatment for cystitis. Marked colonic wall thickening and mucosal hyperenhancement were present (arrows), consistent with *Clostridium difficile* pancolitis. (B) Transverse noncontrast CT in a patient on coumadin for atrial fibrillation who presented with abdominal pain, showing mesenteric hematoma (arrowhead) and bowel wall thickening (arrow) with a density consistent with hemorrhage.

**TABLE 9.1 Medications That May Result in Acute Abdominal Findings at Computed Tomography**

| Medication | Drug-Induced Complication |
|---|---|
| NSAIDs | Gastritis, peptic ulcer disease, NSAID enteropathy |
| Any cytotoxic chemotherapy | Gastritis, enterocolitis (including neutropenic) |
| ACE inhibitors | Angioedema |
| Corticosteroids | Pneumatosis intestinalis, adrenal insufficiency (if withdrawn) |
| Tyrosine kinase inhibitors | Pneumatosis intestinalis |
| α-glucosidase inhibitors | Pneumatosis intestinalis |
| Oxaliplatin, cisplatin | Venoocclusive disease |
| Antibiotics (any) | *Clostridium difficile* colitis |
| Azathioprine | Pancreatitis, cholestatic liver injury |
| L-asparaginase | Pancreatitis |
| Anticoagulants | Spontaneous retroperitoneal, rectus, bowel wall hematomas |
| Opioids | Constipation, stercoral colitis, ileus, acute colonic pseudoobstruction |
| 5-fluorouracil, irinotecan, methotrexate, tamoxifen, corticosteroids, antipsychotics | Steatohepatitis |

*ACE*, Angiotensin-converting enzyme; *NSAID*, nonsteroidal antiinflammatory drug.

## REFERENCES


1. Magidson PD, Martinez JP. Abdominal pain in the geriatric patient. *Emerg Med Clin N Am*. 2016;34(3):559–574.
2. Leuthauser A, McVane B. Abdominal pain in the geriatric patient. *Emerg Med Clin N Am*. 2016;34(2):363–375.
3. Hendrickson M, Naparst TR. Abdominal surgical emergencies in the elderly. *Emerg Med Clin N Am*. 2003;21(4):937–969.
4. Potts FE, Vukov LF. Utility of fever and leukocytosis in acute surgical abdomens in octogenarians and beyond. *J Gerontology Ser*. 1999;54(2):M55–M58.
5. Marco CA, Schoenfeld CN, Keyl PM, Menkes ED, Doehring MC. Abdominal pain in geriatric emergency patients: variables associated with adverse outcomes. *Acad Emerg Med*. 1998;5(12):1163–1168.
6. Gardner CS, Jaffe TA, Nelson RC. Impact of CT in elderly patients presenting to the emergency department with acute abdominal pain. *Abdom Imaging*. 2015;40(7):2877–2882.
7. Lewis LM, Klippel AP, Bavolek RA, Ross LM, Scherer TM, Banet GA. Quantifying the usefulness of CT in evaluating seniors with abdominal pain. *Eur J Radiol*. 2007;61(2):290–296.
8. Raman SP, Mahesh M, Blasko RV, Fishman EK. CT scan parameters and radiation dose: practical advice for radiologists. *J Am Coll Radiol*. 2013;10(11):840–846.
9. Takayanagi T, Suzuki S, Katada Y, Ishikawa T, Fukui R, Yamamoto Y, et al. Comparison of motion artifacts on CT images obtained in the ultrafast scan mode and conventional scan mode for unconscious patients in the emergency department. *Am J Roentgenol*. 2019;213(4):W153–W161.
10. Liang T, McLaughlin P, Arepalli CD, Louis L, Bilawich A, Mayo J, et al. Dual-source CT in blunt trauma patients: elimination of diaphragmatic motion using high-pitch spiral technique. *Emerg Radiology*. 2016;23(2):127–132.
11. Nakayama Y, Awai K, Funama Y, Hatemura M, Imuta M, Nakura T, et al. Abdominal CT with low tube voltage: preliminary observations about radiation dose, contrast enhancement, image quality, and noise. *Radiology*. 2005;237(3):945–951.
12. Kromrey M-L, Funayama S, Tamada D, Ichikawa S, Shimizu T, Onishi H, et al. Clinical evaluation of respiratory-triggered 3D MRCP with navigator echoes compared to breath-hold acquisition using compressed sensing and/or parallel imaging. *Magn Reson Med Sci*. 2020;19(4):318–323.
13. Duffy PB, Stemmer A, Callahan MJ, Cravero JP, Johnston PR, Warfield SK, et al. Free-breathing radial stack-of-stars three-dimensional Dixon gradient echo sequence in abdominal magnetic resonance imaging in sedated pediatric patients. *Pediatr Radiol*. 2021:1–9.

14. Kaltenbach B, Bucher AM, Wichmann JL, Nickel D, Polkowski C, Hammerstingl R, et al. Dynamic liver magnetic resonance imaging in free-breathing. *Invest Radiol*. 2017;52(11):708–714.
15. Bae KT. Intravenous contrast medium administration and scan timing at CT: considerations and approaches. *Radiology*. 2010;256(1):32–61.
16. Fleischmann D, Kamaya A. Optimal vascular and parenchymal contrast enhancement: the current state of the art. *Radiol Clin N Am*. 2009;47(1):13–26.
17. Aycock RD, Westafer LM, Boxen JL, Majlesi N, Schoenfeld EM, Bannuru RR. Acute kidney injury after computed tomography: a meta-analysis. *Ann Emerg Med*. 2018;71(1):44–53. e4.
18. McDonald RJ, McDonald JS, Bida JP, Carter RE, Fleming CJ, Misra S, et al. Intravenous contrast material–induced nephropathy: causal or coincident phenomenon? *Radiology*. 2015;267(1):106–118.
19. Hinson JS, Ehmann MR, Fine DM, Fishman EK, Toerper MF, Rothman RE, et al. Risk of acute kidney injury after intravenous contrast media administration. *Ann Emerg Med*. 2017;69(5):577–586. e4.
20. American College of Radiology. Manual on contrast media. Version 2021. Reston, VA: American Colelge of Radiology, 2021. https://www.acr.org/-/media/ACR/Files/Clinical-Resources/Contrast_Media.pdf. Accessed May 6, 2021.
21. Davenport MS, Perazella MA, Yee J, Dillman JR, Fine D, McDonald RJ, et al. Use of intravenous iodinated contrast media in patients with kidney disease: consensus statements from the American College of Radiology and the National Kidney Foundation. *Radiology*. 2020;294(3):192094.
22. Gurm HS, Dixon SR, Smith DE, Share D, LaLonde T, Greenbaum A, et al. Renal function-based contrast dosing to define safe limits of radiographic contrast media in patients undergoing percutaneous coronary interventions. *J Am Coll Cardiol*. 2011;58(9):907–914.
23. Laskey WK, Jenkins C, Selzer F, Marroquin OC, Wilensky RL, Glaser R, et al. Volume-to-creatinine clearance ratio: a pharmacokinetically based risk factor for prediction of early creatinine increase after percutaneous coronary intervention. *J Am Coll Cardiol*. 2007;50(7):584–590.
24. Jensen CT, Blair KJ, Wagner-Bartak NA, Vu LN, Carter BW, Sun J, et al. Comparison of abdominal computed tomographic enhancement and organ lesion depiction between weight-based scanner software contrast dosing and a fixed-dose protocol in a tertiary care oncologic center. *J Comput Assist Tomo*. 2019;43(1):155–162.
25. George AJ, Manghat NE, Hamilton MCK. Comparison between a fixed-dose contrast protocol and a weight-based contrast dosing protocol in abdominal CT. *Clin Radiol*. 2016;71(12). 1314. e1-1314.e9.
26. Davenport MS, Parikh KR, Mayo-Smith WW, Israel GM, Brown RKJ, Ellis JH. Effect of fixed-volume and weight-based dosing regimens on the cost and volume of administered iodinated contrast material at abdominal CT. *J Am Coll Radiol*. 2017;14(3):359–370.
27. Benbow M, Bull RK. Simple weight-based contrast dosing for standardization of portal phase CT liver enhancement. *Clin Radiol*. 2011;66(10):940–944.
28. Kessner R, Barnes S, Halpern P, Makrin V, Blachar A. CT for acute nontraumatic abdominal pain—is oral contrast really required? *Acad Radiol*. 2017;24(7):840–845.
29. Kielar AZ, Patlas MN, Katz DS. Oral contrast for CT in patients with acute non-traumatic abdominal and pelvic pain: what should be its current role? *Emerg Radiology*. 2016;23(5):477–481.
30. Shriki JE, Shinbane J, Lee C, Khan AR, Burns N, Hindoyan A, et al. Incidental myocardial infarct on conventional nongated CT: a review of the spectrum of findings with gated CT and cardiac MRI correlation. *Am J Roentgenol*. 2012;198(3):496–504.
31. Jacobs JM, Hill MC, Steinberg WM. Peptic ulcer disease: CT evaluation. *Radiology*. 1991;178(3):745–748.
32. Aguirre DA, Santosa AC, Casola G, Sirlin CB. Abdominal wall hernias: imaging features, complications, and diagnostic pitfalls at multi–detector row CT. *Radiographics*. 2005;25(6):1501–1520.
33. Geloven AAW, van, Biesheuvel TH, Luitse JSK, Hoitsma HFW, Obertop H. Hospital admissions of patients aged over 80 with acute abdominal complaints. *Eur J Surg*. 2000;166(11):866–871.
34. Sugi MD, Sun DC, Menias CO, Prabhu V, Choi HH. Acute diverticulitis: key features for guiding clinical management. *Eur J Radiol*. 2020;128:109026.
35. Sheiman L, Levine MS, Levin AA, Hogan J, Rubesin SE, Furth EE, et al. Chronic diverticulitis: clinical, radiographic, and pathologic findings. *Am J Roentgenol*. 2008;191(2):522–528.
36. Verheyden C, Orliac C, Millet I, Taourel P. Large-bowel obstruction: CT findings, pitfalls, tips and tricks. *Eur J Radiol*. 2020;130(9):1–10.
37. Lips LMJ, Cremers PTJ, Pickhardt PJ, Cremers SEH, Janssen-Heijnen MLG, de Witte MT, et al. Sigmoid cancer versus chronic diverticular disease: differentiating features at CT colonography. *Radiology*. 2015;275(1):127–135.
38. Peterson CM, Anderson JS, Hara AK, Carenza JW, Menias CO. Volvulus of the gastrointestinal tract: appearances at multimodality imaging. *Radiographics*. 2009;29(5):1281–1293.
39. Batke M, Cappell MS. Adynamic ileus and acute colonic pseudo-obstruction. *Med Clin N Am*. 2008;92(3):649–670.
40. Unal E, Mehmet RO, Balci S, Aysegul G, Erhan A, Medine B. Stercoral colitis: diagnostic value of CT findings. *Diagn Interv Radiol*. 2016;23(1):5–9.
41. Kirkpatrick IDC, Kroeker MA, Greenberg HM. Biphasic CT with mesenteric CT angiography in the evaluation of acute mesenteric ischemia: initial experience. *Radiology*. 2003;229(1):91–98.
42. Garzelli L, Nuzzo A, Copin P, Calame P, Corcos O, Vilgrain V, et al. Contrast-enhanced CT for the diagnosis of acute mesenteric ischemia. *Am J Roentgenol*. 2020;215(1):29–38.
43. Sinha D, Kale S, Kundaragi NG, Sharma S. Mesenteric ischemia: a radiologic perspective. *Abdom Radiol*. 2020:1–15.
44. Bird JR, Brahm GL, Fung C, Sebastian S, Kirkpatrick IDC. Recommendations for the management of incidental hepatobiliary findings in adults: endorsement and adaptation of the 2017 and 2013 ACR Incidental Findings Committee white papers by the Canadian Association of Radiologists Incidental Findings Working Group. *Can Assoc Radiologists J*. 2020;71(4):437–447.
45. Runner GJ, Corwin MT, Siewert B, Eisenberg RL. Gallbladder wall thickening. *Am J Roentgenol*. 2014;202(1):W1–W12.
46. Wells ML, Fenstad ER, Poterucha JT, Hough DM, Young PM, Araoz PA, et al. Imaging findings of congestive hepatopathy. *Radiographics*. 2016;36(4):1024–1037.
47. Gandhi D, Ojili V, Nepal P, Nagar A, Hernandez-Delima FJ, Bajaj D, et al. A pictorial review of gall stones and its associated complications. *Clin Imag*. 2019;60(2):228–236.
48. Mentzer RM, Golden GT, Chandler JG, Horsley JS. A comparative appraisal of emphysematous cholecystitis. *Am J Surg*. 1975;129(1):10–15.
49. Oyedeji FO, Voci S. Emphysematous cholecystitis. *Ultrasound Q*. 2014;30(3):246–248.

50. Huffman JL, Schenker S. Acute acalculous cholecystitis: a review. *Clin Gastroenterol H*. 2010;8(1):15–22.
51. Hanbidge AE, Buckler PM, O'Malley ME, Wilson SR. From the RSNA refresher courses: imaging evaluation for acute pain in the right upper quadrant. *Radiographics*. 2004;24(4):1117–1135.
52. Levy AD, Murakata LA, Rohrmann Jr. CA. Gallbladder carcinoma: radiologic-pathologic correlation. *Radiographics*. 2001;21(2):295–314.
53. Halabi WJ, Kang CY, Ketana N, Lafaro KJ, Nguyen VQ, Stamos MJ, et al. Surgery for gallstone ileus. *Ann Surg*. 2014;259(2):329–335.
54. Nijs ELF, Callahan MJ. Congenital and developmental pancreatic anomalies: ultrasound, computed tomography, and magnetic resonance imaging features. *Seminars Ultrasound Ct Mri*. 2007;28(5):395–401.
55. Wang Q, Swensson J, Hu M, Cui E, Tirkes T, Jennings SG, et al. Distribution and correlation of pancreatic gland size and duct diameters on MRCP in patients without evidence of pancreatic disease. *Abdom Radiol*. 2019;44(3):967–975.
56. Glaser J, Högemann B, Krummenerl T, Schneider M, Hultsch E, Van N, et al. Sonographic imaging of the pancreatic duct. *Dig Dis Sci*. 1987;32(10):1075–1081.
57. Tirkes T, Shah ZK, Takahashi N, Grajo JR, Chang ST, Venkatesh SK, et al. Reporting standards for chronic pancreatitis by using CT, MRI, and MR cholangiopancreatography: the consortium for the study of chronic pancreatitis, diabetes, and pancreatic cancer. *Radiology*. 2019;290(1):207–215.
58. Andersen PL, Madzak A, Olesen SS, Drewes AM, Frøkjaer JB. Quantification of parenchymal calcifications in chronic pancreatitis: relation to atrophy, ductal changes, fibrosis and clinical parameters. *Scand J Gastroentero*. 2017;53(2):1–7.
59. Campisi A, Brancatelli G, Vullierme M-P, Levy P, Ruzniewski P, Vilgrain V Are pancreatic calcifications specific for the diagnosis of chronic pancreatitis? A multidetector-row CT analysis. *Clin Radiol*. 2009;64(9):903–911.
60. Matsuda Y. Age-related morphological changes in the pancreas and their association with pancreatic carcinogenesis. *Pathol Int*. 2019;69(8):450–462.
61. Matsumoto S, Mori H, Miyaki H, Takaki H, Maeda T, Yamada Y, et al. Uneven fatty replacement of the pancreas: evaluation with CT. *Radiology*. 1995:453–458.
62. Hommos MS, Glassock RJ, Rule AD. Structural and functional changes in human kidneys with healthy aging. *J Am Soc Nephrol*. 2017;28(10):2838–2844.
63. Craig WD, Wagner BJ, Travis MD. Pyelonephritis: radiologic-pathologic review. *Radiographics*. 2008;28(1):255–276.
64. Tonolini M, Ippolito S. Cross-sectional imaging of complicated urinary infections affecting the lower tract and male genital organs. *Insights Imaging*. 2016;7(5):689–711.
65. Nepal P, Ojili V, Kaur N, Tirumani SH, Nagar A. Gas where it shouldn't be! Imaging spectrum of emphysematous infections in the abdomen and pelvis. *Am J Roentgenol*. 2021;216(3):812–823.
66. Huang J-J, Tseng C-C. Emphysematous pyelonephritis: clinicoradiological classification, management, prognosis, and pathogenesis. *Arch Intern Med*. 2000;160(6):797–805.
67. Rushworth RL, Torpy DJ, Falhammar H. Adrenal crises in older patients. *Lancet Diabetes Endocrinol*. 2020;8(7):628–639.
68. Mellnick VM, Heiken JP. The acute abdominal aorta. *Radiol Clin North Am*. 2015;53(6):1209–1224.
69. Chaikof EL, Dalman RL, Eskandari MK, Jackson BM, Lee WA, Mansour MA, et al. The Society for Vascular Surgery practice guidelines on the care of patients with an abdominal aortic aneurysm. *J Vasc Surg*. 2018;67(1):2–77. e2.
70. Halliday KE, al-Kutoubi A. Draped aorta: CT sign of contained leak of aortic aneurysms. *Radiology*. 1996;199(1):41–43.
71. Mehard WB, Heiken JP, Sicard GA. High-attenuating crescent in abdominal aortic aneurysm wall at CT: a sign of acute or impending rupture. *Radiology*. 1994;192(2):359–362.
72. Sever A, Rheinboldt M. Unstable abdominal aortic aneurysms: a review of MDCT imaging features. *Emerg Radiology*. 2016;23(2):187–196.
73. Rakita D, Newatia A, Hines JJ, Siegel DN, Friedman B. Spectrum of CT findings in rupture and impending rupture of abdominal aortic aneurysms. *RadioGraphics*. 2007;27(2):497–507.
74. Arita T, Matsunaga N, Takano K, Nagaoka S, Nakamura H, Katayama S, et al. Abdominal aortic aneurysm: rupture associated with the high-attenuating crescent sign. *Radiology*. 1997;204(3):765–768.
75. Siegel CL, Cohan RH, Korobkin M, Alpern MB, Courneya DL, Leder RA. Abdominal aortic aneurysm morphology: CT features in patients with ruptured and nonruptured aneurysms. *Am J Roentgenol*. 1994;163(5):1123–1129.
76. Sadro CT, Sandstrom CK, Verma N, Gunn ML. Geriatric trauma: a radiologist's guide to imaging trauma patients aged 65 years and older. *Radiographics*. 2015;35(4):1263–1285.
77. Yoshikawa T, Hayashi N, Maeda E, Matsuda I, Sasaki H, Ohtsu H, et al. Peritoneal fluid accumulation in healthy men and postmenopausal women: evaluation on pelvic MRI. *Am J Roentgenol*. 2013;200(6):1181–1185.
78. McGettigan MJ, Menias CO, Gao ZJ, Mellnick VM, Hara AK. Imaging of drug-induced complications in the gastrointestinal system. *Radiographics*. 2016;36(1):71–87.

Chapter 10

# Imaging of Musculoskeletal Infections Related to Recreational Drug Use

Joshua Gu, Saagar Patel, and Manickam Kumaravel

## Outline



## Key Points

- Imaging evaluation of musculoskeletal infections in recreational drug use is usually performed using radiographs, which are frequently nonspecific but may guide early treatment and can be used for subsequent monitoring of treatment algorithms.
- Magnetic resonance imaging (MRI) is often the imaging modality of choice for evaluating musculoskeletal infections, manifesting as increased T2 signal, correspondingly low T1 signal, and enhancement with intravenous contrast.
- In necrotizing fasciitis, early recognition of fascial edema and interfascial fluid on MRI is essential. These signs are detected before soft tissue gas and will facilitate prompt treatment and dramatically impact prognosis.
- Prompt diagnosis of osteomyelitis is essential to the initial early administration of antibiotics to prevent osteonecrosis, which leads to significant long-term pain and disability.

## Introduction

Recreational drug abuse is a significant problem worldwide, resulting in substantial morbidity and mortality, as well as economic impact. The United Nations Office on Drugs and Crime estimates that, in 2017, 271 million people, constituting 5.5% of the global population aged 15 to 64 years, had used drugs in the previous year.[1] This was similar to recent years but represented a 30% increase from 2009, when an estimated 210 million people had used drugs in the previous year. In addition, the economic impacts of recreational drug use are significant, with 585,000 deaths and 42 million years of "healthy" life lost in 2017.[1]

Injected drug abuse is particularly problematic: of those who abused drugs, an estimated 11.3 million worldwide injected them, with a large proportion of those people residing in the United States, China, and Russia. Injected drug abuse leads to significant health consequences. For instance, human immunodeficiency virus (HIV) and hepatitis C infections are highly prevalent among people who inject drugs (PWID), affecting 1.4 million and 5.6 million people, respectively.[2] More acute infectious sequelae of injected drug use are numerous, including localized soft tissue infections such as cellulitis, abscess, and necrotizing fasciitis; local and distant bone and joint infections such as osteomyelitis and septic arthritis; and distant vascular pathologies such as septic thrombophlebitis and mycotic aneurysm.

Because the clinical presentation of musculoskeletal infections may overlap, histories are often unreliable with PWID, and prompt treatment of pathologies such as necrotizing fasciitis and septic arthritis are critical, imaging plays a crucial role in the diagnosis of infections. Diagnosis often starts with radiographs, which, aside from being inexpensive and readily available, provide important anatomic information and may guide subsequent imaging and treatment decisions.

Ultrasound (US) is helpful in evaluating fluid collections such as abscesses and joint effusions. If a collection is identified, it may be used to guide aspiration. It is especially beneficial in the pediatric population, as it produces no ionizing radiation and does not require sedation. However, it is heavily user-dependent and provides little additional value in older patients.[3]

Computed tomography (CT) is fast, relatively inexpensive, and widely available in emergency departments, and provides high spatial resolution and bony detail. CT with intravenous (IV) contrast can be used to evaluate for any enhancing lesions or areas of inflammation and can detect changes of osteomyelitis earlier than conventional radiography, but not as early as magnetic resonance imaging (MRI). The most significant drawback of CT is its use of ionizing radiation.

MRI is the modality of choice in diagnosing most musculoskeletal infections because of its superior soft tissue resolution and sensitivity for pathologic fluid.[3] It is the most sensitive modality for acute osteomyelitis. However, MRI is relatively costly and time-consuming, may not always be available, and can possibly be contraindicated due to incompatible implanted devices/hardware.[3]

## Soft Tissue Infections

### CELLULITIS

Cellulitis is defined as an infection of the dermis and subcutaneous soft tissues. Diagnosis is typically clinical; however, imaging may be beneficial in PWID due to the increased risk of complications, such as an abscess or venous thrombosis. Clinically, cellulitis presents as a painful, poorly defined area of inflammatory skin changes, such as edema, erythema, and warmth. Systemic symptoms such as fever and chills may be present.

Radiographic findings of cellulitis are nonspecific and include indirect signs of infection, such as generalized swelling and obliteration of fascial planes (Fig. 10.1). Radiography may reveal retained radiopaque foreign bodies such as needles in drug abusers, which may serve as a nidus for infection (Fig. 10.2).[4] Cellulitis demonstrates soft tissue edema, resulting in a "cobblestone" appearance of subcutaneous fat on US (Fig. 10.3), as well as increased echogenicity of the soft tissues. This is a nonspecific appearance on grayscale US and may be present with other causes of subcutaneous edema, such as congestive heart failure or fluid overload. One distinguishing feature of edema due to infection is the presence of hyperemia on Doppler imaging (Fig. 10.4). On CT, cellulitis demonstrates increased attenuation of the subcutaneous fat with inflammatory changes, such as stranding and skin thickening (Figs. 10.5, 10.6).[3]

MRI investigation of cellulitis typically includes pre- and postcontrast T1-weighted images, T2-weighted

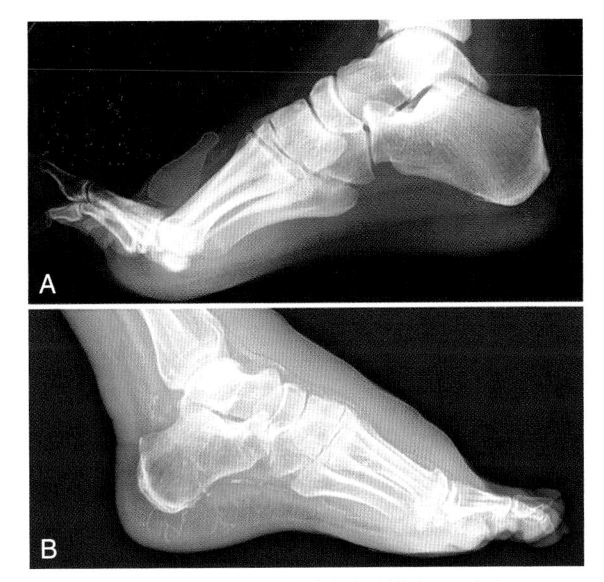


**Fig. 10.1** Lateral radiograph of the right foot (A) demonstrates an area of soft tissue swelling (blue shaded area) along the dorsum of the foot, without periosteal bone reaction, representing cellulitis. Lateral radiograph of the left foot (B) in a different patient demonstrates more extensive soft tissue swelling (green shaded area) along the dorsum of the foot.

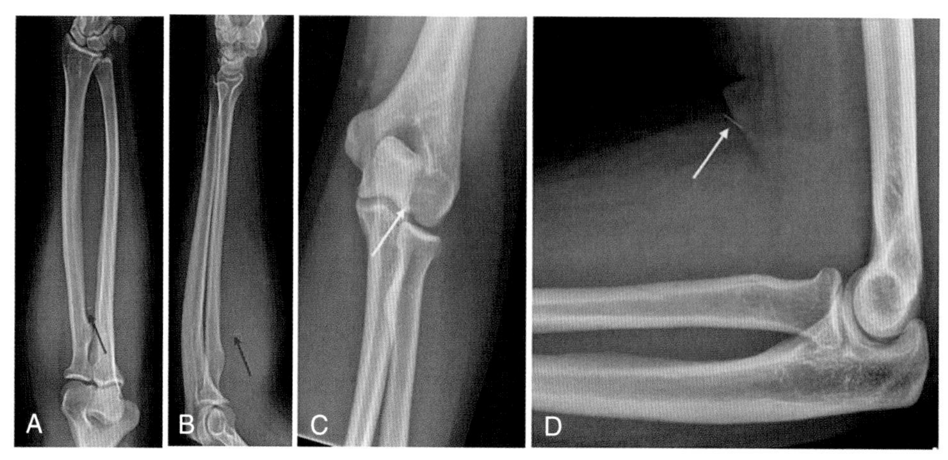


Fig. 10.2 Anteroposterior (AP) (A) and lateral (B) radiographs of the right forearm in a patient with history of heroin abuse demonstrates a thin, linear, radiodense object in the proximal volar soft tissues (red arrows), representing a retained needle. AP (C) and lateral (D) radiographs of the left elbow in a separate patient, also with history of heroin abuse, demonstrate a similar thin, linear, radiodense object in the antecubital fossa (yellow arrows), representing a retained needle.

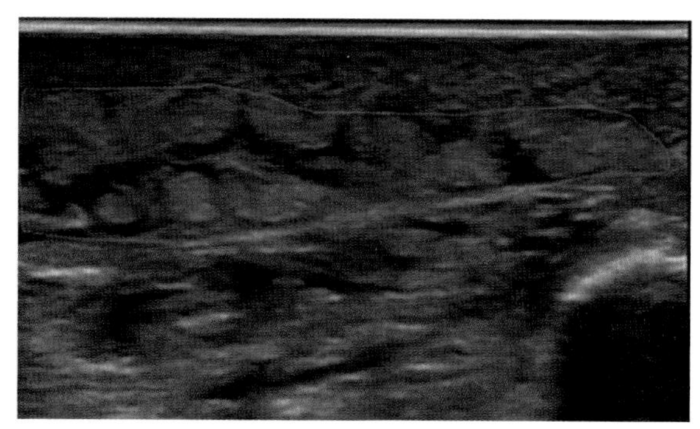

Fig. 10.3 Greyscale ultrasound image of the palmar surface of the hand demonstrates the characteristic "cobblestone" appearance of subcutaneous edema (blue shaded area), consistent with cellulitis.

images, and fluid-sensitive sequences such as short tau inversion recovery (STIR).[5] Diffusion-weighted imaging (DWI) may be added to assess for abscess formation, which will restrict diffusion. Cellulitis appears as a high T2 and STIR signal within the subcutaneous tissues with corresponding low T1 signal and contrast enhancement (Fig. 10.7).

Treatment of cellulitis involves antibiotics and supportive measures.

## ABSCESS

A potential complication of cellulitis is the formation of an abscess, an encapsulated purulent fluid collection, which may be located in superficial or deep soft tissues. Abscesses may form via direct extension from injection sites or due to hematogenous seeding from distant sites. Abscesses are more likely to form around retained foreign bodies and in immunocompromised states, both of which are more prevalent among PWID. Clinical presentation of abscesses depends somewhat on location and depth. Systemic signs and symptoms such as fever, chills, leukocytosis, and elevated inflammatory markers are common.

Abscesses are difficult to visualize on conventional radiographs because, aside from soft tissue swelling, the sequelae of abscesses may be the only indicator, such as adjacent joint effusions or periosteal reactions (Fig. 10.8). On US, abscesses appear as well-defined anechoic cavitary collections with peripheral hyperemia (Fig. 10.9). Mobile internal debris or septae are often seen within abscesses. US is also a useful tool to guide abscess aspiration and drainage.

When abscesses are located in deep soft tissues, US may be inadequate for evaluation, and CT may be required. Abscesses appear on CT as fluid collections with rim enhancement and adjacent inflammatory changes (Fig. 10.10). Like US, CT may be used to guide aspiration and drainage.

On MRI, abscesses exhibit increased T2 and STIR signal with corresponding low T1 signal and peripheral enhancement (Figs. 10.11 and 10.12). DWI will

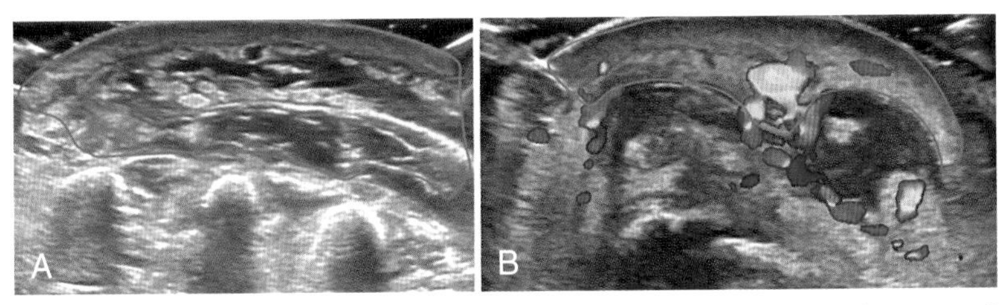


Fig. 10.4 Greyscale (A) and color Doppler (B) ultrasound of the wrist demonstrates complex, edematous subcutaneous tissue (blue shaded area) and hyperemia, consistent with cellulitis.

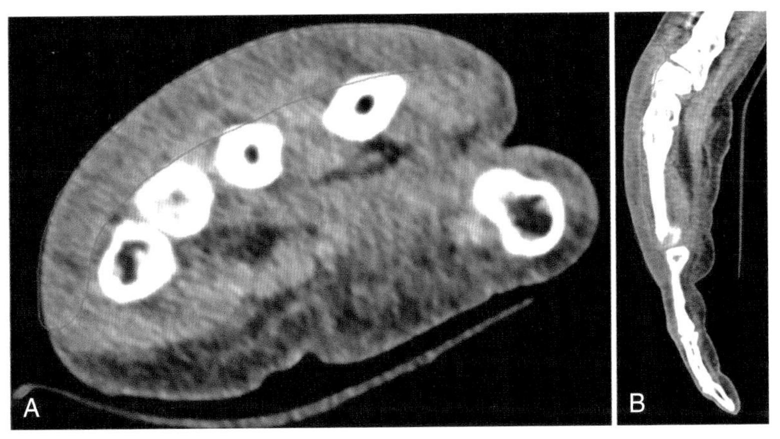


Fig. 10.5 Contrast-enhanced axial (A) and sagittal (B) computed tomography of the right hand in soft tissue window demonstrate diffuse soft tissue swelling and subcutaneous fat stranding of the dorsum of the hand (blue shaded area) representing cellulitis.

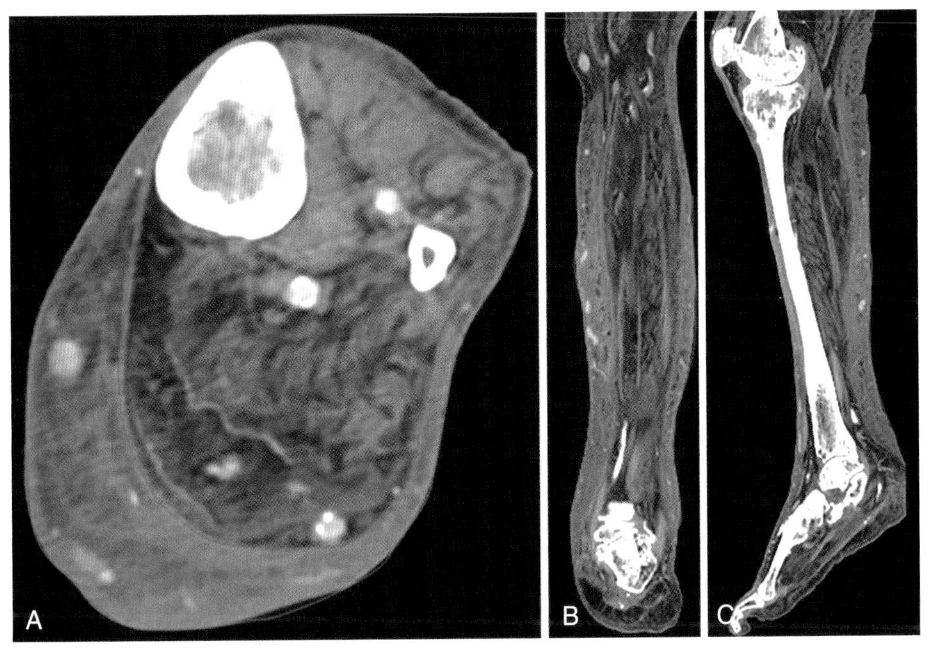


Fig. 10.6 Contrast-enhanced axial (A), coronal (B), and sagittal (C) computed tomography of the left lower extremity in soft tissue window demonstrate diffuse severe superficial soft tissue swelling and subcutaneous fat stranding (blue shaded area) without drainable collection or deep fascial involvement, consistent with cellulitis.

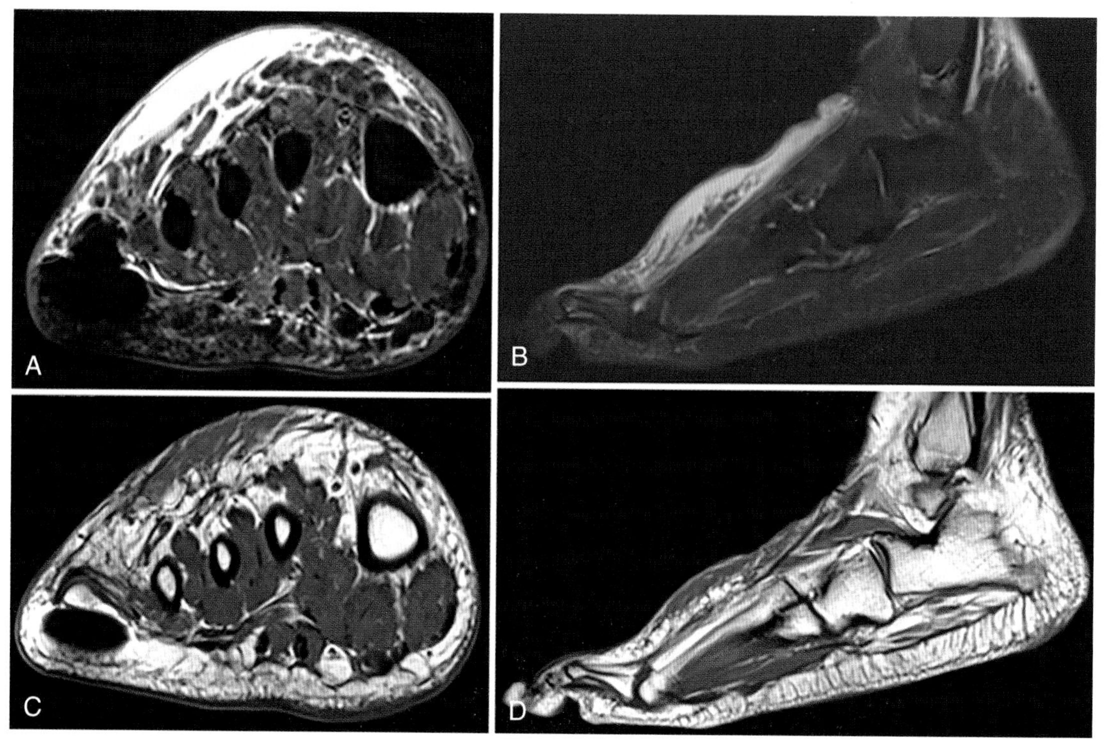


**Fig. 10.7** Axial (A) and sagittal (B) T2-weighted magnetic resonance imaging (MRI) with fat saturation of the right foot demonstrate diffuse T2 hyperintensity along the dorsal cutaneous and subcutaneous soft tissues. Axial (C) and sagittal (D) T1-weighted MRI of the same region demonstrate a smaller region of T1 hypointensity along the dorsal soft tissues. Findings are consistent with cellulitis.

show restricted diffusion internally. Apparent diffusion coefficients of 0.6 to $1.1 \times 10^{-3}$ $mm^2/s$ generally indicate true restricted diffusion seen with abscesses.

In addition to antibiotics and supportive measures, drainage of abscesses may be required. Simple abscesses may be drained percutaneously via imaging guidance. However, complex or multiloculated abscesses may require surgical drainage.

## INCLUSION CYST

Epidermoid or implantation dermoid is an encapsulation of keratin- and lipid-rich debris from inoculation of the hair follicle or epithelial cells to the underlying dermis, often secondary to penetrating trauma, such as IV drug abuse. Over time, PWID lose access to superficial veins and introduce drugs and toxins via subcutaneous or intradermal routes, or through a practice referred to as "skin popping," which may lead to depressed lesions with central pallor and occasional surrounding ecchymosis. Epidermoid cysts are usually asymptomatic but can become a nidus for infection, especially with repeated localized trauma and the introduction of bacteria. Superficial lesions may be evaluated with US, which will show a lipid-rich cyst. CT may be employed for deeper cysts, which will show an encapsulated lesion without peripheral enhancement in the absence of superimposed infection.[4]

Treatment is relatively simple, with no intervention needed unless the patient develops an abscess or localized infection.

## PYOMYOSITIS

Pyomyositis refers to a bacterial infection of skeletal muscle, which may progress to an intramuscular abscess. It is an uncommon entity, as skeletal muscle is relatively resistant to infection.[6] Predisposing factors include the introduction of foreign bodies, such as infected needles, and immunocompromised state, such as HIV infection. Pyomyositis typically presents with acute muscle pain along with typical

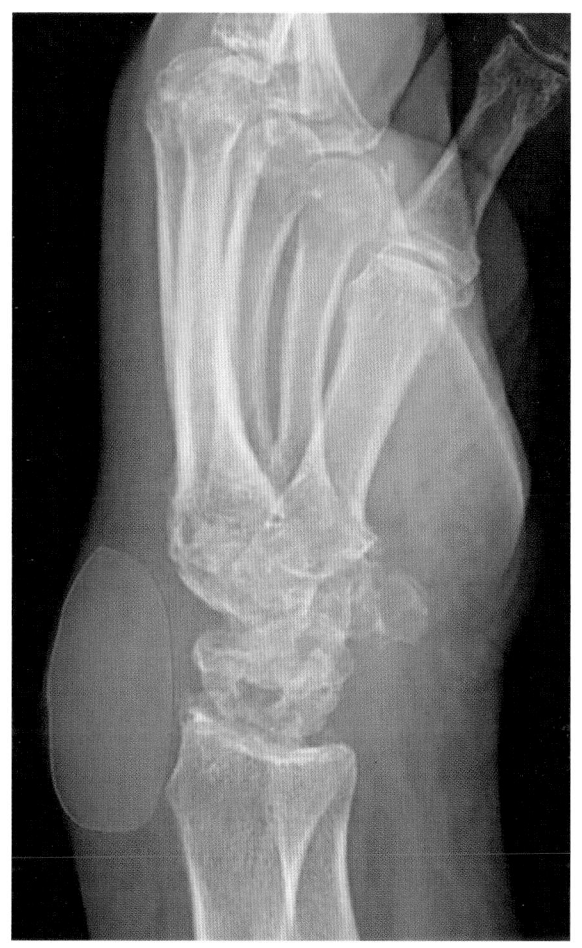

**Fig. 10.8** Lateral radiograph of the wrist demonstrates focal soft tissue swelling of the dorsum of the wrist (blue shaded area) representing an abscess.

inflammatory symptoms, such as edema, warmth, fever, and leukocytosis.

Radiographic findings of pyomyositis are nonspecific, demonstrating only generalized edema and possibly asymmetrically increased muscle bulk. US findings are also limited and include increased muscle volume due to edema or intramuscular fluid collections in the case of progression to an abscess, in which case US may be used to guide aspiration and drainage.

Cross-sectional imaging is critical in the evaluation of pyomyositis. CT will show asymmetric muscle bulk with decreased attenuation indicative of edema, with marginal enhancement after contrast administration (Fig. 10.13). Thickening of regional fascial planes and overlying skin may also be seen. MRI is more sensitive to pyomyositis than CT and will show increased T1- and T2-weighted signal intensity (Figs. 10.14 and 10.15).[7] If an abscess is present, it will demonstrate typical findings, namely a high T2/STIR signal with a surrounding T1 hypointense rim that enhances after contrast administration. Regions of nonenhancement on CT or MRI may indicate muscle necrosis.[4]

Treatment of pyomyositis includes targeted antimicrobial therapy and drainage of any intramuscular abscesses, which may be assisted by imaging guidance.

## NECROTIZING FASCIITIS

One of the most feared infectious processes in recreational drug use is necrotizing fasciitis, a rare necrotic infection of the subcutaneous and superficial soft tissues that rapidly involves the fascial planes and muscles. In addition to IV drug abuse, common risk factors

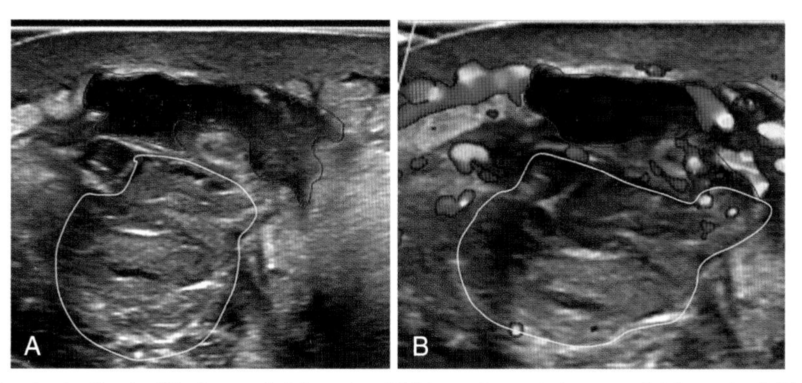


**Fig. 10.9** Grayscale (A) and color Doppler (B) ultrasound of the antecubital fossa demonstrate a superficial complex fluid collection (red outline) representing an abscess and increased regional blood flow representing hyperemia. Mild increased echogenicity of the deeper musculature (yellow outline) suggests a degree of myositis.

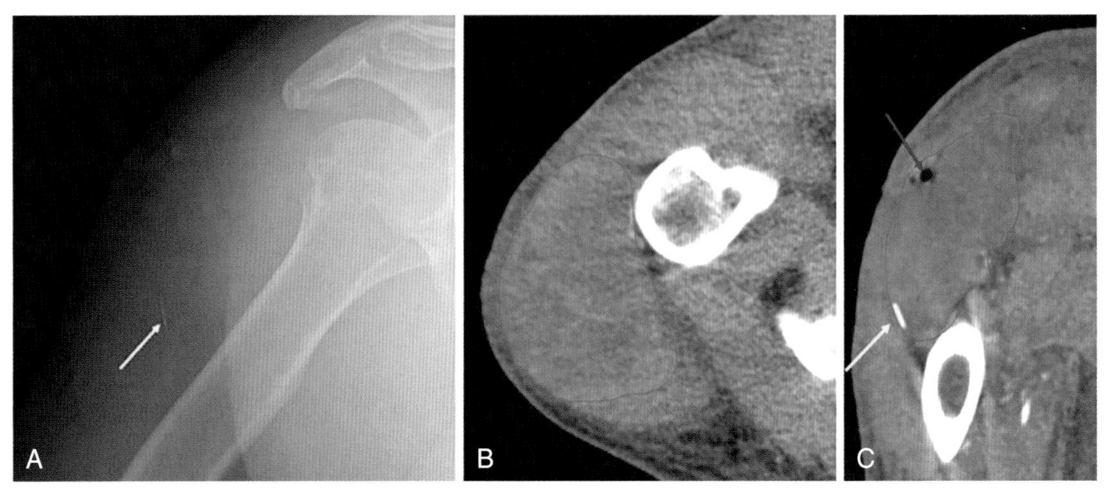


**Fig. 10.10** Anteroposterior radiograph (A) of the humerus demonstrate diffuse soft tissue swelling and a focal, linear, radiodense object (yellow arrow) representing a retained needle. Contrast-enhanced axial (B) and coronal (C) computed tomography in soft tissue window of the same patient show a heterogeneous area of mass-like density (blue shaded area) and a small focus of soft tissue gas (red arrow). The linear density (yellow arrow) representing the retained needle is redemonstrated.

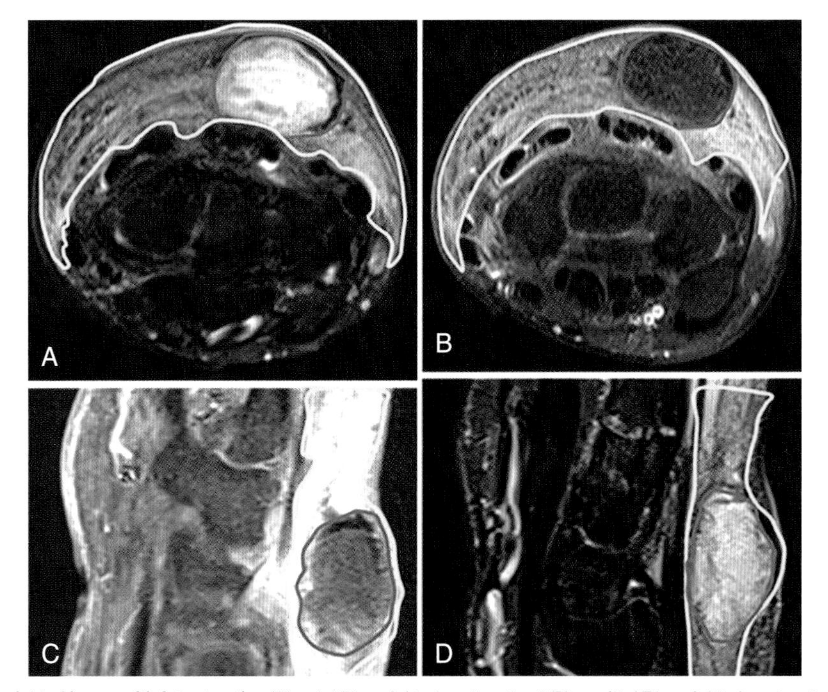


**Fig. 10.11** Axial T2-weighted image with fat saturation (A), axial T1-weighted postcontrast (B), sagittal T1-weighted postcontrast with fat saturation (C), and short tau inversion recovery (D) magnetic resonance imaging of the wrist demonstrate diffuse T2 hyperintensity and enhancement along the dorsum of the wrist (yellow outline) surrounding a focal area of T1 hypointensity/T2 hyperintensity with peripheral enhancement (blue outline), consistent with focal abscess formation.

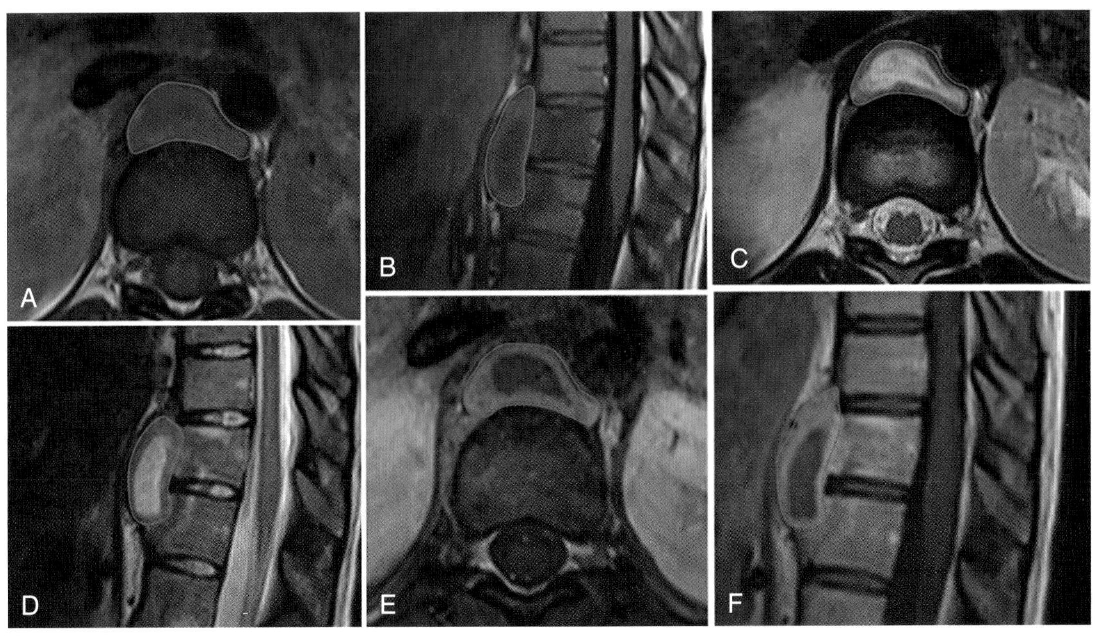


**Fig. 10.12** Axial and sagittal T1-weighted (A, B), T2-weighted (C, D), and T1-weighted postcontrast (E, F) magnetic resonance imaging of the lower thoracic spine demonstrates a T1 hypointense, T2 hyperintense, and peripherally enhancing fluid collection (blue shaded area) anterior to the T11 and T12 vertebral bodies, consistent with a paraspinal abscess.

include diabetes mellitus and peripheral arterial disease. Clinical evaluation is often difficult, because the presentation of necrotizing fasciitis may overlap with more benign soft tissue infections such as cellulitis. Signs and symptoms suggestive of necrotizing fasciitis include severe pain, crepitus indicative of subcutaneous gas, and bullae or blister formation. These may quickly progress to more ominous systemic symptoms such as fever, sepsis, and hypotension/shock.

Imaging plays a critical role in diagnosing and evaluating necrotizing fasciitis, as prompt surgical debridement is required. Findings of conventional radiographs and US are similar to those seen with cellulitis, with subcutaneous gas occasionally seen as lucencies within the soft tissues on the radiograph (Fig. 10.16) and linear echogenic foci, referred to as "ring-down artifact" on US (Figs. 10.17 and 10.18). Cross-sectional imaging is helpful to show deep fascial thickening, fluid collections tracking along fascial planes, and regional inflammation of the fat and muscle. Soft tissue gas will also be seen if a gas-forming anaerobe is present (Fig. 10.19). MRI will demonstrate increased fluid signal (T2/STIR) and loss of the normal T1 muscle texture (Figs. 10.20–10.22).[5] If gas is present, it will be visualized as a signal loss on gradient-echo images. Necrotic tissue is indicated by abnormal hypoenhancement after contrast administration.

Treatment of necrotizing fasciitis involves prompt, aggressive surgical debridement with broad-spectrum antibiotics, including anaerobic coverage.

## INFECTIOUS TENOSYNOVITIS

Infectious tenosynovitis is defined as an infection of a synovial membrane and underlying tendon, which often results from localized penetrating trauma. In recreational drug users, open wounds or needle ("track") marks may introduce pathogens to the tendon or sheath, which causes localized inflammation and infection.

The initial clinical presentation of tenosynovitis may resemble cellulitis, septic arthritis, or abscess, but a characteristic finding on physical examination is pain with muscle contraction. Erythema and edema may follow along tendon sheath planes and involve adjacent muscle bellies and bursae. A common site of infection in the hand is the flexor tendons, leading to pyogenic flexor tenosynovitis. This may manifest as a

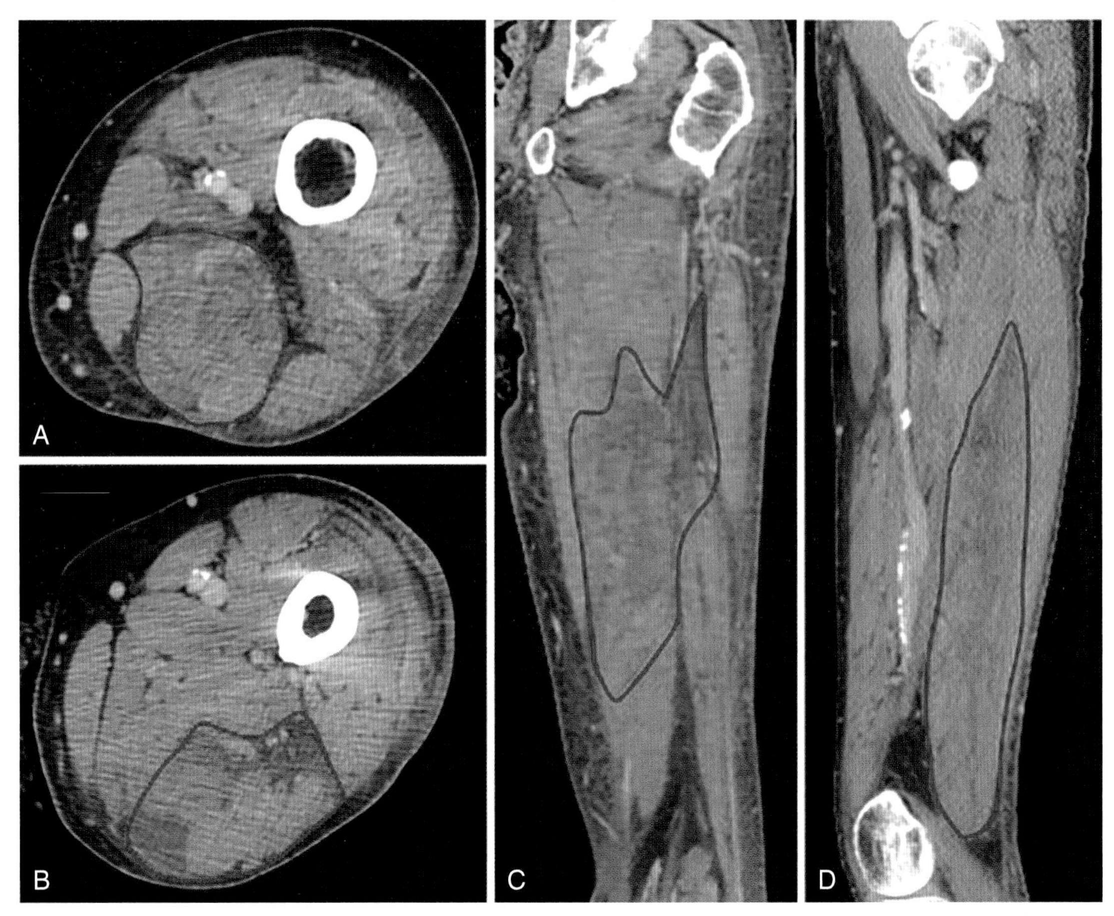


**Fig. 10.13** Contrast-enhanced axial (A and B), coronal (C), and sagittal (D) computed tomography of the left thigh demonstrate enlargement and heterogeneous enhancement of the hamstring muscles, most prominently affecting the semimembranosus muscle (red outline), representing pyomyositis.

"horseshoe abscess," which is an infection of the tendon sheath that is typically shared between the first and fifth metacarpals.[8]

The tendon sheath is not usually visible on US unless there is abnormal swelling. In tenosynovitis, US will show thickening of the synovial sheath and increased fluid tracking within. Using color Doppler may differentiate between chronic and acute disease: an acute process will have frank fluid, rather than just synovial thickening. These US findings have been reported to be 94% sensitive and 65% specific.

MRI is the preferred imaging modality and will show hypointense T1-weighted signal, hyperintense T2-weighted signal, and distension of the tendon sheath with areas of thickening (Fig. 10.23).

Clinically, the Kanavel criteria may be used to stage or grade cases of flexor tenosynovitis of the hand. These criteria include fusiform swelling, tenderness to palpation, pain with passive extension, and a flexed posture of the affected finger. The Michon classification may also be used to stage the infection. Stage I refers to increased fluid within the sheath, stage II refers to purulent synovial fluid, and stage III refers to necrosis of the involved structures.

Initial treatment of infectious tenosynovitis includes intravenous antibiotic therapy and observation.[9] If the infection does not improve within days of antibiotic administration, surgical intervention may be necessary, which involves tendon sheath irrigation and drainage, with or without debridement of surrounding

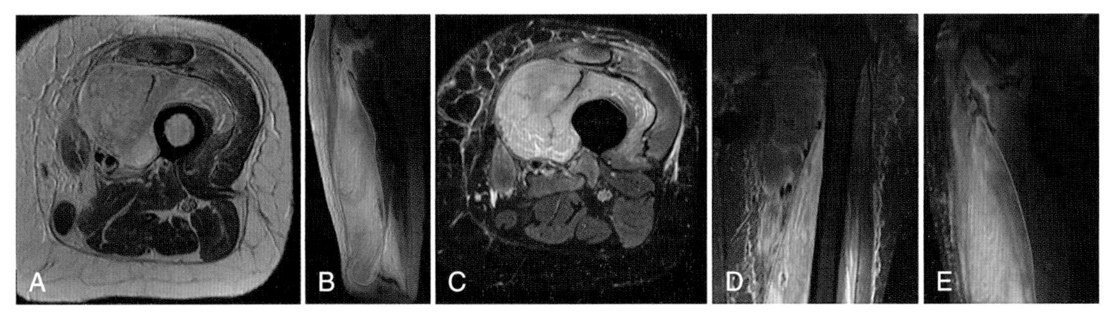


**Fig. 10.14** Axial (A) and sagittal (B) T1-weighted and axial (C), coronal (D), and sagittal (E) T2-weighted magnetic resonance imaging of the left thigh demonstrates mild T1 hyperintensity and heterogeneous T2 hyperintensity (blue shaded areas) of the quadriceps musculature representing edema, most severely involving the vastus medialis muscle, consistent with pyomyositis.

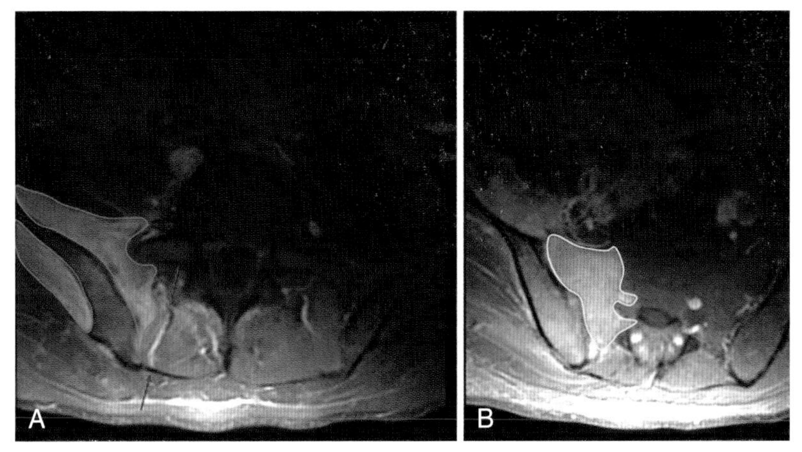


**Fig. 10.15** Multiple axial T2-weighted magnetic resonance images of the lumbosacral spine demonstrate hyperintensity within the right sacroiliac joint (red arrows) indicating joint effusion and hyperintensity of the adjacent musculature (blue shaded area). Hyperintense T2-weighted signal in the sacrum (yellow shaded area) represents bone marrow edema. Findings are consistent with sacroiliitis with adjacent myositis.

necrotic tissue and the sheath itself, depending on the stage of infection.[10]

### CHONDRITIS

Multiple cases of chondritis secondary to drug use have been reported. The most common complications include nasal chondritis from snorting and smoking cocaine. Patients often are seen to have a loss of turbinates, maxillary sinus mucosal thickening, and severe thinning or loss of the nasal septum. Cocaine is known to cause micronecrosis of the surrounding bone and cartilaginous tissue leading to extensive erosion. Physical examination findings include epistaxis, crusting, nasal obstruction, and saddle nose deformity. Examination findings can be correlated to drug use or rarely granulomatosis with polyangiitis.

Distinguishing factors can be seen on imaging with MRI, which can show hypointense T2-weighted signal involving the inferior turbinate and nasal septum for chronic drug use patients. Involvement tends to follow a "centrifugal" pattern, with progression of the necrosis from the nasal septum to the nasal walls.[11]

Treatment depends on severity of symptoms, with occasional surgical intervention to improve obstruction and/or vasculopathy.

## Bone and Joint Infections

### OSTEOMYELITIS

Osteomyelitis refers to inflammation of the bone, almost always due to infection, which may be acute or chronic. Clinically, acute osteomyelitis presents with

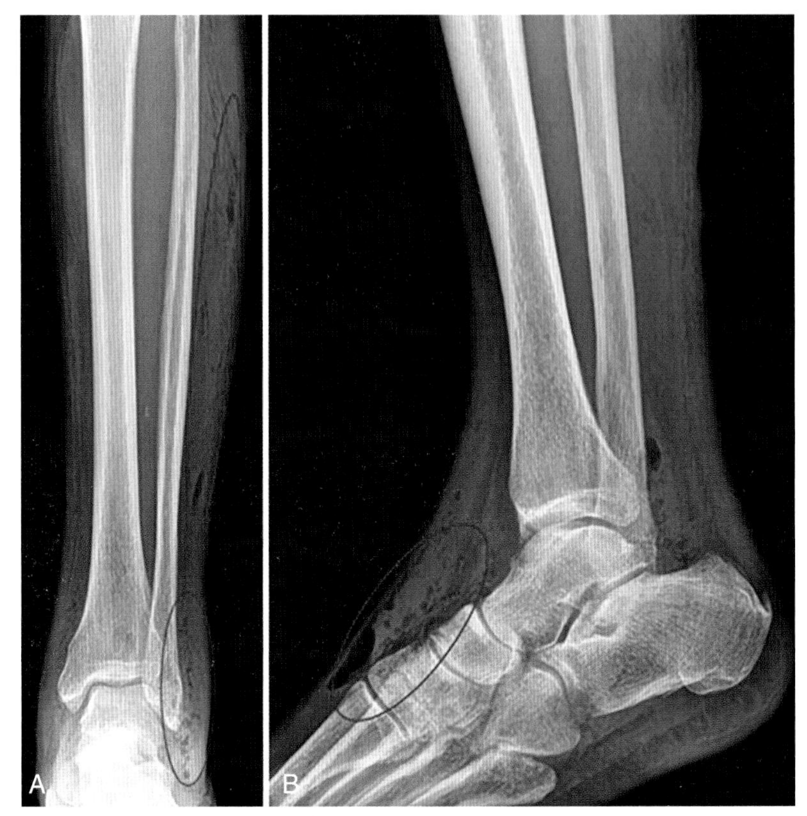


**Fig. 10.16** Anteroposterior (A) and lateral (B) radiographs of the left tibia-fibula and ankle demonstrate mild soft tissue swelling and scattered linear subcutaneous/interfascial gas (red ovals), suggestive of necrotizing fasciitis.

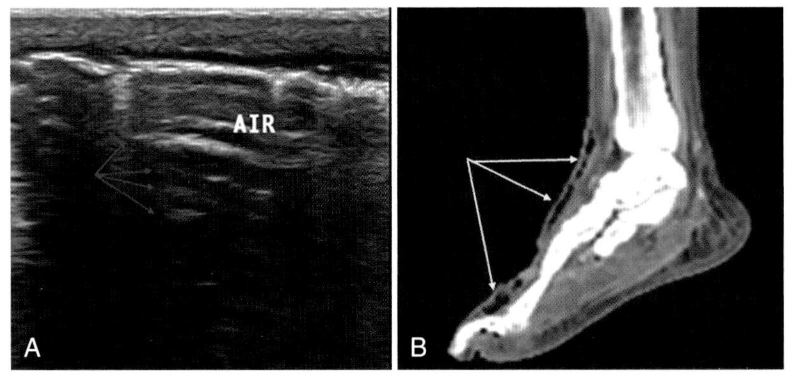


**Fig. 10.17** Greyscale (A) ultrasound of the dorsal aspect of the right foot demonstrate multiple ill-defined layering linear hyperechoic foci (red arrows) representing "ring-down artifact," suggestive of subcutaneous gas. Contrast-enhanced sagittal computed tomography (B) of the right foot in soft tissue window in the same patient confirms subcutaneous gas (yellow arrows), as well as significant soft tissue edema.

focal symptoms such as bone pain, erythema, and draining sinus tracts and more nonspecific symptoms such as fever, chills, and elevated inflammatory markers. Generally, osteomyelitis due to hematogenous spread will cause a slow, progressive condition, while infection from direct local extension will result in a more acute, pronounced presentation. Moreover, hematogenous osteomyelitis most often involves the

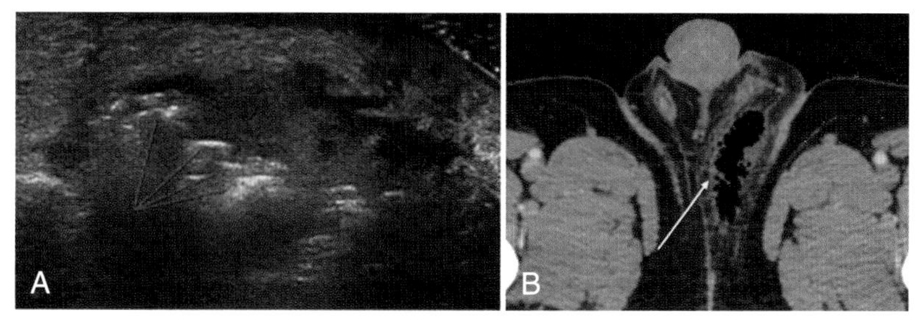


**Fig. 10.18** Greyscale ultrasound (A) of the groin demonstrates curvilinear echogenic foci (red arrows) with posterior dirty shadowing, indicative of subcutaneous gas. Contrast-enhanced axial computed tomography (B) of the same patient in soft tissue window confirms a large amount of gas (yellow arrow) within the left perineum/groin.

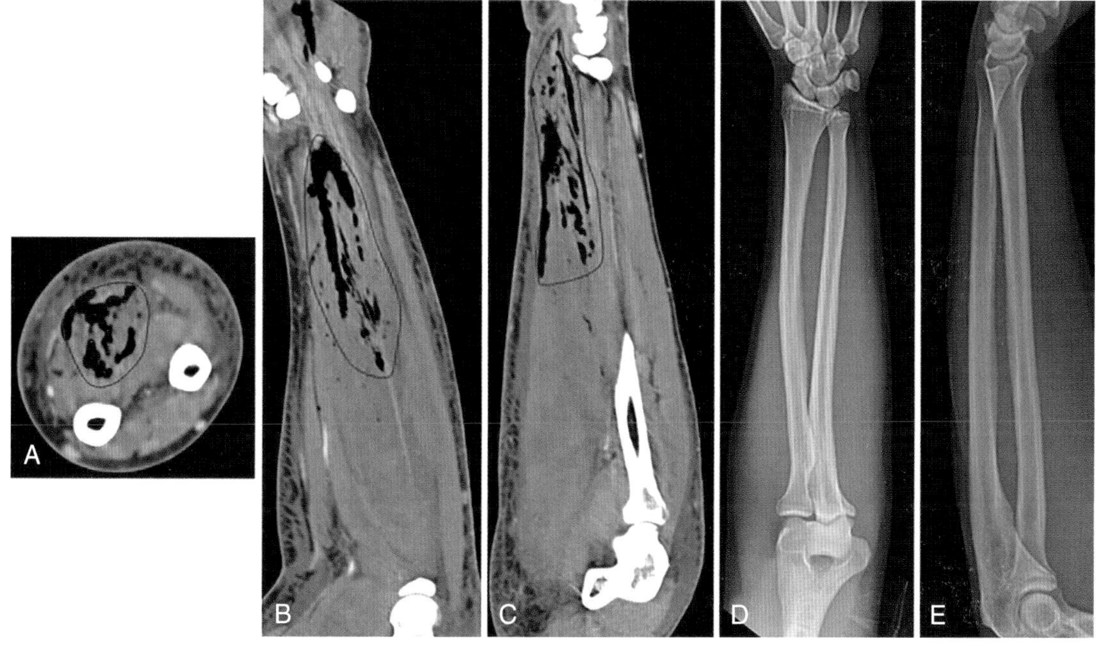


**Fig. 10.19** Contrast-enhanced axial (A), coronal (B), and sagittal (C) computed tomography (CT) of the left forearm demonstrate diffuse deep soft tissue edema with extensive linear anterior compartment soft tissue gas in the intermuscular and interfascial compartment (red outline), consistent with necrotizing fasciitis. Of note, anteroposterior (D) and lateral (E) radiographs were normal 9 hours prior to the CT, illustrating the potential for rapid progression of disease.

spine in adults, whereas local spread may infect any bone, particularly those near injection sites.[12]

Prompt diagnosis of osteomyelitis is essential to facilitate early administration of antibiotics and to prevent osteonecrosis, which may lead to significant long-term pain and disability. Evaluation of patients with suspected osteomyelitis in the emergency setting typically begins with radiographs to provide supporting evidence for osteomyelitis or suggest alternative diagnoses. Radiographs will show soft tissue changes such as edema and blurring of fascial planes. Specific bony changes include periosteal reaction, focal osteopenia, cortical erosion, and endosteal scalloping. While these early radiographic findings are relatively specific, they are rather insensitive, as erosions involving up to 30% of bone may be required to be visible on radiographs,

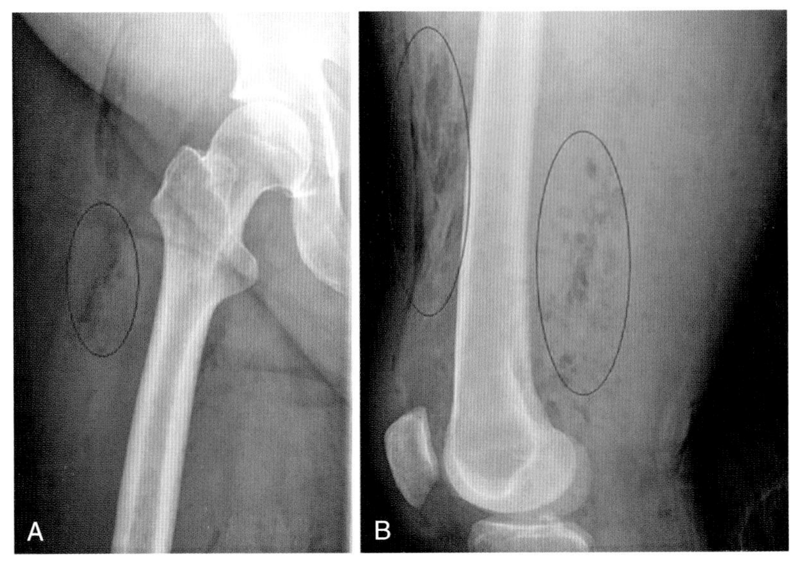


**Fig. 10.20** Anteroposterior (A) and lateral (B) radiographs of the right thigh demonstrate extensive intramuscular and subcutaneous linear gas shadows (red ovals) consistent with necrotizing fasciitis.

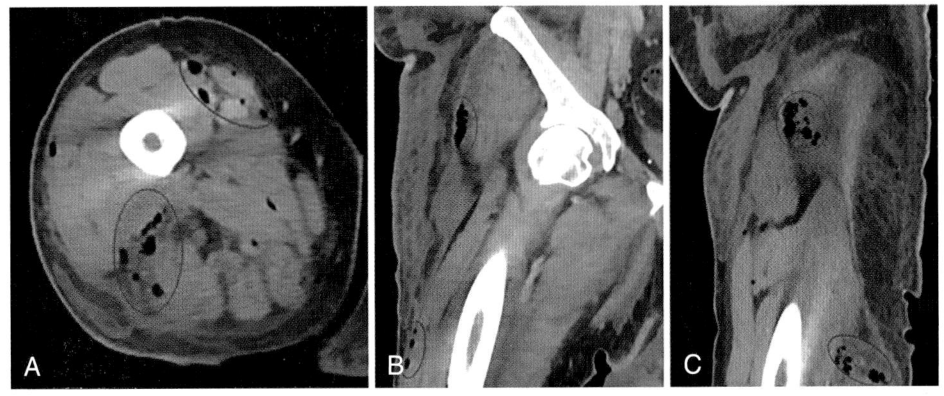


**Fig. 10.21** Axial (A), coronal (B), and sagittal (C) computed tomography images of the right hip and thigh in the same patient further demonstrate the subcutaneous edema (blue shaded area) and intramuscular gas (red ovals).

which can take up to 3 weeks to develop. During the subacute and chronic phases of osteomyelitis, Brodie abscesses may form, appearing as well-circumscribed lucent lesions that typically involve the extremities.[13]

US may be used to detect osteomyelitis several days earlier than conventional radiographs. An additional advantage of US is that it may be used in patients whose evaluation by cross-sectional imaging would be limited, such as those with orthopedic hardware causing beam hardening artifact on CT, or those with implanted devices that contraindicate MRI. On US, acute osteomyelitis causes elevation of the periosteum with a hypoechoic layer of infectious debris. Soft tissue abscesses may also be visible in the case of subacute or chronic osteomyelitis.

While CT provides superior anatomic detail, especially of the bones, it will show similar findings of osteomyelitis to those seen on conventional radiographs; namely, soft tissue swelling, local osteopenia, cortical erosions, and periosteal reaction. CT is particularly useful in cases of chronic osteomyelitis, as it may better show cortical thickening, sclerotic

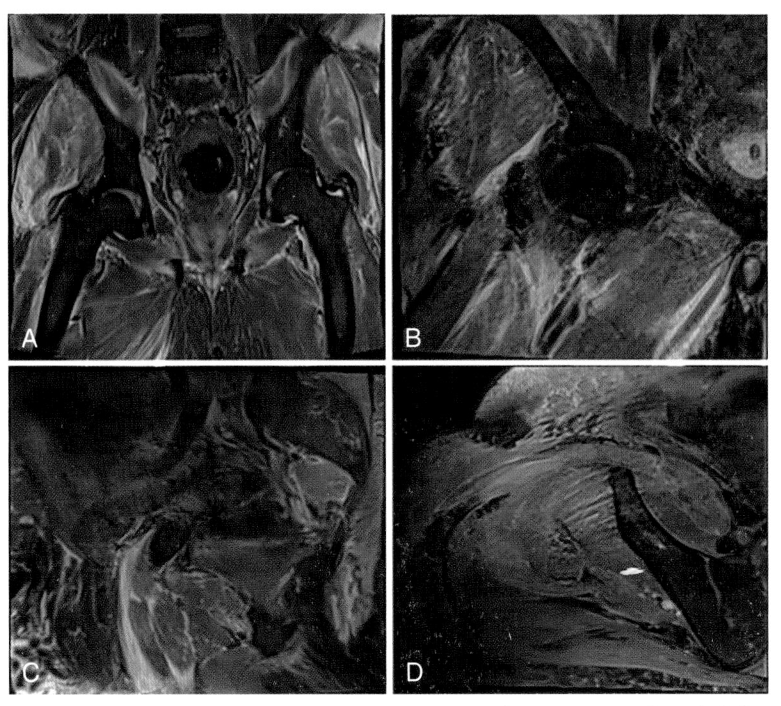


**Fig. 10.22** Coronal T2-weighted magnetic resonance (MR) image of the pelvis (A) and focused coronal (B), sagittal (C), and axial (D) T2-weighted MR images of the right hip in the same patient demonstrate multifocal fascial thickening, muscle edema, and interfascial fluid (blue shaded area) consistent with necrotizing fasciitis.

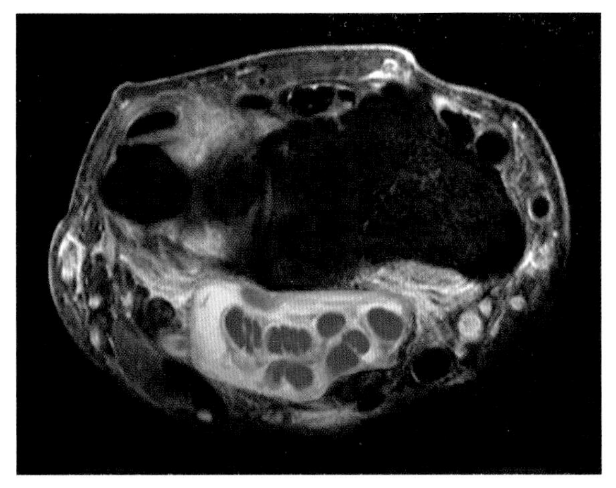

**Fig. 10.23** Axial T2-weighted image of the wrist demonstrates hyperintensity and thickening of the flexor tenosynovium (blue shaded area), consistent with tenosynovitis.

changes, draining sinuses, and sequestra that would be obscured on radiographs.[14]

MRI is the imaging modality of choice for the diagnosis of osteomyelitis because of its superior soft tissue resolution and sensitivity for the earliest changes of osteomyelitis, such as bone marrow edema, which manifest as early as 1 to 2 days after infection onset. MRI protocol should include fluid-sensitive sequences such as STIR, T2, or proton density and T1-weighted sequences in at least two planes. Bone marrow edema demonstrates fluid signal within the bone: high T2 and STIR signal with corresponding low T1 signal. Affected bone will enhance with contrast (Fig. 10.24). If low T1 signal is absent, findings may represent reactive osteitis rather than acute osteomyelitis.[15]

Despite the high sensitivity of MRI to acute osteomyelitis, bone biopsy is the gold standard for diagnosis. However, yield of positive cultures from bone biopsy is low. A recent study found that only 21% of bone biopsies yielded positive cultures, most of which grew *Staphylococcus aureus* and *Escherichia coli*, which were frequently also grown from wound cultures.[14] Administration of empiric antibiotics prior to biopsy may lower yield; however, this is controversial. One possible reason for

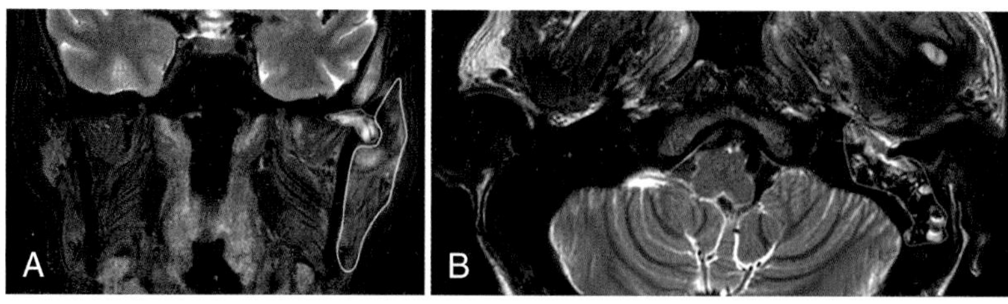


**Fig. 10.24** Coronal T2-weighted magnetic resonance image (A) of the midface demonstrate asymmetric hyperintense signal (blue outline) of the left temporomandibular joint with erosive changes of the mandibular condyle (not imaged), consistent with septic temporomandibular joint arthritis and osteomyelitis. Also note asymmetric hyperintensity of the adjacent preauricular soft tissues (yellow outline) and temporalis muscle (red outline), indicating inflammation. Axial T2-weighted image (B) at the level of the skull base demonstrates increased signal within the left mastoid air cells (green outline), indicating a mastoid effusion.

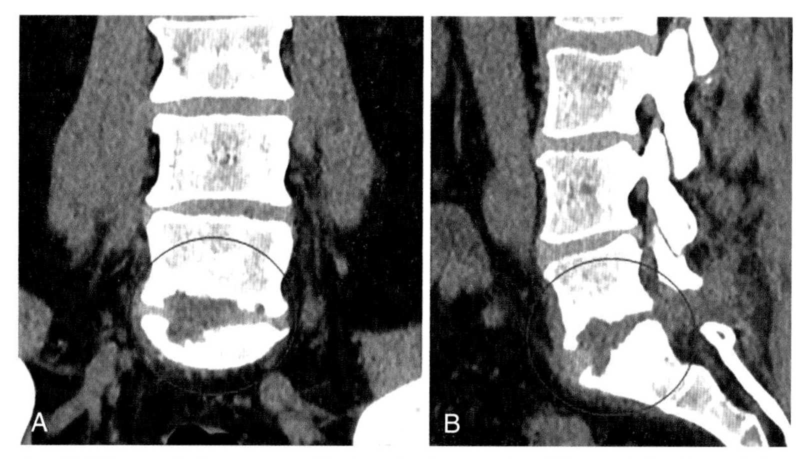


**Fig. 10.25** Coronal (A) and sagittal (B) computed tomography of the lower lumbar spine in soft tissue window demonstrate endplate erosive changes at L5–S1 (red circles) with prevertebral fat stranding, consistent with discitis-osteomyelitis. Also note protrusion of the intervertebral disc into the epidural space and laminectomy changes at this level.

the low yield of bone biopsy is the heterogeneous distribution of infection in the bone. Due to frequently poor yield, bone biopsy results seldom alter patient management.

Treatment of osteomyelitis involves intravenous antibiotics, typically for extended time periods. Surgical debridement is often necessary. If medical and local debriment treatment fails, amputation may be required.

## DISCITIS

Discitis refers specifically to infection of the intervertebral disc spaces of the spine. Diagnosis is often difficult, because symptoms of discitis are nonspecific and frequently overlap with other causes of back pain. Symptoms include insidious, nonmechanical back pain that is not relieved by rest. Early infection will usually not demonstrate neurologic symptoms, although these may develop later. Laboratory tests often reveal leukocytosis and elevated inflammatory markers. Infection typically arises via hematogenous spread from distant sites in PWID. Infectious pathogens may follow an anterograde course through the vertebral bodies' nutrient arterioles, or a retrograde course through the paravertebral Batson plexus. As with other musculoskeletal infections, prompt diagnosis is imperative, because delayed treatment may lead to significant long-term sequelae.

Radiographic findings of discitis are nonspecific and may resemble degenerative changes, such as narrowed intervertebral disc spaces and endplate irregularity. CT will show similar findings at an earlier stage but may still be indeterminate for discitis without noticeable soft tissue inflammatory changes such as edema or associated abscess (Fig. 10.25).

Much like osteomyelitis in the body, MRI is the most sensitive and specific modality for diagnosing acute discitis. The protocol should include sagittal pre- and postcontrast T1-weighted images, T2-weighted images, and STIR. If abnormal levels are noted on sagittal images, focused axial T2-weighted images and postcontrast T1-weighted images should be obtained. MRI demonstrates increased T2 signal and corresponding low T1 signal in the affected intervertebral disc spaces. High b-value DWI will also show hyperintense signal. Bone edema of adjacent vertebral bodies will follow a similar pattern to that seen elsewhere: high T2/STIR signal and low T1 signal. Postcontrast T1-weighted images will demonstrate diffuse enhancement of the intervertebral disc, as well as adjacent paravertebral soft tissues (Figs. 10.26 and 10.27).

A vital differential consideration is Modic type 1 changes, which are degenerative changes that manifest as low T1 and high T2 vertebral endplate signal, similar to those seen in vertebral osteomyelitis.[16,17] A distinguishing feature will be the lack of a high T2 signal in the intervertebral disc, as seen in true discitis. The clinical history may also help distinguish spondylosis versus infection.

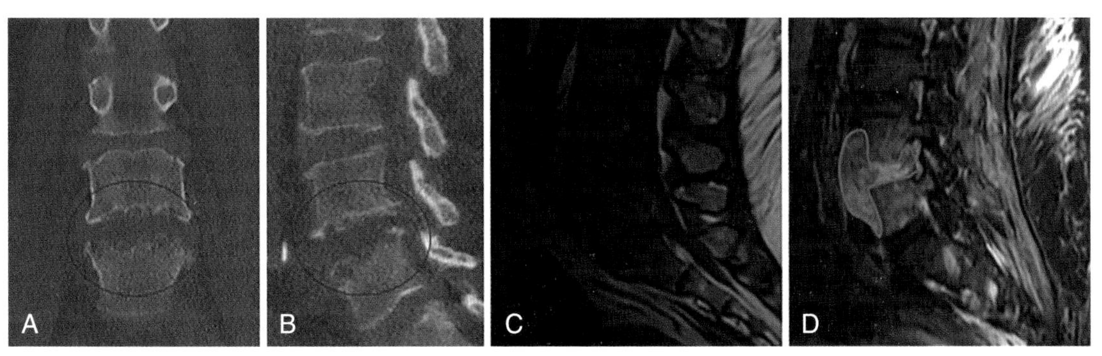


**Fig. 10.26** Coronal (A) and sagittal (B) computed tomography in bone window of the lumbar spine demonstrate destructive changes of the adjacent L4 and L5 endplates (red circles). Concurrent T1-weighted (C) and T2-weighted (D) sagittal magnetic resonance at the same level demonstrate decreased T1-weighted bone marrow signal in the affected vertebral bodies, as well as increased T2-weighted signal in and around the L4–L5 intervertebral disc (blue shaded area). Findings are consistent with L4–L5 discitis-osteomyelitis with associated prevertebral/epidural phlegmon.

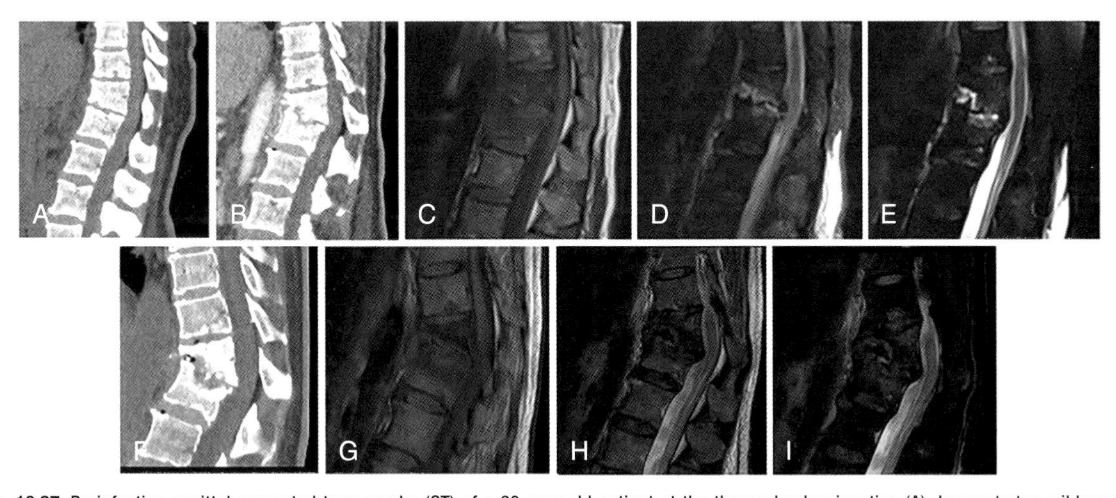


**Fig. 10.27** Preinfection sagittal computed tomography (CT) of a 60-year-old patient at the thoracolumbar junction (A) demonstrates mild wedge compression deformity at T12–L1. Sagittal CT (B) and T1-weighted (C), T2-weighted (D), and T2-weighted with fat saturation (E) magnetic resonance images at the same level obtained at infection onset demonstrate intervertebral disc space narrowing and endplate destruction, resulting in acute kyphotic angulation and spinal canal stenosis. Subsequent images obtained at 13 (F) and 16 (G, H, I) weeks after onset demonstrate further progression of these findings.

Similar to osteomyelitis, treatment of discitis involves extended intravenous antibiotic therapy.

## SEPTIC ARTHRITIS

Septic arthritis may occur due to instrumentation, direct penetrating trauma, or seeding via hematogenous spread (especially in large joints with rich blood supply). In PWID, it may result from complications of nearby injection, particularly in joints not usually associated with septic arthritis, such as the pubic symphysis, acromioclavicular, sacroiliac, and sternoclavicular joints. The sternoclavicular joint, in particular, may be involved due to injection of the upper extremity and passage of pathogens via the subclavian vein (Figs. 10.28 and 10.29). Prompt diagnosis and treatment are critical, because infection may progress rapidly and cause permanent joint damage.

Imaging is not typically required for the diagnosis of septic arthritis, which may be confirmed by synovial fluid sampling. However, if the joint in question is difficult to evaluate clinically or difficult to aspirate, then imaging may provide important information. Radiographs are typically the first image modality and may be normal with hyperacute infections. Joint effusion with regional soft tissue swelling will develop in the acute phase. In the case of later infections, bony

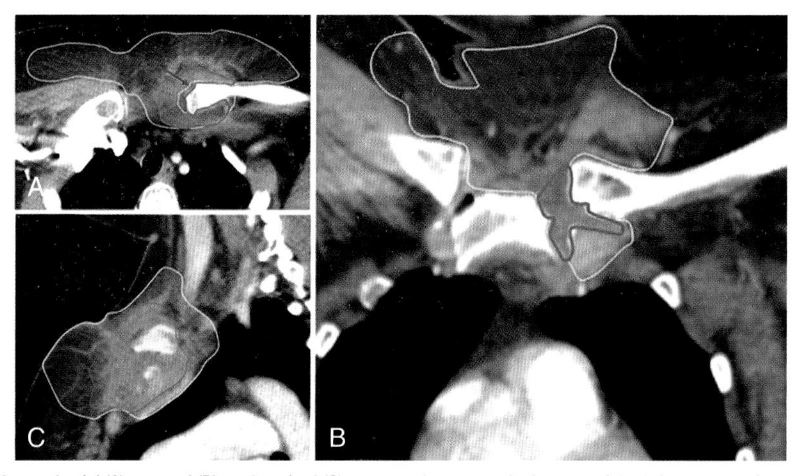


**Fig. 10.28** Contrast-enhanced axial (A), coronal (B), and sagittal (C) computed tomography images of the left sternoclavicular joint demonstrate erosive changes of the proximal clavicle (red arrows) with a sternoclavicular joint effusion (blue shaded area) and surrounding inflammatory changes (yellow shaded area), consistent with septic arthritis.

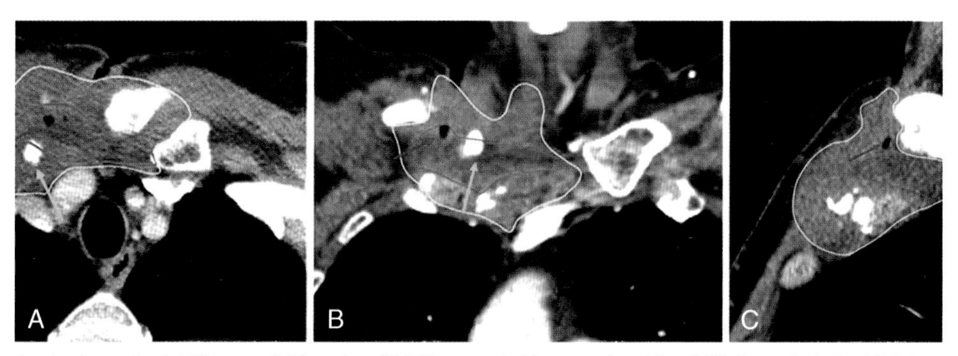


**Fig. 10.29** Contrast-enhanced axial (A), coronal (B), and sagittal (C) computed tomography of the right sternoclavicular joint demonstrate an ill-defined joint effusion (blue outline) containing a small focus of air (red arrows), surrounded by soft tissue density and subcutaneous fat stranding (yellow outline), representing phlegmonous changes. Additional note is made of a focal outpouching of the subclavian vein (green arrows), representing a mycotic aneurysm.

findings such as periarticular osteoporosis or erosions and joint space narrowing due to cartilaginous destruction may occur.[15] If untreated, chronic septic arthritis will result in the destruction of periarticular structures with deformity and sclerosis.

CT will show similar findings to radiographs, with the benefit of higher resolution and greater sensitivity for small effusions in joints not well assessed by radiographs and retained foreign bodies. It may also be used to guide joint aspiration. Similarly, US may be used to evaluate joint effusions and guide aspiration.

Like osteomyelitis, MRI is extremely sensitive for septic arthritis. However, findings may overlap with other inflammatory arthritides. Protocols include pre- and postcontrast T1-weighted images, T2-weighted images, and STIR sequences. MRI shows a joint effusion with synovial thickening and enhancement on postcontrast images, indicating synovitis.

If untreated, the inflammatory response incited by the white blood cells in the infected synovial space may cause rapid, permanent joint damage. Prompt drainage of the purulent synovial fluid and appropriate antibiotic therapy are the mainstays of septic arthritis treatment. In cases of infection of small joints, needle aspiration may be sufficient. If larger joints are involved, however, surgical washout and debridement may be necessary.

### VERTEBRAL BODY INFECTION

Immunocompromised states such as HIV infection, often encountered in patients who use recreational drugs, may lead to granulomatous infections. Three of the most common infectious diseases leading to granulomatous infections of the spine are coccidiomycosis, brucellosis, and tuberculosis.

As discussed above, MRI is the imaging modality of choice in the evaluation of osteomyelitis. This is especially true in evaluating infections of the spine, because US would be interfered with by the multiple bony prominences of the spine, and CT, while able to delineate cortical and vertebral body disruption, lacks the soft tissue resolution of MRI.

MRI protocol for evaluation of vertebral body infections should include T1-weighted images and fluid-sensitive sequences such as T2-weighted images and STIR. Brucellosis and tuberculosis will manifest as high fluid signal (T2/STIR) with corresponding low T1-weighted signal within the vertebral body.[18] Brucellosis typically causes mild osteomyelitis of the lower lumbar spine and spares the vertebral bodies and cortical margins; deformity is rarely seen.[19] Tuberculosis, on the other hand, results in severe vertebral body damage with involvement of the adjacent paraspinal soft tissues, particularly the anterior longitudinal ligament; spinal deformity is seen more frequently. This type of infection is given the eponym "Pott disease" and presents with back pain, kyphotic deformity, and "cold" intradural abscesses (a late finding), which are abscesses that lack associated pain, frank inflammation, or pus formation.[20] Involvement of contiguous vertebral bodies via the anterior longitudinal ligament may result in an acute short segment kyphosis, termed "Gibbus deformity." Vertebral coccidiomycosis may result in similar findings (Fig. 10.30).

Treatment of vertebral body infections involves source control and appropriate antibiotic therapy. Surgical intervention may be necessary in patients with severe spine deformity or large abscesses.

## Vascular Infections

### MYCOTIC ANEURYSM

Mycotic aneurysms are defined as infected balloon-like dilatations of the arterial wall, usually bacterial. They develop because of disruption of the arterial wall due to preexisting infectious arteritis rather than direct trauma. Like other infectious processes in PWID, they may occur at injection sites or due to hematogenous seeding. Mycotic aneurysms are false aneurysms and are prone to rupture due to instability.[15] They may also progress to form arteriovenous fistulae and produce septic emboli.

US of mycotic aneurysm will reveal inflammatory soft tissue changes around the infected artery, although it cannot reliably differentiate between infectious and noninfectious aneurysms.

MRI will demonstrate high T2 signal and corresponding low T1 signal, with postcontrast enhancement of the periarterial soft tissues.

CT is the modality of choice for detection of mycotic aneurysms. Common features include a lobulated vascular mass, irregularity and poor definition of the arterial wall, and regional soft tissue inflammation and edema (Fig. 10.31). An uncommon but specific finding is gas within an arterial aneurysm.

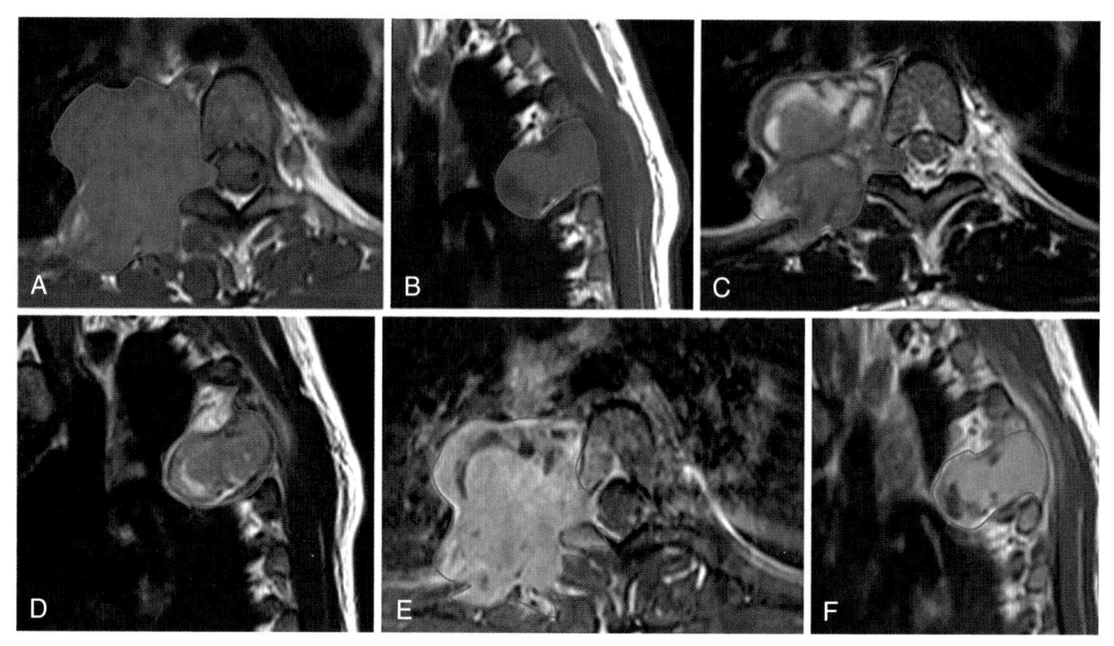


**Fig. 10.30** Axial and sagittal T1-weighted (A, B), T2-weighted (C, D), and T1-weighted postcontrast (E, F) magnetic resonance images of the upper thoracic spine demonstrate a T1 isointense, T2 heterogeneous, enhancing mass-like lesion (blue shaded area) involving the right T4 costovertebral junction. This mass was resected and cultured, and grew *Coccidioides* species.

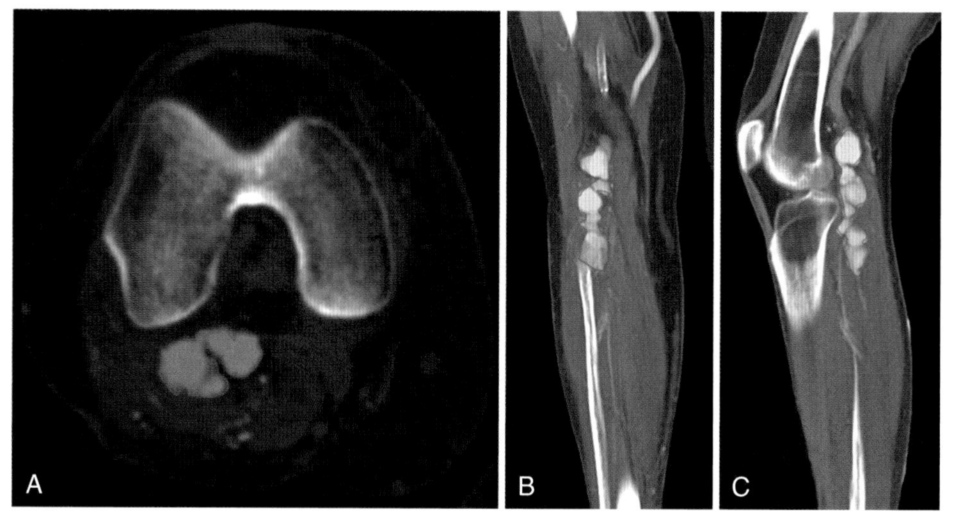


**Fig. 10.31** Axial (A), coronal (B), and sagittal (C) computed tomography angiogram in vascular window demonstrate multifocal aneurysmal dilatation of a long segment of the popliteal artery (blue shaded area) in a patient with bacteremia, suggestive of a mycotic aneurysm.

Treatment of mycotic aneurysms includes antibiotic therapy with surgical debridement of adjacent infected tissues and possible vascular reconstruction. Potential complications of mycotic aneurysm include a high risk of rupture and embolus production.

## Conclusion

Recreational drug use, especially intravenous drug use, is becoming an increasingly serious problem worldwide, leading to significant morbidity, mortality, and economic impact. Drug abuse in its many forms may affect virtually every system of the body, particularly the musculoskeletal system via direct trauma or introduction of pathogens, which may progress to acute and chronic infectious processes. As with other disease processes, radiology plays multiple integral roles in the diagnosis and management of musculoskeletal infections related to drug use. Prompt recognition of infectious processes may direct care and lead to life- or limb-saving treatments. Imaging may also assist in obtaining tissue or fluid collection so as to tailor antimicrobial therapy. Knowledge of the possible infectious manifestations of recreational drug use and a high degree of suspicion are critical in the evaluation and treatment of such patients.

### REFERENCES

1. UNODC. World drug report 2019, Booklet 1, Executive Summary. 2020. Vienna, Austria: United Nations Office on Drugs and Crime; 2020.
2. Roy É, Arruda N, Bruneau J, Jutras-Aswad D. Epidemiology of injection drug use: new trends and prominent issues. *Can J Psychiatry*. 2016;61(3):136–144.
3. Simpfendorfer CS. Radiologic approach to musculoskeletal infections. *Infect Dis Clin North Am*. 2017;31(2):299–324.
4. Johnston C, Keogan MT. Imaging features of soft-tissue infections and other complications in drug users after direct subcutaneous injection ('skin popping'). *AJR*. 2004;182(5):1195–1202.
5. Hayeri MR, Ziai P, Shehata ML, Teytelboym OM, Huang BK. Soft-tissue infections and their imaging mimics: from cellulitis to necrotizing fasciitis. *Radiographics*. 2016;36(6):1888–1910.
6. Gordon BS, Martinez S, Collins AJ. Pyomyositis: characteristics at CT and MR imaging. *Radiology*. 1995;197(1):279–286.
7. Fayad LM, Carrino JA, Fishman EK. Musculoskeletal infection: role of CT in the emergency department. *Radiographics*. 2007;27(6):1723–1736.
8. Small LN, Ross JJ. Suppurative tenosynovitis and septic bursitis. *Infect Dis Clin North Am*. 2005;19(4):991–1005.
9. Turecki MB, Taljanovic MS, Stubbs AY, Graham AR, Holden DA, Hunter TB, et al. Imaging of musculoskeletal soft tissue infections. *Skelet Radiology*. 2010;39(10):957–971.
10. Jardin E, Delord M, Aubry S, Loisel F, Obert L. Usefulness of ultrasound for the diagnosis of pyogenic flexor tenosynovitis: A prospective single-center study of 57 cases. *Hand Surg Rehabil*. 2018;37(2):95–98.
11. Mirzaei A, Zabihiyeganeh M, Haqiqi A. Differentiation of cocaine-induced midline destructive lesions from ANCA-associated vasculitis. *Iran J Otorhinolaryngol*. 2018;30(5):309–313.
12. Allison DC, Holtom PD, Patzakis MJ, Zalavras CG. Microbiology of bone and joint infections in injecting drug abusers. *Clin Orthop Relat Res*. 2010;468(8):2107–2112.
13. Pineda C, Espinosa R, Pena A. Radiographic imaging in osteomyelitis: the role of plain radiography, computed tomography, ultrasonography, magnetic resonance imaging, and scintigraphy. *Semin Plas Surg*. 2009;23:80–89.
14. Ang MT, Wong GR, Wong DR, Clements W, Joseph T. Diagnostic yield of computed tomography–guided biopsy and aspiration for vertebral osteomyelitis. *J Med Imaging Radiat Oncol*. 2019;63(5):589–595.
15. Delaney FT, Stanley E, Bolster F. The needle and the damage done: musculoskeletal and vascular complications associated with injected drug use. *Insights into Imaging*. 2020;11(1):1–14.
16. Hong SH, Choi J-Y, Lee JW, Kim NR, Choi J-A, Kang HS. MR imaging assessment of the spine: infection or an imitation? *Radiographics*. 2009;29(2):599–612.
17. Laur O, Mandell JC, Titelbaum DS, Cho C, Smith SE, Khurana B. Acute nontraumatic back pain: infections and mimics. *Radiographics*. 2019;39(1):287–288.
18. Sharif HS, Clark DC, Aabed MY, Haddad MC, al Deeb SM, Yaqub B, et al. Granulomatous spinal infections: MR imaging. *Radiology*. 1990;177(1):101–107.
19. Crete RN, Gallmann W, Karis JP, Ross J. Spinal coccidioidomycosis: MR imaging findings in 41 patients. *AJNR*. 2018;39(11):2148–2153.
20. Diehn FE. Imaging of spine infection. *Radiol Clin North Am*. 2012;50(4):777–798.

Chapter 11

# Emergency Department Neuroimaging for the Sick Child

Elka Miller and Neetika Gupta

## Outline



## Key Points

- Acute neuro emergencies in children require a low imaging threshold.
- Emphasize the role of imaging in pediatric neuroemergencies and the promising role of rapidly evolving ultrafast magnetic resonance imaging.
- Describe the key imaging findings of commonly encountered pediatric neurological emergencies.
- Highlight the common challenges and imaging pitfalls faced by the emergency radiologist.
- It is critical to identify the key imaging findings and commonly-encountered pitfalls in the assessment of pediatric neuro emergencies.
- Outline a reporting checklist facilitating the rapid and appropriate communication of the critical findings.
- The imaging modality of choice in pediatric neuro emergencies is guided by the patient status, availability of the modality, and requirement of contrast and/or sedation.
- Ultrafast MRI is a rapidly evolving technique that addresses the progressive imaging requirement of an acutely sick child without radiation exposure.

## Introduction

Acute neurological emergencies in children can present with a wide variety of symptoms and signs such as fever, vomiting, headache, poor feeding, seizures, and altered consciousness, ultimately leading to encephalopathy and deep coma.[1] Often, an inevitable deficiency of relevant clinical history and lack of dependable neurological examination in an acutely sick child pose a challenge to the emergency team in delivering a precise diagnosis and instituting the appropriate management as early as possible.[2]

The roles of the radiologist in these emergencies are manifold. The first and foremost role is to determine whether neuroimaging is indicated, as well as which imaging modality is preeminent to answer the clinical question. The choice of imaging modality may also be guided by its availability, the condition of the child, and the requirement for contrast and/or sedation in an emergency setting. Secondly, the radiologist should be cognizant of the key imaging findings to provide a timely and appropriate diagnosis, consider pertinent differentials, and detect complications that warrant urgent medical attention.[3] Any critical imaging findings that can affect the immediate management and prognosis must also be promptly conveyed to the emergency department (ED) physician.

## Imaging Techniques

Different imaging modalities can be considered based on clinical status, age, provisional diagnosis, and institutional availability. Radiographs are practically limited to the trauma of the spine.[4] Skull radiographs, once used frequently, are now obsolete and only used as a part of the skeletal survey in suspected nontraumatic brain injury.[3] Transcranial ultrasound is a good initial imaging modality of choice in neonates or infants with open fontanelle to evaluate ventricular size and exclude intraventricular bleed.[5] Computed tomography (CT) is the most commonly used imaging modality due to the easy accessibility, intermediate cost, and rapid acquisition time, which obviates the need for anesthesia.[1] However, CT is of concern in children given the higher radiation susceptibility of rapidly dividing cells and longer life span, during which they may develop long-term cumulative effects of radiation. Cautious optimization of the CT examination using the As Low As Reasonably Achievable (ALARA) principle, based on the age and weight of the child, allows effective acquisition of the best-quality image with the lowest radiation dose possible.[6] While CT may be superior for the evaluation of bone, magnetic resonance imaging (MRI) does not utilize ionizing radiation and allows excellent tissue contrast to assess intracranial pathology.[7] MRI acquisition time is longer and potentially requires anesthesia depending on the age and clinical status of the patient. The introduction of ultrafast MRI offers some flexibility, allowing shorter acquisition time and decreasing the need for sedation.[8] This has come in handy in children with ventriculoperitoneal shunts, where the use of ultrafast MRI protocols has played an important role in avoiding multiple CT examinations for suspected shunt dysfunction.[9] Recently, with improved image resolution, ultrafast MRI protocols have been introduced as the initial imaging modality of choice whenever possible instead of CT. Previously limited to T2-wieghted sequences using single-shot fast spin-echo (SSFSE) or Half-Fourier-Acquired Single-shot Turbo spin Echo, newer ultrafast MRI protocols have additional sequences such as fluid-attenuated inversion recovery (FLAIR), T1-weighted imaging (T2*WI), diffusion-weighted imaging (DWI), and T2-weighted imaging (T2WI) that demonstrate sufficient image quality in comparison with routine brain MRI, with acquisition time ranging from 1 to 5 minutes.[10–12] The most common pediatric neurological emergencies requiring ED visits are trauma, stroke, and infections, along with headaches.

## Traumatic Brain Injury

The impact of traumatic injury on the developing brain mostly depends on the severity of the trauma and the age of the child: the younger the age, the higher the risk.[13,14] Causes of trauma are also variable and age-dependent, such as an accidental drops in infants and falls in toddlers and older children, while adolescents commonly suffer from sports-related injuries or motor vehicle accidents.[13]

Head injuries are clinically classified as mild,[13,14] moderate,[8–12] or severe[3–7] based on the Glasgow coma scale (GCS) and on the pediatric GCS for nonverbal children (under 2 years of age).[15] Patients with moderate to severe injury undergo a CT examination after clinical stabilization.[16] In mild injury, the need for imaging in children follows further clinical criteria. The clinical tool that is most often used is the Pediatric Emergency Care Applied Research Network (PECARN). PECARN helps ED physicians decide which children require urgent CT and who can be managed conservatively without imaging.[17,18] The most important pediatric traumatic entities are described below.

### SCALP INJURY

Soft tissue injuries including scalp hematomas and lacerations are common.[19] Scalp hematomas that can cross midline or sutures are caput succedaneum (superficial to the galea aponeurotica), and subgaleal hematoma (deep to the galea aponeurotica)[20] (Fig. 11.1). Cephalhematoma is often a birth-related finding, located deep to the periosteum, and does not cross suture or midline (Fig. 11.2).

### SKULL FRACTURES

Skull fractures are common in children due to the thin calvaria from underdeveloped diploe. Sutural diastasis is also a known complication in children (Fig. 11.3). Calvarial fractures can be linear, comminuted, nondepressed, and depressed. Ping-pong fracture is a unique depressed skull fracture (Fig. 11.4) seen in newborns and infants due to inward buckling

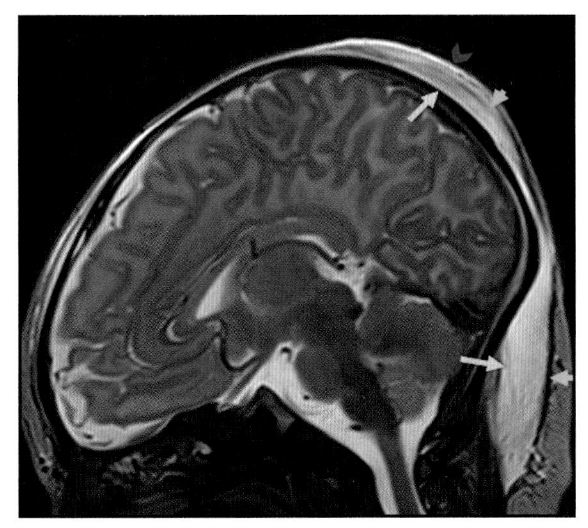

**Fig. 11.1** A 2-week-old girl born after 24 hours of prolonged and difficult labor. Sagittal T2 image demonstrates a subgaleal hematoma (yellow arrows) deep to galea aponeurotica (green arrows) extending from parietal bone to the neck. Mild fluid was also noted in subcutaneous tissue (chevron) in the high parietal region, representing resolving caput succedaneum.

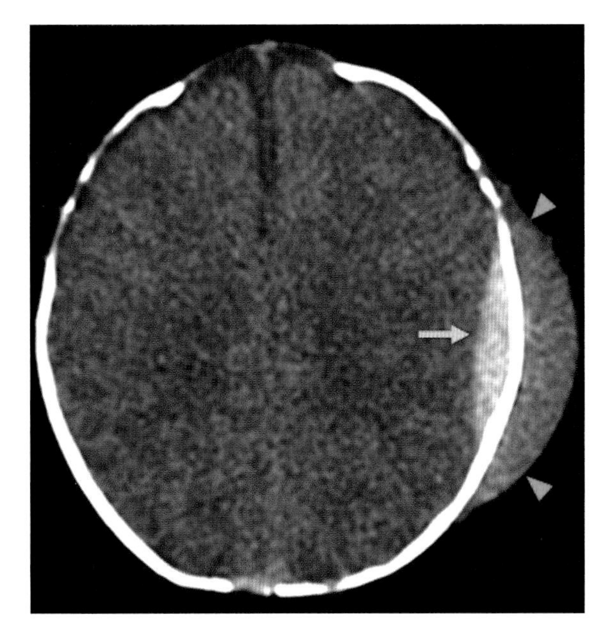

**Fig. 11.2** A 1-week-old boy who underwent forceps delivery. Axial computed tomography image demonstrates a left parietal cephalhematoma (arrowheads) confined by the sutures and periosteal attachment. A small biconvex epidural hematoma (arrow) along the left parietal region causing a slight mass effect and sulcal effacement of the underlying left frontoparietal lobe was also noted.

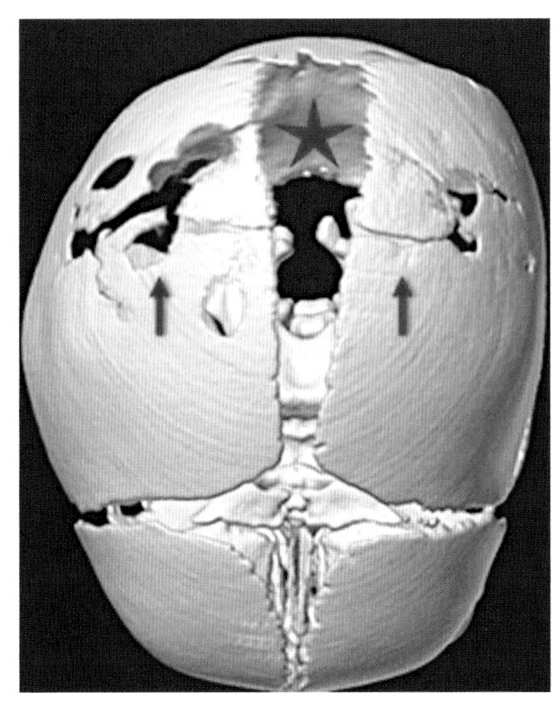

**Fig. 11.3** A 2-month-old girl with suspected nonaccidental injury. Three-dimensional reformat shows sagittal suture diastasis (star) and multiple bilateral parietal bone fractures (arrows), with mild separation of the fracture fragments on the right side.

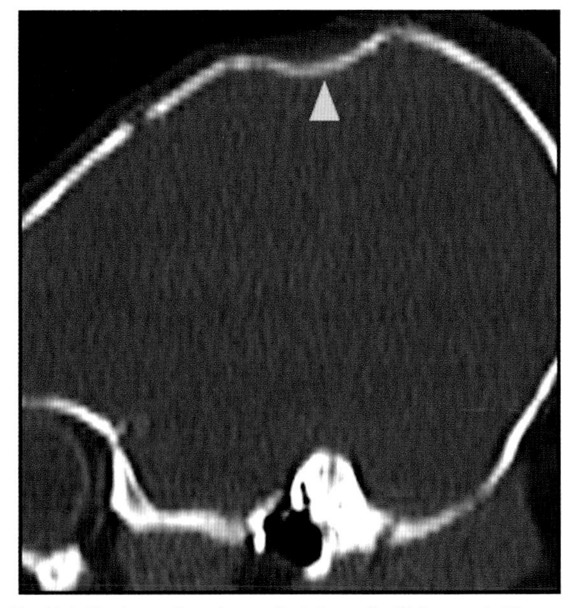

**Fig. 11.4** Newborn after a traumatic delivery. Sagittal computed tomography head in the bone window shows a ping-pong fracture as a smooth depression (arrowhead) of the left parietal bone with intact cortex.

of the under mineralized calvaria (analogous to buckle fracture of the appendicular skeleton).[21] Skull base fractures are often related to severe injury and should be suspected with orbitofacial trauma (Fig. 11.5). Vascular injuries involving caroticojugular vessels (Fig. 11.6) and cranial nerve injuries causing facial palsy and hearing loss are common with skull base fractures and may present as an immediate or delayed complication.[20]

### Growing Skull Fracture

This is a delayed complication of calvarial fracture with a dural tear, typically seen in children under 3 years of age. The parietal bone is the most common site.[22] Due to dural tear, there is constant transmission of cerebrospinal fluid (CSF) pulsations to the fracture site, resulting in progressive widening and scalloping (Fig. 11.7). This results in herniation of pia-arachnoid, formation of a leptomeningeal cyst, and encephalomalacia of the underlying brain parenchyma.[20]

### Imaging Pitfalls

Linear undisplaced fractures can be confused with primary and accessory sutures. Helpful clues that favor sutures are sclerotic borders, interdigitated margins, expected course and location, and the fact that they are frequently bilateral.[23]

### Imaging Requisites

All fractures should be evaluated in all three planes, and, when possible, imaging should reconstruct a three-dimensional shaded surface display of the skull.[24] Always rule out a skull base fracture in the presence of pneumocephalus.

### Reporting Checklist

Fracture location, extension, crossing the suture or midline, depressed or nondepressed, displaced or undisplaced, width of displacement, and depth of depression. Look for the involvement of orbitofacial,

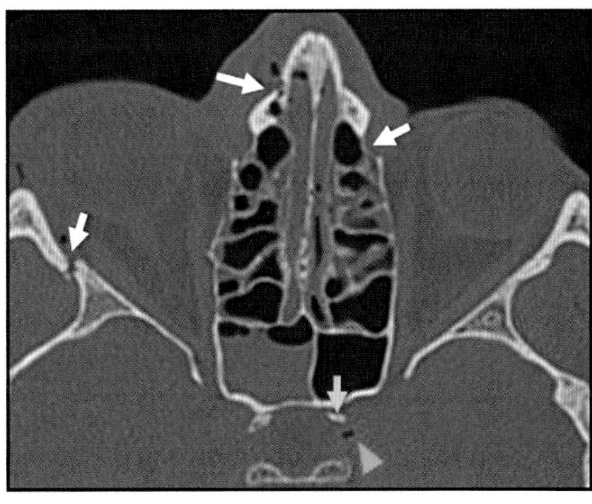

**Fig. 11.5** A 9-year-old girl with pedestrian injury. Axial computed tomography image shows multiple orbitofacial fractures (arrows) and a small pneumocephalus (arrowhead) in the sella, concerning for a skull base fracture. On close inspection, there was a fracture of the left anterior clinoid process (yellow arrow).

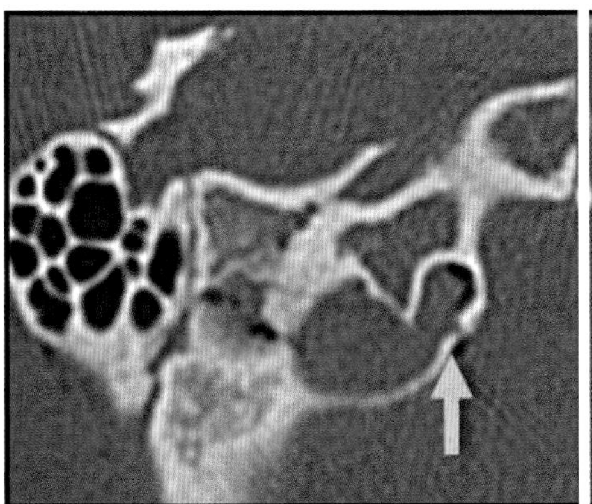

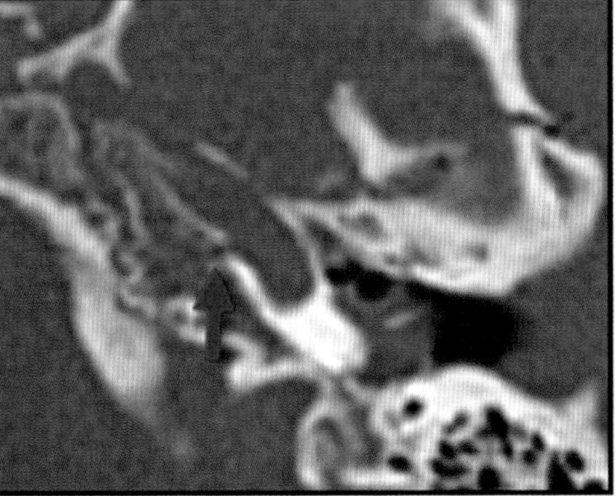

**Fig. 11.6** A 12-year-old boy presented to the emergency room with hemotympanum following a motor vehicle accident. Axial computed tomography scan of the head in bone window demonstrates right temporal and basiocciput fractures involving the right jugular foramen (yellow arrow) and a few tiny air foci in and around the jugular fossa. On the left side, an oblique fracture of the left temporal bone was noted, with extension and involvement of left carotid canal (red arrow) but no carotid dissection on computed tomography angiography (not shown).

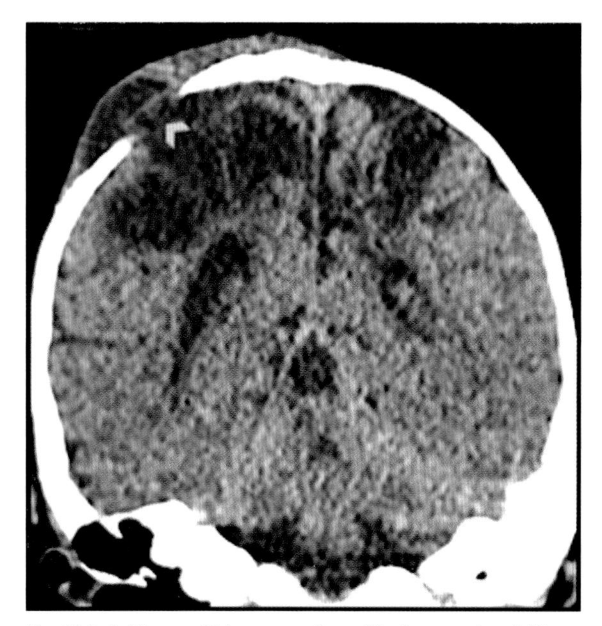

**Fig. 11.7** A 10-year-old boy presenting with slow-growing right parietal scalp swelling, history of a severe head trauma 3 years ago. Coronal computed tomography of the head shows a small right parietal bone defect (chevron) with herniation of the cystic encephalomalacic parenchyma and leptomeninges—leptomeningeal cyst with a growing skull fracture.

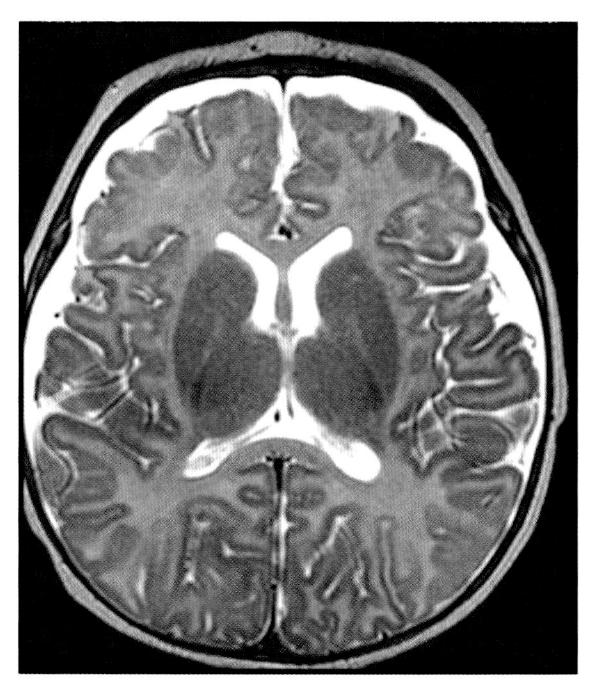

**Fig. 11.8** A 2.5-month-old girl with suspected nonaccidental injury. T2-weighted axial image reveals subdural collections (arrows) along the bilateral frontoparietal region with no significant mass effect on the underlying brain parenchyma. Susceptibility weighted images (not shown) show multiple blooming foci in the subdural collection, in keeping with subdural bleeding.

petromastoid, and caroticojugular canal with skull base fractures.

## EXTRAAXIAL HEMORRHAGE

There are three types of extraaxial hemorrhage (EAH), and the imaging appearance depends upon age and location of the hemorrhage, admixing of CSF, preexisting collection, and the presence of underlying bleeding diathesis.[20,25]

### Epidural Hematoma

Typical biconvex hematoma (Fig. 11.2) in the epidural space, do not cross suture but may cross the midline (dural venous sinus bleed). Unlike adults, these are commonly venous in origin and can occur without fracture due to malleable bones and unsupported meningeal vessels.[2,20]

### Subdural Hematoma

Classic concavoconvex collection (Fig. 11.8) of blood in the potential subdural space. May cross the suture, but do not cross the midline. The commonest intracranial hematoma in children, particularly in infants and toddlers; unlike in adults, it is frequently bilateral.[26]

### Subarachnoid Hemorrhage

Focal and linear hyperdensity along the sulci and cisterns (Fig. 11.9) within subarachnoid space.[27] The most common site is Sylvian fissure.[20]

### Imaging Pitfalls

Subarachnoid hemorrhage (SAH) should not be confused with pseudo-SAH secondary to cerebral edema or bilateral subdural hematoma (SDH).[28] Venous epidural hematoma is common in pediatric patients and can cross the midline.

### Imaging Requisites

EAHs can be missed with the routine parenchymal window and are best evaluated at subdural window

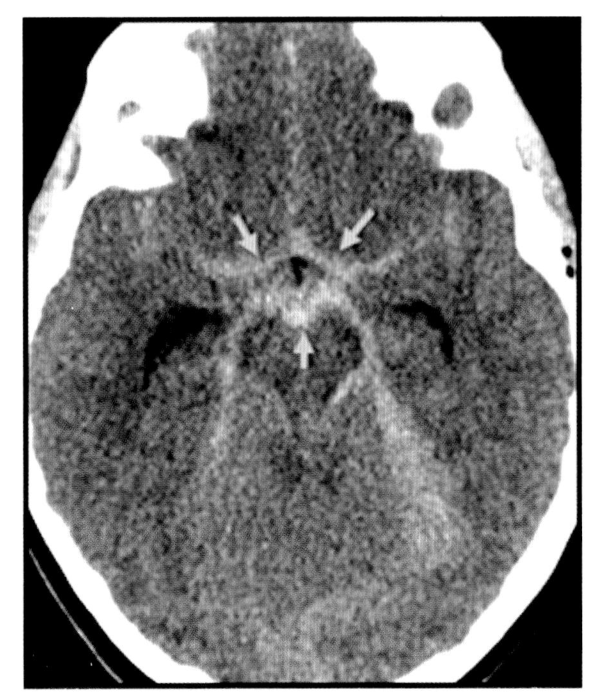

**Fig. 11.9** A 17-year-old boy presented with a Glasgow coma scale score of 7 following an all-terrain vehicle accident. Computed tomography of the head shows skull base fractures (not shown) and blood filling the basal cisterns (arrows) in keeping with subarachnoid hemorrhage.

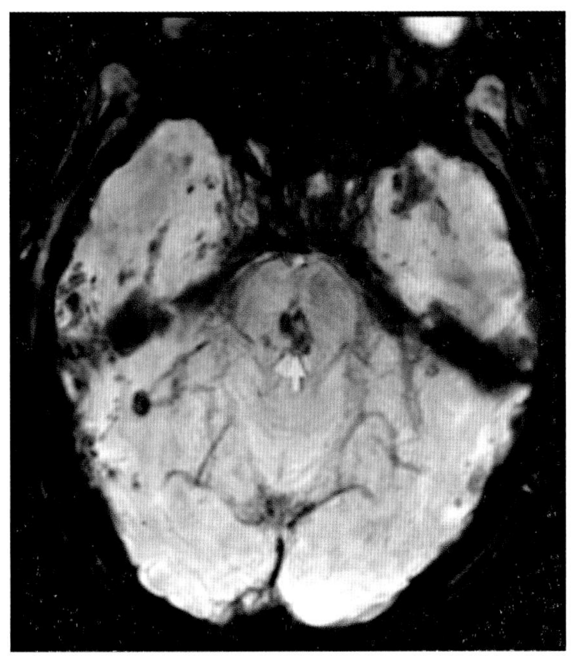

**Fig. 11.10** A 17-year-old old boy following head injury after collision of motorbike with stationary truck shows hemorrhagic contusion in the left anterior temporal region (red arrow) and multiple blooming foci in bilateral temporal lobes, brainstem (yellow arrow), and cerebellum (grade 3 diffuse axonal injury) on susceptibility-weighted magnetic resonance imaging.

130 and level 30 (standard brain window 75 and level 20).[29] Triplanar evaluation is necessary.

#### Reporting Checklist

Hematoma location, extension, size, maximum width, mass effect, midline shift, and brain herniation.

## INTRAAXIAL INJURY

### Cortical Contusions

Occur due to collision of the brain and skull at the site of impact (Fig. 11.10) or opposite to it (coup-countercoup). Usually less common and less severe in children due to smooth and softer calvaria.[30]

#### Diffuse Axonal Injury

Occurs due to sudden acceleration and deceleration. The younger the age, the more severe and extensive the injury. Typically presents as multifocal hemorrhagic foci with surrounding edema (Figs. 11.10 and 11.11) and can be divided into: grade I: lobar white matter involvement at the grey-white matter junction; grade II: corpus callosum involvement; grade III: involvement of brainstem and posterior fossa structures (Fig. 11.10).[31]

## ABUSIVE HEAD TRAUMA

Typically seen in children below 2 years of age, with maximum risk in the first 6 months of life.[32] Shaking injury from violent motion of the head results in SDH (Fig. 11.8), SAH, generalized parenchymal injury (cytotoxic edema, laceration, axonal injury), and bridging vein injury (Fig. 11.12), with or without thrombosis.[33] Fractures that are multiple, complex, bilateral, or unexplained with the mechanism of trauma should raise suspicion for abusive head trauma (AHT). CT is usually the primary imaging tool, but MRI is superior for determining the full extent of the injury.[33] A concern of AHT should be raised when there is discordance between the clinical history and

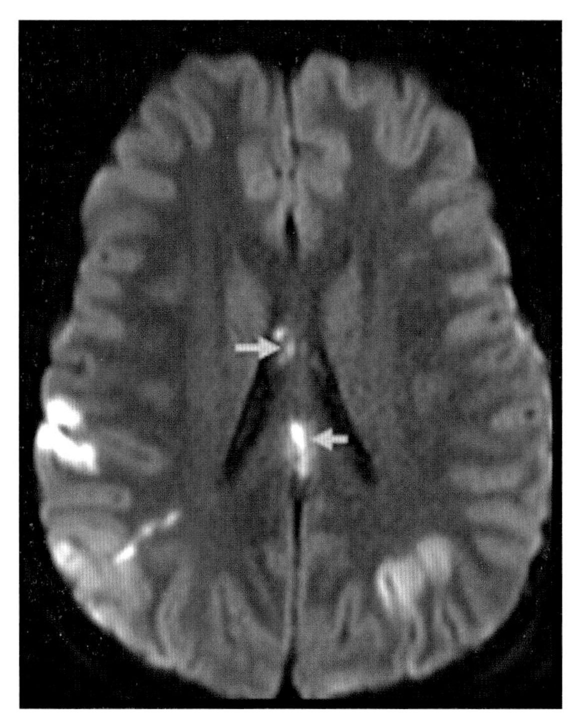

Fig. 11.11 A 15-year-old girl presented with a Glasgow coma scale score of 9 following a road traffic accident. Axial fluid-attenuated inversion recovery magnetic resonance imaging shows multiple hyperintense foci at the grey-white matter junction and at the level of body and splenium (arrows) of the corpus callosum, representing diffuse axonal injury (grade 2 diffuse axonal injury).

the degree of injury. However, AHT is not an imaging diagnosis and requires a multidepartmental approach.

### Imaging Pitfalls

In clinically significant trauma with normal-appearing CT, look for secondary signs of edema such as sulcal effacement and cisternal narrowing and herniation.

### Imaging Requisites

Diffuse axonal injury and nonhemorrhagic contusions can be difficult to detect on CT. An MRI is to be considered when there are discrepancies between the clinical findings and CT examination.

### Reporting Checklist

Document the location, extent, and size of the injury. Look for mass effect, midline shift, or herniation.

## PEDIATRIC STROKE

Pediatric strokes, including perinatal (20 weeks gestation to 28th day after birth) or childhood (29th day to 18 years) strokes, are less frequent than adult strokes but have an equal propensity for ischemic and hemorrhagic types.[34] Timely diagnosis and management of pediatric stroke can be challenging due to its relative rarity, numerous etiologies, and vague presentations, which can include headache, seizure, lethargy, and neurological deficit.[35]

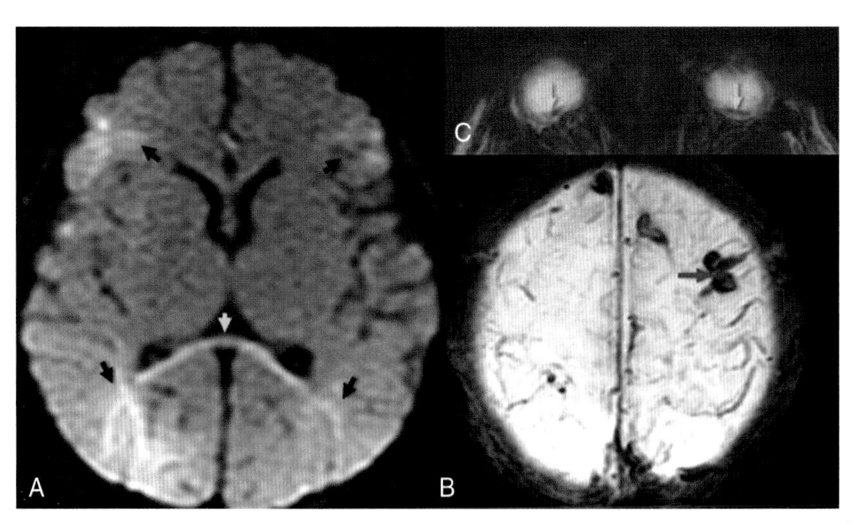


Fig. 11.12 A 2.5-month-old girl with suspected nonaccidental injury. Magnetic resonance imaging shows multiple areas of restricted diffusion (A); some of them have watershed distribution (black arrows) as well as cortical and splenium (green arrow) involvement. Susceptibility-weighted imaging (B) of the same patient shows multiple blooming foci and typical lollipop/tadpole sign (red arrow) due to disruption and thrombosis of the bridging veins. There is also blooming artifact in the posterior retina from retinal hemorrhages (C) (yellow arrows). There were also associated mild bilateral subdural collections, which are shown in Fig. 11.8.

## Acute Ischemic Stroke

The most common causes of childhood acute ischemic stroke (AIS) are cerebral arteriopathies, followed by cardioembolic (Fig. 11.13), prothrombotic, and idiopathic diseases.[36] Other less common causes are dissection, vasculitis, and infections. The cerebral arteriopathies can further be subdivided into transient (reversible cerebral vasoconstriction syndrome, post-varicella, postinfection) and progressive (Moya-Moya, sickle cell disease, fibromuscular dysplasia).[34,37]

The role of imaging is to confirm the diagnosis, find the possible etiology, and exclude stroke mimics. MRI is the preferred imaging modality.[38] Recommended sequences include DWI/apparent diffusion coefficient (ADC) map to diagnose acute ischemia, susceptibility-weighted imaging (SWI) to detect hemorrhage and occasionally intravascular thrombus (susceptibility-vessel sign),[35] and the T1WI and FLAIR/T2*WI sequences to assess edema, bleeding, and myelination. Magnetic resonance angiography (MRA) and magnetic resonance venography (MRV) help evaluate the craniocervical vessels.

Additional sequences such as magnetic resonance (MR) perfusion can help identify the penumbra, a salvageable hypoperfused tissue without diffusion restriction (diffusion-perfusion mismatch) compared to the non-salvageable hypoperfused ischemic tissue with restricted diffusion (matched area).[35] This is important in guiding treatment. Arterial spin labeling MR perfusion is desirable in children due to the inherently high signal-to-noise ratio and lack of contrast requirement.[39] Vessel wall imaging (VWI), also known as black blood imaging, is starting to play a role in the imaging of various arteriopathies.[40]

## Cerebral Sinovenous Thrombosis

Venous infarcts are a common complication of pediatric cerebral sinovenous thrombosis (CSVT). Common pediatric risk factors are infection, trauma, dehydration, and prothrombotic states.[41]

### Imaging Findings

CSVT should be suspected in cases of nonarterial distribution of infarction and or hemorrhage.[34] The most common sites for thrombosis are the superior sagittal sinus, followed by the transverse sinus (Fig. 11.14). Hemorrhagic transformation of venous infarct is seen in up to 50% of cases. MRV and/or postcontrast three-dimensional T1-weighted gradient echo (GRE) sequences are preferred to detect venous filling defects. CT venography is a good alternative.[42] GRE and SWI images are of particular value to detect the low signal from cortical vein thrombosis.

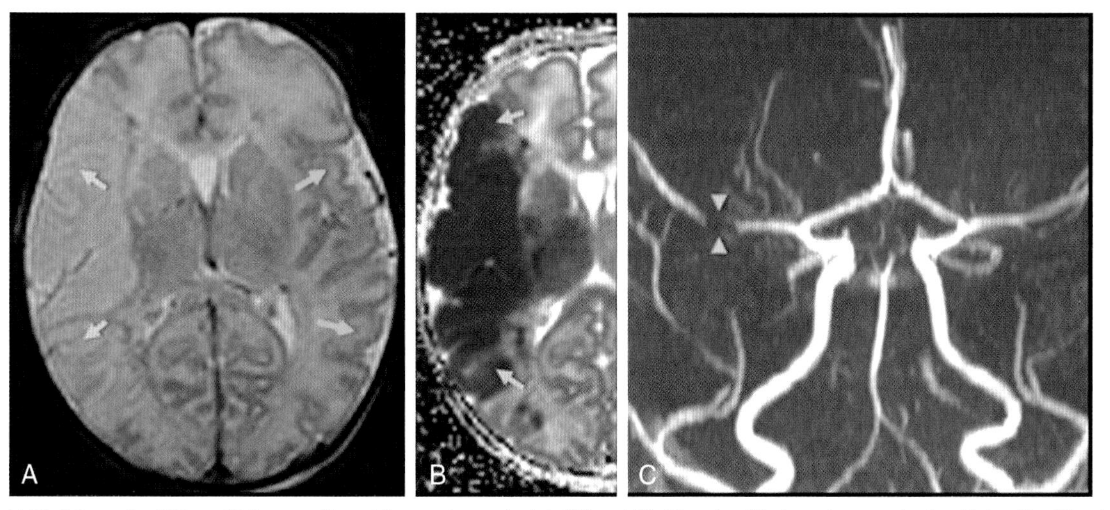


**Fig. 11.13** A 3-month-old boy with transposition of the great vessels. Axial T2-weighted imaging (A) shows increase in signal intensity of the right frontoparietal region with poor grey-white matter differentiation and loss of cortical ribbon (arrows) compared with the left side (green arrows). The apparent diffusion coefficient map (B) shows restricted diffusion and corresponding hypointensity of the right frontoparietal and right gangliothalamic region. The time-of-flight magnetic resonance angiography (C) shows mild attenuation of the right middle cerebral artery with complete focal signal loss at the M1/M2 junction (arrowheads) due to cardioembolic phenomenon.

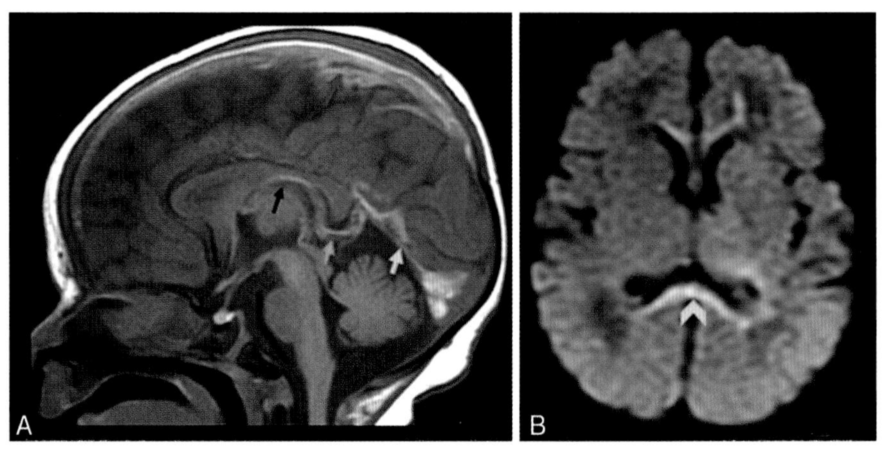


**Fig. 11.14** A 4-year-old girl with acute lymphoblastic leukemia. (A) Sagittal T1 image shows extensive cerebral dural venous sinus thrombosis in the superior sagittal sinus (red arrow), straight sinus (yellow arrow), vein of Galen (green arrow), and internal cerebral vein (black arrow). (B) Axial diffusion-weighted imaging of the same patient shows restricted diffusion in the corpus callosum (chevron) and surrounding white matter, posterior more than anterior (not shown) from venous infarcts.

### Imaging Pitfalls

The typical DWI, T1WI, and T2*WI appearance a of stroke may be less obvious in infants due to the undermyelinated brain. Loss of the normal cortical ribbon in T2 weighted images and corresponding hypointensity on ADC map help in diagnosis (Fig. 11.13).

### Stroke Mimics

Hypoglycemia, hemiplegic migraine, and postictal paresis commonly mimic stroke and can be distinguished on MRI.[43]

### Imaging Requisites

The MRI stroke protocol must begin with DWI to detect sites of infarction, especially in cases where the child is unstable or uncooperative. The protocol should include SWI, MRA (craniocervical), and in many cases MRV, allowing rapid differentiation of AIS from other causes such as CSVT. MR perfusion should be considered when a child is presented within the treatment window. VWI can be carried out in suspected arteriopathy.

### Reporting Checklist

The extent of the infarction, presence of hemorrhage, vessel involvement (arterial/venous) and distribution, mass effect, and presence of diffusion-perfusion mismatch. Comment on the involvement of critical structures such as the corticospinal tract and optic radiation. This involvement is helpful in predicting long-term disability.

## NONTRAUMATIC INTRACRANIAL HEMORRHAGE

Intracranial hemorrhage (ICH) is a frequent cause of morbidity and mortality in children. Common etiologies include vascular malformations (arteriovenous malformations [Fig. 11.15] and cavernous malformations), brain tumors, and coagulopathies.[44,45] A ruptured aneurysm is a relatively uncommon cause of ICH in children compared with adults.[44]

### Imaging Findings

The role of imaging is to evaluate the extent and phase of ICH, complications, and causative etiology. Imaging of ICH reflects temporal evolution, with distinctive MR appearance of each phase: hyperacute, acute, early or late-subacute, and chronic. GRE and SWI are the most sensitive sequences in the detection of ICH (Fig. 11.10).

### Imaging Pitfalls

The T1WI and T2*WI appearance of ICH depends on the phase, etiology, and admixing of CSF and should always be considered while assessing the ICH. Nonvisualization of the nidus of an arteriovenous malformation (AVM) in acute hemorrhage can occur due to

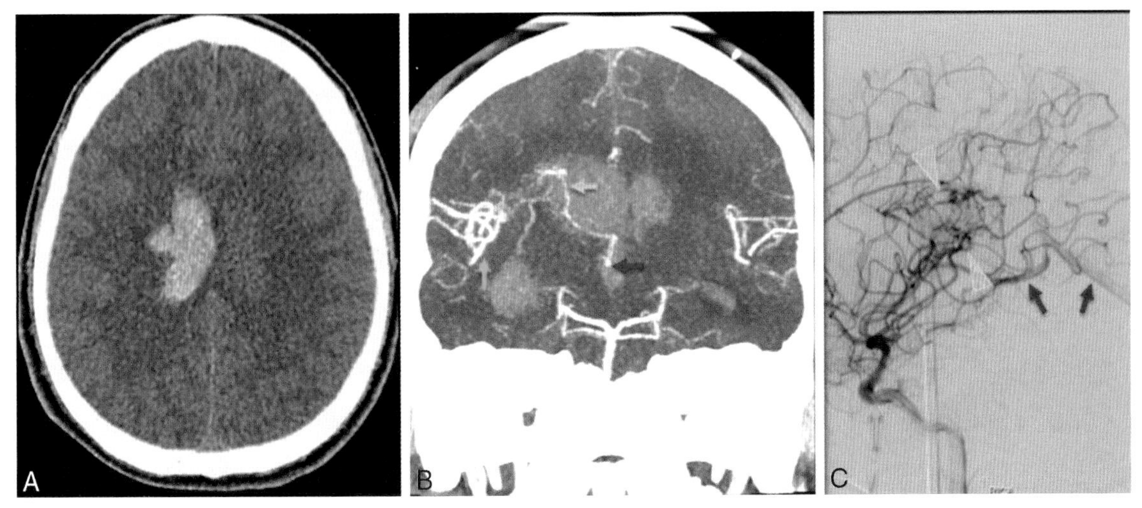


**Fig. 11.15** A 17-year-old boy presents with seizure and Glasgow coma scale score of 8. (A) Axial non enhanced computed tomography (CT) image shows diffuse intraventricular hemorrhage in all the ventricles and a small triangular bleed (chevron) in the right high frontal periventricular white matter. The CT angiogram (B) shows multiple arterial channels (green arrow) arising from the M3 and M4 segments of the right middle cerebral artery supplying the right high frontal periventricular white matter lesion associated with early arterial filling of the right thalamostriate vein (yellow arrow) and internal cerebral vein (red arrow), suggestive of arteriovenous malformation (AVM). Findings were further confirmed by digital subtraction angiography (C) that showed a somewhat diffuse nidus (arrowhead) of AVM supplied by distal branches of the right middle cerebral artery (green arrow) and draining into the deep venous system (red arrows).

mass effect. Early venous filling (Fig. 11.15B) from arteriovenous shunting is an indirect sign that helps to establish etiology.[46]

Turbulent flow in tortuous vessels and large aneurysms can result in underestimation of flow on nonenhanced MRA (time-of-flight [TOF]) and MRV (phase-contrast). Contrast-enhanced MRA and MRV are superior and avoid any misinterpretation.[47]

### Imaging Requisites

The MRI protocol should include a GRE or SWI and a craniocervical MRA and MRV in suspected vascular malformation. A contrast-enhanced study helps diagnose and differentiate various vascular malformations and to evaluate a neoplasm.

### Reporting Checklist

Size and location of the bleeding, vessel involvement (arterial or venous), mass effect, and temporal evolution. Look for the "spot sign" (progressive enlargement of the hematoma in enhanced scan), which is a predictor of hemorrhagic progression.[48]

## Infections

Central nervous system (CNS) infections are among the common causes of neurological emergencies and should be considered in every child presenting with an altered mental status with fever.[1] The role of imaging is to assess the extent of CNS involvement and evaluate for any life-threatening complications requiring urgent management.[42]

### MENINGITIS

Leptomeningeal inflammation can occur secondary to bacterial, viral, fungal, tubercular, or aseptic (autoimmune/drug/chemical) causes.[42] The diagnosis of uncomplicated meningitis is usually confirmed with CSF analysis, and neuroimaging is not routinely performed unless complications are suspected. MRI with contrast is the investigation of choice to demonstrate enhancing membranes and exudates (Fig. 11.16A), empyema (epidural or subdural), cerebritis, and ventriculitis. DWI/ADC allows evaluation of infarctions (Fig. 11.16B) and abscesses (Fig. 11.19B), and MRA and MRV are helpful for the assessment of

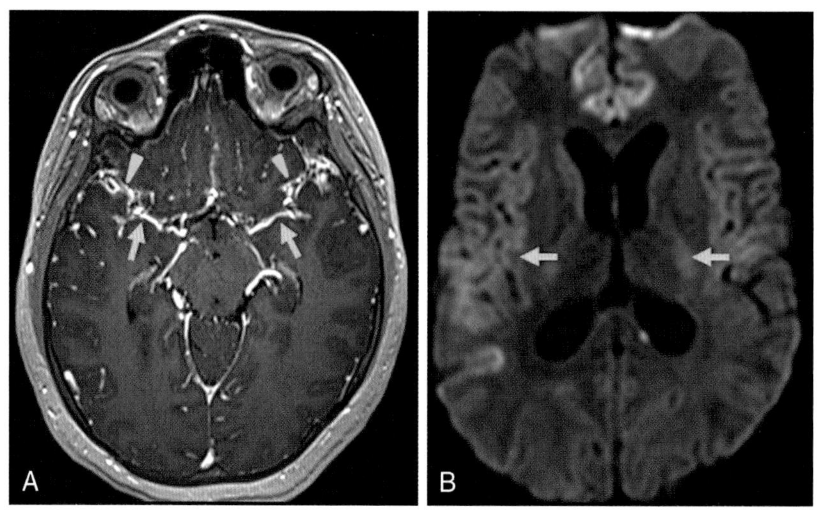


**Fig. 11.16** An 11-year-old girl with acute group B streptococcal meningitis. (A) Axial T1 postcontrast image shows diffuse leptomeningeal and basal exudate (green arrowheads) enhancement with attenuation of the bilateral middle cerebral and anterior cerebral arteries (arrows), suggestive of vasculitis. (B) Multiple areas of restricted diffusion in the bilateral frontoparietal region and internal capsule (arrows) are also noted in keeping with secondary vasculitic infarcts.

secondary vasculitis or cerebral venous thrombosis.[42] Ventriculitis, which is rare in adults, can be seen as a complication of neonatal meningitis, as ependymal enhancement, intraventricular debris, and septations.

## ENCEPHALITIS

Parenchymal inflammation can occur secondary to viruses, bacteria, parasites, autoimmune etiology, or demyelination. Herpetic encephalitis is common in neonates and young children, while enteroviral encephalitis is frequent in toddlers.[49] MRI with contrast is the modality of choice and can suggest the diagnosis based on the typical distribution of the findings: mesial temporal, subfrontal, insular, and cingular cortex in herpes simplex virus (HSV)-1 encephalitis (Fig. 11.17), diffuse or scattered white matter and cortical involvement with or without basal ganglia in HSV-2 encephalitis (Fig. 11.18), limbic involvement in autoimmune encephalitis, and thalamic involvement with flavivirus. Note that HSV-2 encephalitis in the neonate usually spares the mesial temporal and subfrontal lobes.[50]

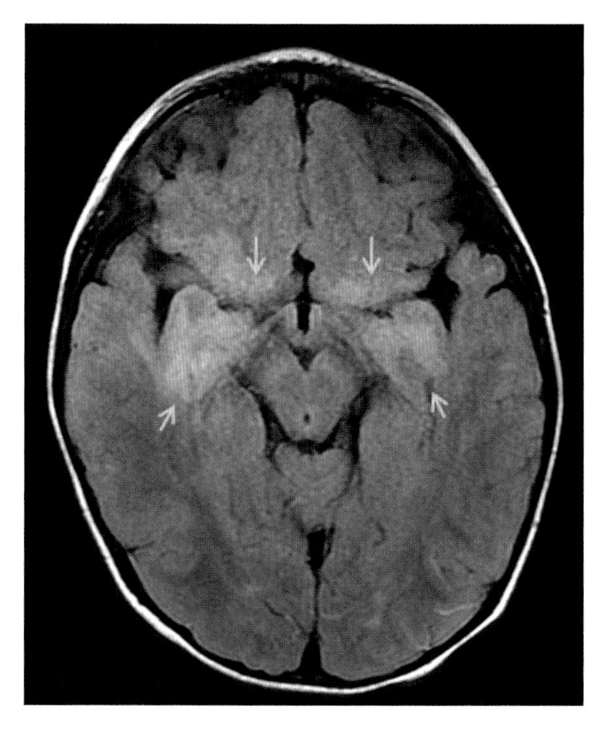

**Fig. 11.17** A 5-year-old boy with febrile encephalopathy. Axial fluid-attenuated inversion recovery images showed bilateral asymmetrical basifrontal, and mesial temporal hyperintensities (arrows) in proven herpes simplex virus–1 encephalitis.

## BRAIN ABSCESS

Frequently develops from an adjacent infective focus, including sinusitis, mastoiditis, dental infections, or

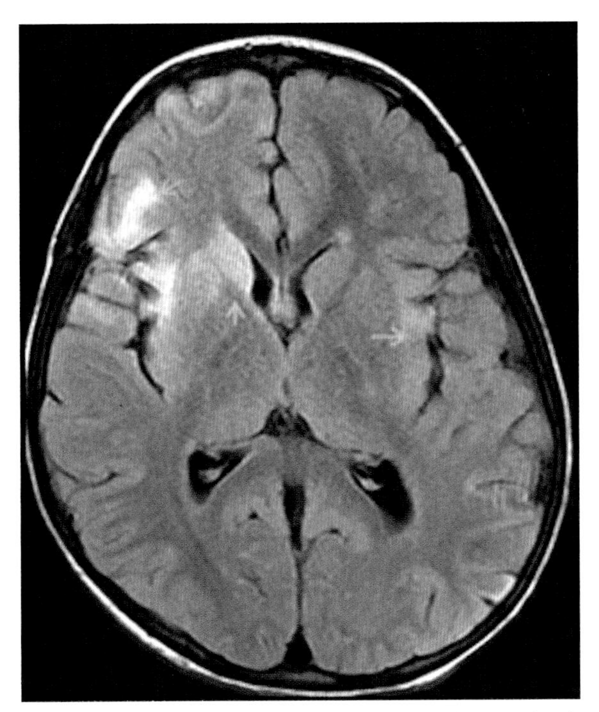

Fig. 11.18 A 2.5-month-old girl with complex febrile seizures and positive herpes simplex virus–2 titer shows multiple fluid-attenuated inversion recovery hyperintensities in the right basal ganglia, right frontotemporal cortical-subcortical, and right insular regions (arrows), with relative sparing of the medial temporal (not shown) and basi-frontal region.

meningitis, or secondary to congenital heart defect, tubercular and fungal infections.[51] Fungal CNS infections are most commonly seen in premature or immunocompromised children. FLAIR/T2*WI show extensive surrounding vasogenic edema and ring-like enhancement (Fig. 11.19A) on postcontrast T1WI.[52] The ring or wall of pyogenic and tubercular abscesses appears relatively smooth compared with the fungal abscess, which frequently shows intracavitary projections.[52] DWI/ADC helps differentiate fungal abscess by the presence of diffusion restriction predominantly in the wall, compared with pyogenic and tubercular abscesses, which also demonstrate restriction in the cavity (Fig. 11.19B).

## TUBERCULOSIS

More than 25% of children show extrapulmonary presentation of tuberculosis, most frequently tuberculous meningitis.[53] Contrast-enhanced MRI is the imaging modality of choice and typically shows enhancing basal exudates and thick irregular meninges.[42] Vasculitis, infarcts, and hydrocephalus are common complications of tuberculous meningitis. Tuberculomas (Fig. 11.20) are small parenchymal lesions, usually multiple. The MR features of tuberculoma depend upon the extent of caseation and necrosis. Caseating tuberculomas are

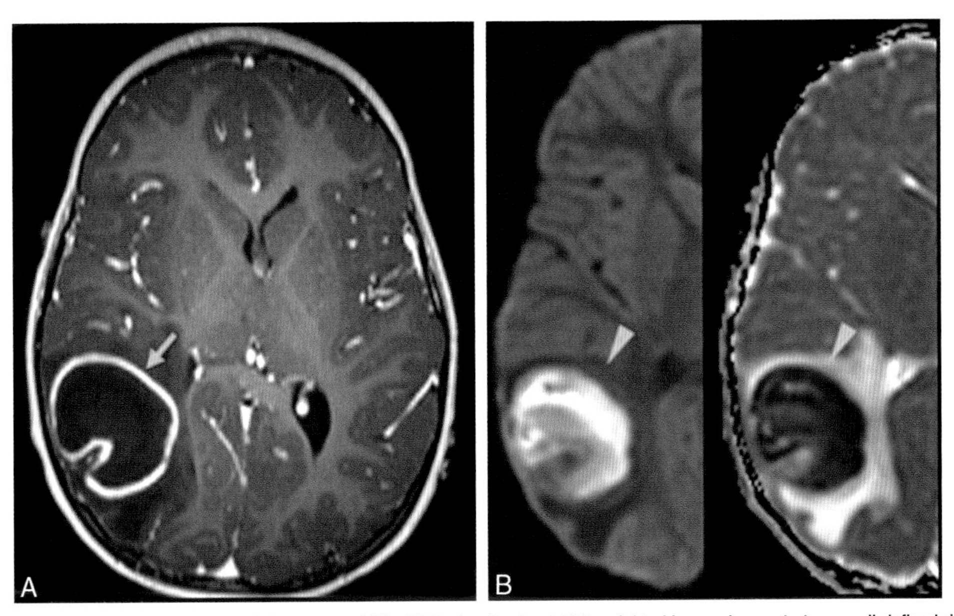


Fig. 11.19 A 9-year-old boy with complicated right otomastoiditis. (A) Postcontrast axial T1-weighted image demonstrates a well-defined ring-enhancing lesion (arrow) in the right parietooccipital region with surrounding edema. (B) On diffusion-weighted imaging, the lesion shows restricted diffusion (arrowheads) within the lesion, appearing hyperintense on B1000 and hypointense on the apparent diffusion coefficient map, favoring a cerebral abscess.

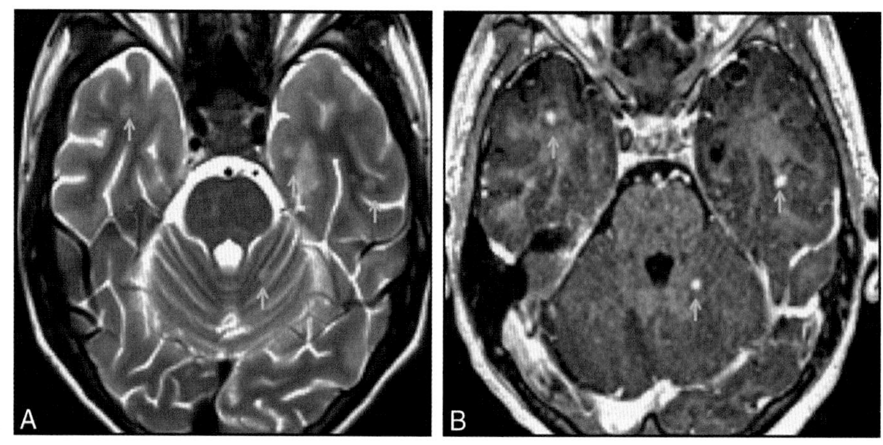


Fig. 11.20 A 17-year-old girl with known pulmonary tuberculosis. (A) T2-weighted axial magnetic resonance image demonstrates multiple small, rounded, hyperintense lesions (yellow arrows) in the brain parenchyma, predominantly at the corticomedullary junction, with mild surrounding edema. (B) On postcontrast T1-weighted imaging, these lesions show disc-like enhancement (arrows), in keeping with tuberculomas without caseous necrosis.

hypo-isointense on T1 and hypointense on T2 with a T1 hyperintense rim and ring-like enhancement, while noncaseating and necrotic caseous tuberculomas are hypointense on T1, hyperintense on T2 with disc-like enhancement in noncaseous, and ring-like enhancement in necrotic caseous tuberculoma. Calcified tuberculomas are hypointense on all sequences with no contrast enhancement.[54]

### SARS-COV-2

There is a relative paucity of literature for pediatric brain involvement in SARS-CoV-2 infection in children because children are less affected and do not frequently exhibit CNS involvement.[55] Based on the limited publications, a few patterns such as immune-mediated inflammation of the brain (acute demyelinating encephalomyelitis [ADEM]-like), spine (myelitis), cranial nerves, and spinal nerve roots (neuritis and or cauda equine syndrome) have been identified.[56] Other imaging findings include thromboischemic infarction, microhemorrhages, splenial lesions, cerebellitis, and facial myositis.[56]

#### Imaging Pitfalls

Uncomplicated meningitis can present as normal on MRI, and CSF analysis is the key to diagnosis. ADEM can mimic infective encephalitis, but encephalopathic presentation and history of recent infection/vaccination favors ADEM.

#### Imaging Requisites

Postcontrast T1WI, preferably with fat saturation, should be obtained. Magnetization prepared rapid gradient-echo imaging (MP-RAGE)/spoiled gradient recalled (SPGR) acquisition is desirable over turbo spin-echo when venous sinus thrombosis is suspected. DWI and TOF-MRA should be part of the imaging protocol to evaluate the complications. MR spectroscopy (MRS) helps differentiate from tumor. In presence of empyema, closely evaluate the adjacent calvaria for signs of osteomyelitis.

#### Reporting Checklist

Identify the extent of involvement; look for complications such as cerebritis, abscess, hydrocephalus, vasculitis, infarcts, CSVT, and extra-axial collections. Complicated extracranial infections (sinuses, ear, orbits) should be reported and warrant close evaluation of the surrounding intracranial structures.

## Hydrocephalus

Children with increased intracranial pressure present to the ED either due to the development of acute hydrocephalus or worsening of preexisting hydrocephalus from a shunt malfunction. Clinical presentation varies with age. Infants present with abnormal and rapidly increasing head circumference, irritability, vomiting, and bulging fontanelle, while in older children nausea, vomiting, worsening headache, and diplopia are frequently encountered.[57] Hydrocephalus can occur secondary to obstruction of CSF flow, decreased CSF resorption, or increased CSF production.

Neuroimaging should be directed to evaluate the extent of hydrocephalus and identify the underlying cause. MRI is the investigation of choice. Ultrafast MR protocols are frequently replacing emergency CT in children, as they offer superior anatomic detail of the ventricular system and brain parenchyma, and allow reliable visualization of the ventricular catheter without radiation or anesthesia.[9,58–62]

## NEW-ONSET HYDROCEPHALUS

Noncommunicating obstructive causes are the most common and usually occur secondary to the tumor at a critical location such as foramina of Monroe, aqueduct of Sylvius, and fourth ventricle (Fig. 11.21), followed by less common causes: aqueductal stenosis or web (Fig. 11.22), nonneoplastic cysts, and Chiari malformations.[61] The role of imaging is to determine the site and the cause of obstruction, as well as the extent of ventricular dilatation, and to exclude metastatic disease in presence of malignancy.[1]

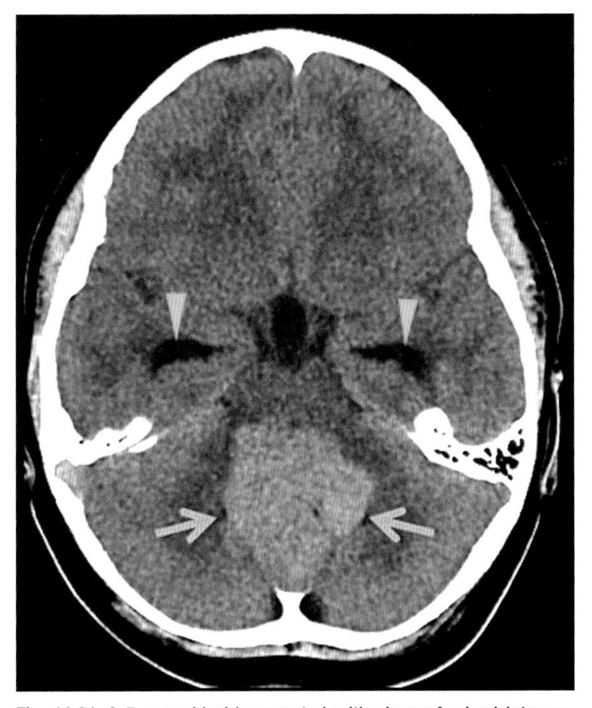

**Fig. 11.21** A 5-year-old girl presented with signs of raised intracranial pressure. Axial computed tomography image shows supratentorial hydrocephalus (arrowheads) and a large, homogeneous, hyperdense mass filling the fourth ventricle (yellow arrow) without definite necrosis, hemorrhage, or calcification. The final diagnosis was medulloblastoma.

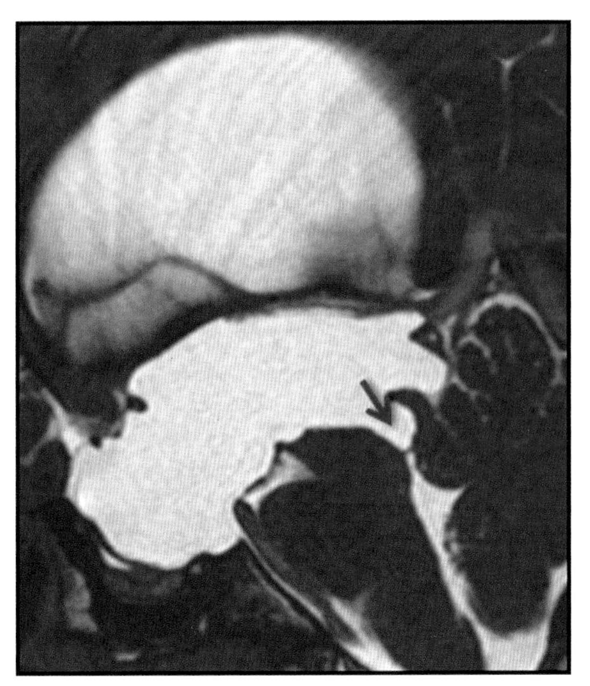

**Fig. 11.22** A 13-year-old boy presented with increasing headache and signs of raised intracranial pressure. Ultrafast sagittal magnetic resonance imaging shows severe dilatation of lateral and third ventricle and prominence of the cranial aqueduct of Sylvius with a thin membrane in the distal aqueduct (arrow). Normal-appearing fourth ventricle. Diagnosis was aqueductal stenosis from aqueductal web.

## HYDROCEPHALUS DUE TO SHUNT MALFUNCTION

Ventricular shunt malfunction (Fig. 11.23) is seen in up to 40% of children, commonly within the first 2 years, and is usually due to mechanical obstruction, requiring replacement of the obstructed component. Failure of endoscopic third ventriculostomy (ETV) is highest in the first 3 months, and delayed dysfunctions of ETV are less frequent than malfunction of the ventricular shunt. Another common complication is the shunt infection, which is more common with ventricular shunt than ETV and is seen in up to 10% of cases, usually within the first 3 months following the surgery.[57]

Imaging in shunted hydrocephalus is performed to determine the change in ventricular size and configuration, to identify intracranial infarction or hemorrhage, and to assess shunt catheter discontinuity, migration, or

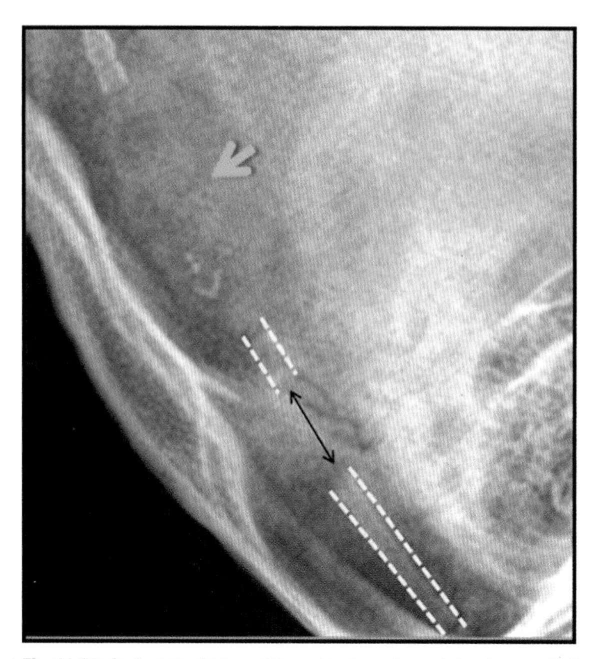

**Fig. 11.23** An 8-year-old boy with ventriculoperitoneal shunt presented with increasing headache and signs of raised intracranial pressure. The lateral skull X-ray taken as part of the shunt survey shows the discontinuity (black arrow line) of the catheter (broken yellow lines) measuring approximately 1.1 cm compared with the previous X-ray (not shown), where it measured 0.3 cm. Normal lucency at the level of the reservoir (green arrow).

infection.[3] Although MRI is the modality of choice, low-dose CT along with radiographs of skull, neck, chest, and abdomen (shunt survey) may be required in certain cases to evaluate shunt catheter integrity (Fig. 11.23).[62] When abdominal symptoms are present, an ultrasound of the abdomen to evaluate for peritoneal CSF collection is useful in the assessment of these patients.[3]

### Imaging Pitfalls

Pulsatile CSF flow may be confused with lesions on MRI due to flow voids. On shunt series, the lucency between the radiopaque markers and reservoir (green arrow in Fig. 11.23) should not be considered discontinuity of the catheter.[3] *Ex vacuo* dilatation of the ventricle with parenchymal volume loss is not hydrocephalus.

### Imaging Requisites

An ultrafast MR protocol must include three planes of T2 SSFSE and additional T1WI to exclude hemorrhage in patients with shunt surgery.[9] Evaluation of the shunt catheter integrity must be part of the routine assessment in children with suspected shunt malfunction; a CT scanogram may be helpful.[3,62]

### Reporting Checklist

Size and configuration of the ventricles, interval change, presence of transependymal CSF leak, and level and cause of obstruction. Presence of any complication (hemorrhage, herniation, or mass lesion). Carefully inspect the shunt catheter within the field of view for any discontinuity.

The reporting radiologist must review all the available previous scans to evaluate serial changes in the size and configuration of the ventricular system. Measurements of the ventricular size may not necessarily correlate with intracranial pressure, and the frontal or occipital horn ratios have not proven to be reliable in assessing the effectiveness of the treatment. Clinical assessment in combination with the imaging findings remains the most accepted method.[63]

## NEW-ONSET AFEBRILE SEIZURE

According to the International League Against Epilepsy, new-onset seizures/epilepsy with a medical emergency (status epilepticus, focal localization, or neurological deficit) requires emergency neuroimaging, in contrast to first-time simple febrile seizures, which do not warrant emergency neuroimaging.[64] The role of emergent neuroimaging is to assess for intracranial pathologies that require urgent intervention, for example, ICH (Fig. 11.15), space-occupying lesion (Fig. 11.24) (Fig. 11.25), hydrocephalus, encephalitis, hypoxic-ischemic injury (Fig. 11.26), and metabolic conditions (Fig. 11.27), as well as to rule out acute life-threatening complications, such as cerebral herniation.[65] New-onset nontraumatic afebrile seizure in a neonate is almost always associated with a recognizable etiology and should always be followed by emergent neuroimaging.[3] Although CT is often used as a first imaging tool in the ED, MRI is the imaging modality of choice to rule out the structural and metabolic causes associated with the first presentation of an afebrile seizure.

### Imaging Requisites

CT is often the primary imaging modality in the ED, but MR should be embraced whenever possible in a new-onset afebrile seizure with focal localization, neurological deficit, or status epilepticus.

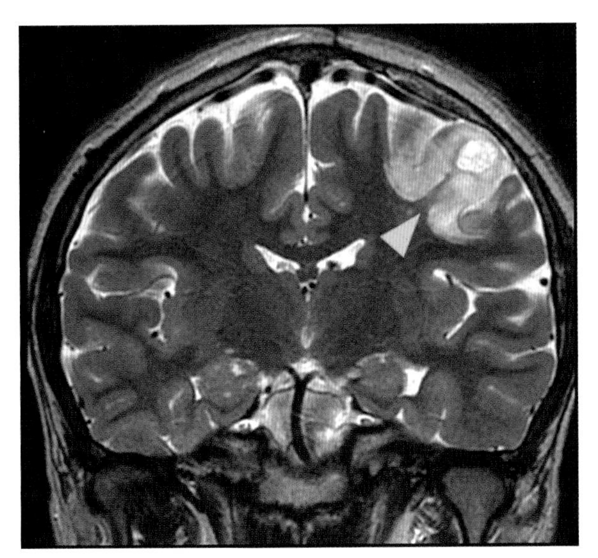

Fig. 11.24 A 16-year-old girl with new-onset seizures. Coronal T2-weighted image shows a T2-hyperintense cortical and subcortical bubbly mass lesion (yellow arrowhead) of the left precentral gyrus suggestive of low-grade glioma or dysembryoplastic neuroepithelial tumor (biopsy not done).

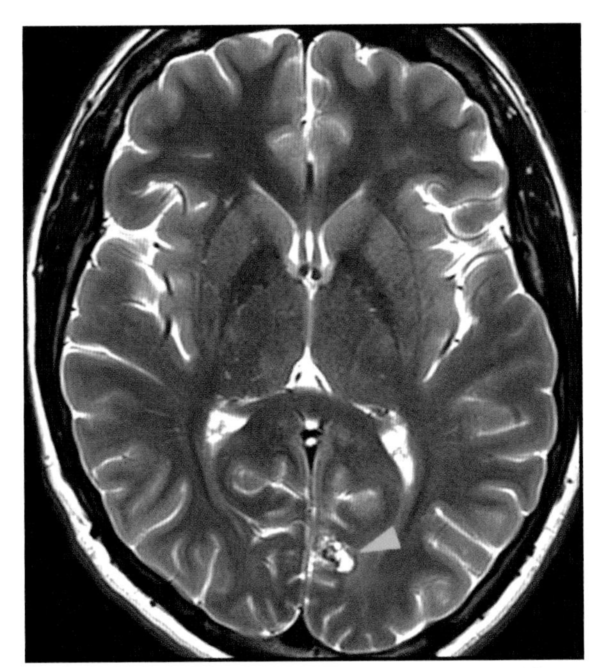

Fig. 11.25 A 7-year-old girl with seizures. Axial T2-weighted image shows a T2-hyperintense cortical lesion in the left medial occipital cortex with typical popcorn appearance (green arrowhead) and blooming on susceptibility-weighted images (not shown), in keeping with a cavernoma.

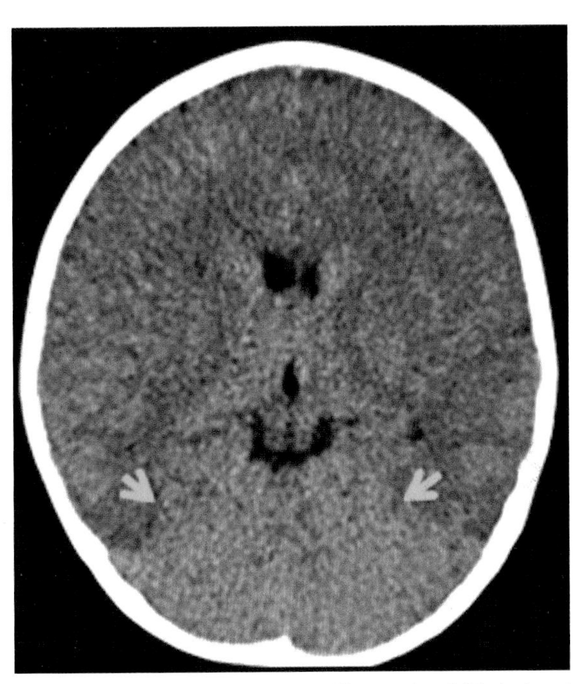

Fig. 11.26 A 6-month-old boy, post-cardiac arrest and 45 minutes of cardiopulmonary resuscitation. Axial nonenhanced computed tomography shows diffuse cerebral hypodensity and loss of grey-white matter differentiation with normal-appearing (arrows) cerebellum (white cerebellar sign), in keeping with severe hypoxic-ischemic encephalopathy.

### Imaging Pitfalls

Postictal or Todd palsy, although rare in children, can mimic focal neurological deficit clinically and space-occupying lesion on imaging, due to mass-like cortical-subcortical involvement, restricted diffusion, and variable postcontrast enhancement.[43]

### Reporting Checklist

Exclude life-threatening complications requiring urgent intervention, such as hydrocephalus, cerebral edema, ICH, or brain herniation. Look for the presence of structural abnormalities, tumors, metabolic and ischemic abnormality, or toxin- or drug-related changes.

## Headache

Pediatric headache is among the most frequent complaints requiring an ED visit. The most common recurrent headaches in childhood are migraines, while tension headaches prevail in adolescence.[66] The

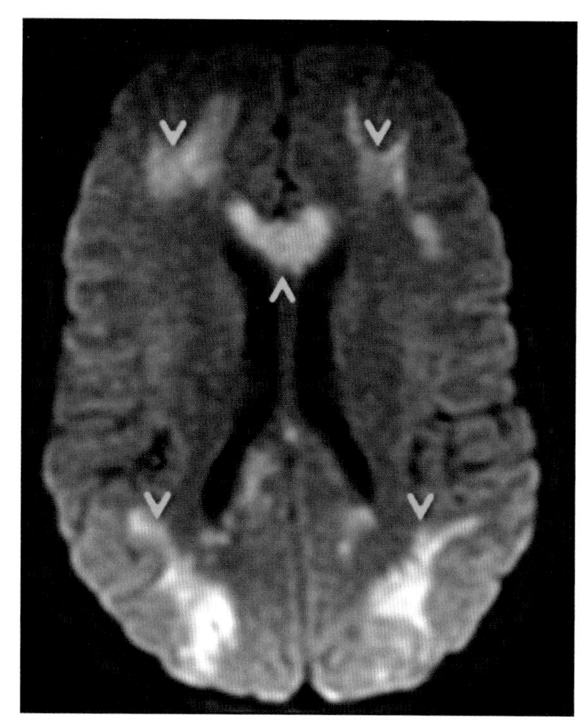

Fig. 11.27 A 15-year-old boy with a history of polysubstance abuse and altered mentation. Axial diffusion-weighted imaging shows multiple areas of restricted diffusion involving the coronary radiata, periventricular white matter, and corpus callosum (arrowheads) from cocaine-induced leukoencephalopathy.

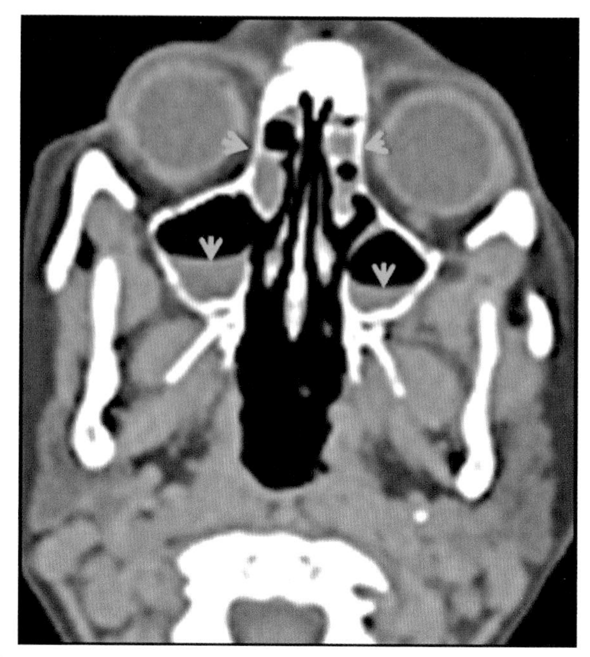

Fig. 11.28 A 12-year-old boy with acute severe headache. Axial unenhanced computed tomography shows opacification of ethmoid and maxillary sinuses with air-fluid levels (arrows), in keeping with acute sinusitis.

International Headache Society published a standardized classification scheme that provides diagnostic criteria for headaches in general, and its most recent update was released in 2018, which divides headaches into primary, secondary, and painful cranial neuropathies.[67] Emergency imaging is not warranted in primary benign-type headaches but is commonly performed in suspected secondary causes, essentially in the presence of warning signs (red flags) like sudden-onset headache, changing pattern of headache, sleep disturbance, associated vomiting, altered mentation, seizure, focal neurological deficit, and papilledema.[68]

CT is the most common initial imaging modality in an emergency. CT examination may include facial bones if sinonasal disease is suspected (Fig. 11.28).[68] Whenever available and feasible, an ultrafast MRI is increasingly used in pediatric patients.[69] Even for SAH, a combination of FLAIR and SWI is equivalent or even found better than CT in few studies.[70] Idiopathic intracranial hypertension (IIH), though a rare cause, may present in the ED with severe headache and shows characteristic findings including empty sella, optic nerve tortuosity, and transverse venous sinuses stenosis.

### Imaging Requisites

CT is helpful in excluding bleeding or space-occupying lesions, but MRI is the investigation of choice. When MRI is performed for the initial assessment of headache, the protocol should include T1, T2, DWI, FLAIR, and SWI sequences. The addition of MRA/MRV helps rule out a vascular cause. Screening of the spine should be considered in suspected Chiari malformations (Fig. 11.29).

### Imaging Pitfalls

When imaging for headaches, be aware of the possibility of unrelated findings such as arachnoid cyst and pineal gland cyst (incidentalomas). Transverse sinus stenosis in IIH should not be confused with venous sinus thrombosis.

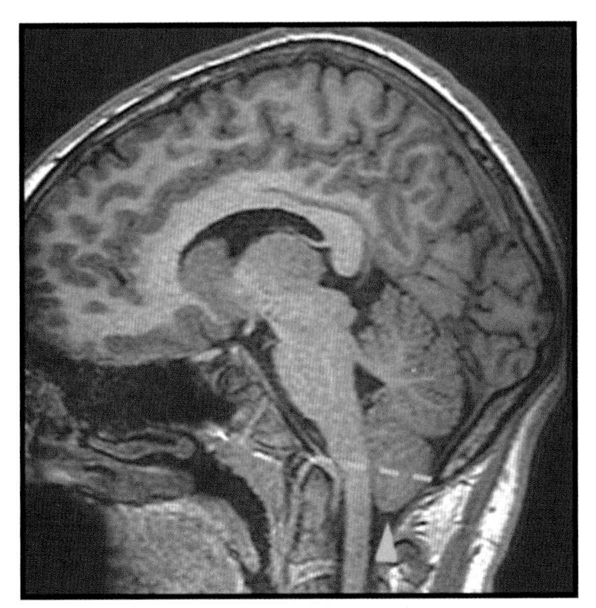

**Fig. 11.29** A 14-year-old boy with chronic headache. Sagittal T1-weighted ultrafast magnetic resonance imaging screening protocol shows low-lying cerebellar tonsils (arrowhead), resulting in crowding of the foramen magnum (dotted line), effaced retrocerebellar, prepontine, and premedullary cisterns representing Chiari I malformation. The spine (not shown) was normal.

### Reporting Checklist

Rule out sinonasal disease, petromastoid pathologies, signs of IIH, and Chiari malformations, along with vascular causes.

## Acute Encephalopathy

Childhood encephalopathy is an uncommon but serious disorder that is associated with significant mortality and long-term morbidity. Encephalopathy is an umbrella diagnosis that encompasses a variety of serious medical conditions presenting with lethargy, drowsiness, and altered consciousness and/or cognition.[71] Acute pediatric encephalopathy can occur from a myriad of conditions, including infection, trauma, hypoxic-ischemic injury, hypertension, demyelination, metabolic dysfunction, toxins, and drugs, or in association with hematooncological disease.[72] After clinical examination and laboratory evaluation to rule out hypoglycemia and ketoacidosis, neuroimaging is often contemplated.[73] In an emergency setting, CT is primarily performed to rule out any life-threatening complications. MRI is the imaging modality of choice, and the protocol should include DWI, SWI, MRA, MRV, and MRS.[72]

### HYPOXIC-ISCHEMIC ENCEPHALOPATHY

Hypoxic-ischemic encephalopathy (Fig. 11.26) is the most common cause of neonatal and infantile encephalopathy.[72] MRI is the investigation of choice,[74] while MRS and DWI/ADC are the most sensitive sequences. MRS may become positive within the first 24 hours (lactate peak at 1.3 ppm), when DWI may underestimate the restriction in the undermyelinated brain. DWI is most diagnostic around 24 hours and should be read with the corresponding ADC map.[74]

#### Toxic-Metabolic

This is a broad category that includes drug-related (therapeutic and illegal) (Fig. 11.27), metabolic (lactic acidosis, organic acidurias, urea cycle disorders, osmotic demyelination), and endocrinal (hyperglycemia, ketoacidosis) causes. Bilateral cerebral edema is a nonspecific finding and is seen in almost all cases.[71] However, in an appropriate clinical setting, specific imaging findings may point to the specific diagnosis. For example, CSVT (Fig. 11.14A) is seen in asparaginase therapy in leukemia, stroke and ICH in cocaine and heroin drug abuse (Fig. 11.27), leukoencephalopathy after methotrexate therapy, and periinsular involvement with urea cycle disorders.[1,43,74]

#### Neonatal Hypoglycemia

Usually presents within the first 3 days of life in term neonates with severe hypoglycemia and can cause extensive brain injury. Prognosis depends on the early recognition and treatment of hypoglycemia. MRI shows edema or infarction, most commonly in the bilateral parietooccipital lobes, splenium (Fig. 11.30), basal ganglia, thalamus, and brainstem. If the diagnosis is made by blood or urine examination, neuroimaging is then carried out to evaluate the extent of the injury.

#### Autoimmune

ADEM is a monophasic demyelinating disorder presenting with encephalopathy 1 to 3 weeks following nonspecific infection, vaccination, or idiopathic causes.[49] Typical imaging findings are multifocal and asymmetric white matter involvement with deep grey matter lesions

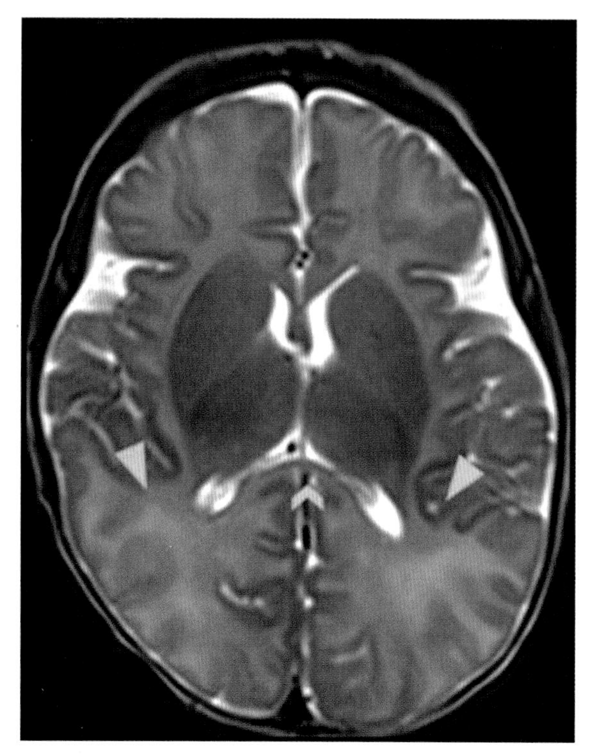

Fig. 11.30 A 5-day-old term boy born to a diabetic mother presented with lethargy and poor feeding. Axial T2-weighted imaging shows bilateral parietooccipital (arrowheads) and splenium (chevron) hyperintensities from neonatal hypoglycemia.

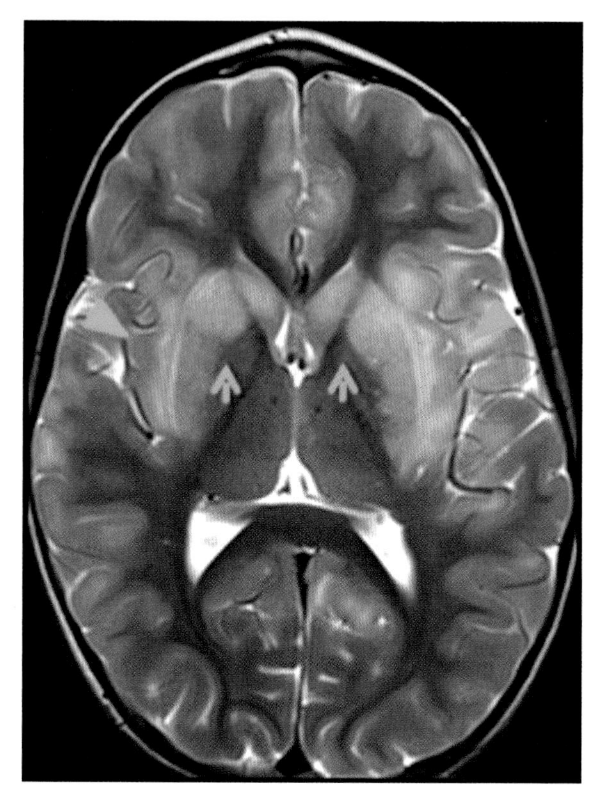

Fig. 11.31 A 6-year-old boy with encephalopathy following 2 weeks of flu-like illness. Axial T2-weighted imaging shows multiple hyperintense areas involving bilateral putamina (arrows), cortical-subcortical white matter, insular regions (arrowheads), and brainstem (not shown). The appearance is typical of acute demyelinating encephalomyelitis. Complete resolution on follow-up images (not shown).

(Fig. 11.31); the brainstem, cerebellum, and cord can also be involved.[42] Acute hemorrhagic encephalomyelitis (Hurst disease), the most severe and frequently fatal variant, presents with classical hemorrhagic leukoencephalitis due to necrotizing vasculitis.[75]

### Posterior Reversible Encephalopathy Syndrome

Hypertensive encephalopathy in the pediatric population usually occurs secondary to drugs (immunosuppressive medication, e.g., tacrolimus, cyclosporine, some chemotherapeutic agents) and renal dysfunction.[72] MRI is the imaging of choice and demonstrates vasogenic edema in the watershed areas, most frequently the parietooccipital. Infrequently, the basal ganglia, pons, and cerebellum can be involved.

### Imaging Requisites

The MRI protocol should include T1WI, T2*WI, DWI, SWI, MRA, MRV, and MRS.[76] Postcontrast T1 and FLAIR imaging improve the ability to diagnose leptomeningeal enhancement.

### Imaging Pitfalls

In ADEM, imaging findings may lag behind the initial symptoms and could persist even after clinical improvement. The differential diagnosis of PRES is cerebral ischemia and hypoglycemia, but DWI is usually negative in PRES. Restriction diffusion, enhancement, and hemorrhages are rare in PRES (atypical PRES) and suggest poorer outcomes.

### Reporting Checklist

Extent and distribution of parenchymal involvement, hemorrhages, presence of diffusion restriction, and parenchymal or leptomeningeal enhancement.

## Conclusion

Children with acute neuroemergencies can have very unpredictable presentations. The unavoidable deficiency in pertinent history and lack of reliable clinical evaluation in the ED implies marked responsibility on the radiologist for delivering a precise diagnosis and calling immediate attention to life-threatening complications requiring urgent intervention.

## REFERENCES


1. Orman G, Rossi A, Meoded A, Huisman TAGM. Children with acute neurological emergency Updated 2020. Accessed. In: Hodler J, Kubik-Huch RA, von Schulthess GK, eds. *Diseases of the Brain, Head and Neck, Spine 2020–2023: Diagnostic Imaging [Internet]*. Springer; April 4, 2021. http://www.ncbi.nlm.nih.gov/books/NBK554331/.
2. Saigal G, Ezuddin NS, de la Vega G. Neurologic Emergencies in pediatric patients including accidental and nonaccidental trauma. *Neuroimaging Clin N Am*. 2018;28(3):453–470.
3. Pediatric Central Nervous System Emergencies - Neuroimaging Clinics [Internet]. https://www.neuroimaging.theclinics.com/article/S1052-5149(10)00080-8/abstract. [Accessed 4 April 2021].
4. McAllister AS, Nagaraj U, Radhakrishnan R. Emergent Imaging of pediatric cervical spine trauma. *RadioGraphics*. 2019;39(4):1126–1142.
5. Visocchi M, Chiaretti A, Genovese O, Di Rocco F. Haemodynamic patterns in children with posttraumatic diffuse brain swelling. A preliminary study in 6 cases with neuroradiological features consistent with diffuse axonal injury. *Acta Neurochir (Wien)*. 2007;149(4):347–356.
6. Kadom N, Vey BL, Frush DP, Broder JS, Applegate KE. Committee Members of the IGTA-HC. Think A-Head Campaign of Image Gently: shared decision-making in pediatric head trauma. *Am J Neuroradiol*. 2018;39(8):1386–1389.
7. Zimmerman RA, Bilaniuk LT, Pollock AN, Feygin T, Zarnow D, Schwartz ES, et al. 3.0 T versus 1.5 T pediatric brain imaging. *Neuroimaging Clin N Am*. 2006;16(2):229–239. ix.
8. Ramgopal S, Karim SA, Subramanian S, Furtado AD, Marin JR. Rapid brain MRI protocols reduce head computerized tomography use in the pediatric emergency department. *BMC Pediatrics*. 2020;20(1):14.
9. Rozovsky K, Ventureyra ECG, Miller E. Fast-brain MRI in children is quick, without sedation, and radiation-free, but beware of limitations. *J Clin Neurosci*. 2013;20(3):400–405.
10. Blystad I, Warntjes JBM, Smedby O, Landtblom A-M, Lundberg P, Larsson E-M. Synthetic MRI of the brain in a clinical setting. *Acta Radiol*. 2012;53(10):1158–1163. 1.
11. Wagner MW, Kontzialis M, Seeburg D, Stern SE, Oshmyansky A, Poretti A, et al. Acute brain imaging in children: can MRI replace CT as a screening tool? *J Neuroimaging*. 2016;26(1):68–74.
12. Ha JY, Baek HJ, Ryu KH, Choi BH, Moon JI, Park SE, et al. One-minute ultrafast brain MRI with full basic sequences: can it be a promising way forward for pediatric neuroimaging? *Am J Roentgenology*. 2020;215(1):198–205.
13. Farrell CA. Canadian Paediatric Society, Acute Care Committee. Management of the paediatric patient with acute head trauma. *Paediatrics & Child Health*. 2013;18(5):253–258.
14. Sookplung P, Vavilala MS. What is new in pediatric traumatic brain injury? *Curr Opin Anaesthesiol*. 2009;22(5):572–578.
15. Holmes JF, Palchak MJ, MacFarlane T, Kuppermann N. Performance of the pediatric glasgow coma scale in children with blunt head trauma. *Acad Emerg Med*. 2005;12(9):814–819.
16. Kuppermann N, Holmes JF, Dayan PS, Hoyle JD, Atabaki SM, Holubkov R, et al. Identification of children at very low risk of clinically-important brain injuries after head trauma: a prospective cohort study. *Lancet*. 2009;374(9696):1160–1170.
17. Maguire JL, Boutis K, Uleryk EM, Laupacis A, Parkin PC. Should a head-injured child receive a head CT scan? A systematic review of clinical prediction rules. *Pediatrics*. 2009;124(1):e145–e154.
18. Educational Modules for Appropriate Imaging Referrals - Paediatric Head Trauma | RANZCR [Internet]. Accessed April 4, 2021. https://www.ranzcr.com/documents/3870-paediatric-head-trauma
19. Themes UFO. Injuries of extracranial, cranial, intracranial, spinal cord, and peripheral nervous system structures [Internet]. Neupsy Key. Updated 2019. Accessed April 4, 2021. https://neupsykey.com/injuries-of-extracranial-cranial-intracranial-spinal-cord-and-peripheral-nervous-system-structures/
20. O'Brien WT, Caré MM, Leach JL. Pediatric emergencies: imaging of pediatric head trauma. *Semin Ultrasound CT MR*. 2018;39(5):495–514.
21. Zia Z, Morris A-M, Paw R. Ping-pong fracture. *Emerg Med J*. 2007;24(10):731.
22. Liu X, You C, Lu M, Liu J. Growing skull fracture stages and treatment strategy: Clinical article. *J Neurosurgery: Pediatrics*. 2012;9(6):670–675.
23. Idriz S, Patel JH, Ameli Renani S, Allan R, Vlahos I. CT of normal developmental and variant anatomy of the pediatric skull: distinguishing trauma from normality. *Radiographics*. 2015;35(5):1585–1601.
24. Orman G, Wagner MW, Seeburg D, Zamora CA, Oshmyansky A, Tekes A, et al. Pediatric skull fracture diagnosis: should 3D CT reconstructions be added as routine imaging? *J Neurosurg Pediatr*. 2015;16(4):426–431.
25. Poussaint TY, Moeller KK. Imaging of pediatric head trauma. *Neuroimaging Clin N Am*. 2002;12(2):271–294. ix.
26. Demaerel PAJ. Barkovich: Pediatric neuroimaging, 3rd edn. *Eur Radiol*. 2001;11(11). 2347-2347.
27. Strub WM, Leach JL, Tomsick T, Vagal A. Overnight preliminary head CT interpretations provided by residents: locations of misidentified intracranial hemorrhage. *AJNR Am J Neuroradiol*. 2007;28(9):1679–1682.
28. Coulier B. Pseudo-subarachnoid hemorrhage. *J Belg Soc Radiol*. 2018;102(1):32.
29. Heit JJ, Iv M, Wintermark M. Imaging of intracranial hemorrhage. *J Stroke*. 2017;19(1):11–27. J.
30. Gentry LR. Imaging of closed head injury. *Radiology*. 1994;191(1):1–17.
31. Abu Hamdeh S, Marklund N, Lannsjö M, Howells T, Raininko R, Wikström J, et al. Extended anatomical grading in diffuse axonal injury using MRI: hemorrhagic lesions in the substantia nigra and mesencephalic tegmentum indicate poor long-term outcome. *J Neurotrauma [Internet]*. 2017;34(2):341–352.
32. Gelineau-Morel RN, Zinkus TP, Le Pichon J-B. Pediatric Head trauma: a review and update. *Pediatr Rev*. 2019;40(9):468–481.
33. Wright JN. CNS injuries in abusive head trauma. *Am J Roentgenol*. 2017;208(5):991–1001.
34. Mirsky DM, Beslow LA, Amlie-Lefond C, Krishnan P, Laughlin S, Lee S, et al. Pathways for neuroimaging of childhood stroke. *Pediatr Neurol*. 2017;69:11–23.

35. Khalaf A, Michael I, Fullerton H, Wintermark M. Pediatric stroke imaging. *Pediatr Neurol*. 2018;86:5–18.
36. Wintermark M, Hills NK, deVeber GA, Barkovich AJ, Elkind MSV, Sear K, et al. Arteriopathy diagnosis in childhood arterial ischemic stroke: results of the vascular effects of infection in pediatric stroke study. *Stroke*. 2014;45(12):3597–3605.
37. Lanni G, Catalucci A, Conti L, Di Sibio A, Paonessa A, Gallucci M. Pediatric stroke: clinical findings and radiological approach. *Stroke Res Treat*. 2011;8:172168.
38. Paonessa A, Limbucci N, Tozzi E, Splendiani A, Gallucci M. Radiological strategy in acute stroke in children. *Eur J Radiol*. 2010;74(1):77–85.
39. Nezamzadeh M, Matson GB, Young K, Weiner MW, Schuff N. Improved pseudo-continuous arterial spin labeling for mapping brain perfusion. *J Magn Reson Imaging*. 2010;31(6): 1419–1427.
40. Stence NV, Pabst LL, Hollatz AL, Mirsky DM, Herson PS, Poisson S, et al. Predicting progression of intracranial arteriopathies in childhood stroke with vessel wall imaging. *Stroke*. 2017;48(8):2274–2277.
41. Ritchey Z, Hollatz AL, Weitzenkamp D, Fenton LZ, Maxwell EC, Bernard TJ, et al. Pediatric cortical vein thrombosis: frequency and association with venous infarction. *Stroke*. 2016;47(3):866–868.
42. Chang PT, Yang E, Swenson DW, Lee EY. Pediatric emergency magnetic resonance imaging: current indications, techniques, and clinical applications. *Magn Reson Imaging Clin N Am*. 2016;24(2):449–480.
43. Lall NU, Stence NV, Mirsky DM. Magnetic resonance imaging of pediatric neurologic emergencies. *Top Magn Reson Imaging*. 2015;24(6):291–307.
44. Goodman S, Pavlakis S. Pediatric and newborn stroke. *Curr Treat Options Neurol*. 2008;10(6):431–439.
45. Smith ER, Butler WE, Ogilvy CS. Surgical approaches to vascular anomalies of the child's brain. *Curr Opin Neurol*. 2002;15(2):165–171.
46. Koenigsberg RA Brain imaging in arteriovenous malformation: practice essentials, radiography, computed tomography [Internet]. Accessed March 07, 2017. https://emedicine.medscape.com/article/337220-overview
47. Yanamadala V, Sheth SA, Walcott BP, Buchbinder BR, Buckley D, Ogilvy CS. Non-contrast 3D time-of-flight magnetic resonance angiography for visualization of intracranial aneurysms in patients with absolute contraindications to CT or MRI contrast. *J Clin Neurosci*. 2013;20(8):1122–1126.
48. Wada R, Aviv RI, Fox AJ, Sahlas DJ, Gladstone DJ, Tomlinson G, et al. CT angiography "spot sign" predicts hematoma expansion in acute intracerebral hemorrhage. *Stroke*. 2007;38(4):1257–1262.
49. Simon DW, Silva YSD, Zuccoli G, Clark RSB. Acute encephalitis. *Crit Care Clin*. 2013;29(2):259–277.
50. Baskin HJ, Hedlund G. Neuroimaging of herpesvirus infections in children. *Pediatr Radiol*. 2007;37(10):949–963.
51. Shachor-Meyouhas Y, Bar-Joseph G, Guilburd JN, Lorber A, Hadash A, Kassis I. Brain abscess in children - epidemiology, predisposing factors and management in the modern medicine era. *Acta Paediatr*. 2010;99(8):1163–1167.
52. Luthra G, Parihar A, Nath K, Jaiswal S, Prasad KN, Husain N, et al. Comparative evaluation of fungal, tubercular, and pyogenic brain abscesses with conventional and diffusion MR imaging and proton MR spectroscopy. *AJNR Am J Neuroradiol*. 2007;28(7):1332–1338.
53. Aulakh R, Chopra S. Pediatric tubercular meningitis: a review. *J Pediatr Neurosci*. 2018;13(4):373–382.
54. Khatri GD, Krishnan V, Antil N, Saigal G. Magnetic resonance imaging spectrum of intracranial tubercular lesions: one disease, many faces. *Pol J Radiol*. 2018;83:e524–e535.
55. Hoang A, Chorath K, Moreira A, Evans M, Burmeister-Morton F, Burmeister F, et al. COVID-19 in 7780 pediatric patients: A systematic review. *E Clinical Medicine*. 2020;24:100423.
56. Lindan CE, Mankad K, Ram D, Kociolek LK, Silvera VM, Boddaert N, et al. Neuroimaging manifestations in children with SARS-CoV-2 infection: a multinational, multicentre collaborative study. *Lancet Child Adolesc Health*. 2021;5(3):167–177.
57. Kahle KT, Kulkarni AV, Limbrick DD, Warf BC. Hydrocephalus in children. *Lancet*. 2016;387(10020):788–799.
58. Ashley WW, McKinstry RC, Leonard JR, Smyth MD, Lee BC, Park TS. Use of rapid-sequence magnetic resonance imaging for evaluation of hydrocephalus in children. *J Neurosurg*. 2005;103(2 Suppl):124–130.
59. Niederhauser BD, McDonald RJ, Eckel LJ, Keating GF, Broomall EM, Wetjen NM, et al. Retrospective review of rapid pediatric brain MR imaging at an academic institution including practice trends and factors affecting scan times. *AJNR Am J Neuroradiol*. 2013;34(9):1836–1840.
60. O'Neill BR, Pruthi S, Bains H, Robison R, Weir K, Ojemann J, et al. Rapid sequence magnetic resonance imaging in the assessment of children with hydrocephalus. *World Neurosurg*. 2013;80(6):e307–e312.
61. Barkovich J, Raybaud C *Pediatric Neuroimaging*. Wolters Kluwer, Lippincott Williams & Wilkins; 2005. Fourth Edition.
62. Orman G, Bosemani T, Tekes A, Poretti A, Huisman TAGM. Scout view in pediatric CT neuroradiological evaluation: do not underestimate! *Childs Nerv Syst*. 2014;30(2):307–311.
63. Nikas DC, Post AF, Choudhri AF, Mazzola CA, Mitchell L, Flannery AM, et al. Pediatric hydrocephalus: systematic literature review and evidence-based guidelines. Part 10: Change in ventricle size as a measurement of effective treatment of hydrocephalus. *J Neurosurg Pediatr*. 2014;14(Suppl 1):77–81.
64. Lyons TW, Johnson KB, Michelson KA, Nigrovic LE, Loddenkemper T, Prabhu SP, et al. Yield of emergent neuroimaging in children with new-onset seizure and status epilepticus. *Seizure*. 2016;35:4–10.
65. Teng D, Dayan P, Tyler S, Hauser WA, Chan S, Leary L, et al. Risk of intracranial pathologic conditions requiring emergency intervention after a first complex febrile seizure episode among children. *Pediatrics*. 2006;117(2):304–308.
66. Cain MR, Arkilo D, Linabery AM, Kharbanda AB. Emergency department use of neuroimaging in children and adolescents presenting with headache. *J Pediatr*. 2018;201:196–201.
67. Headache Classification Committee of the International Headache Society (IHS) The International Classification of Headache Disorders, 3rd edition. *Cephalalgia*. 2018;38(1):1–211.
68. Guryildirim M, Kontzialis M, Ozen M, Kocak M. Acute headache in the emergency setting. *RadioGraphics*. 2019;39(6):1739–1759.
69. Blanco-Baudrit DA, Blanco-Baudrit LF, Yock-Corrales A. Pediatric headache in the emergency department. *Pediatr Neonatal Nurs Open J [Internet]*. 2016;2(3):99–103.
70. Verma RK, Kottke R, Andereggen L, Weisstanner C, Zubler C, Gralla J, et al. Detecting subarachnoid hemorrhage: comparison of combined FLAIR/SWI versus CT. *Eur J Radiol*. 2013;82(9):1539–1545.
71. Davies E, Connolly DJ, Mordekar SR. Encephalopathy in children: an approach to assessment and management. *Arch Dis Child*. 2012;97(5):452–458.
72. McCann JWJ, Phelan E. Pediatric neurological emergencies. In: Marincek B, Dondelinger RF, eds. *Emergency Radiology:*

*Imaging and Intervention*. Berlin, Heidelberg: Springer; 2007:583–599.

73. Lim YXJ, Kwek SY, How CH, Chan WSD. A clinical approach to encephalopathy in children. *Singap Med J*. 2020;61(12):626–632.
74. Huang BY, Castillo M. Hypoxic-Ischemic brain injury: imaging findings from birth to adulthood. *RadioGraphics*. 2008;28(2):417–439.
75. Borlot F, da Paz JA, Casella EB, Marques-Dias MJ. Acute hemorrhagic encephalomyelitis in childhood: Case report and literature review. *J Pediatr Neurosci*. 2011;6(1):48–51.
76. Agarwal A, Kapur G, Altinok D. Childhood posterior reversible encephalopathy syndrome: Magnetic resonance imaging findings with emphasis on increased leptomeningeal FLAIR signal. *Neuroradiol J*. 2015;28(6):638–643.

Chapter 12

# Emergency Department Body Imaging for the Sick Child

Katya Rozovsky, Gali Shapira-Zaltsberg, and Gina Nirula

## Outline



## Key Points

- Abdominal ultrasound serves as a first-line imaging modality in diagnosis of intussusception.
- The first imaging modality in a child with suspicion for foreign body ingestion is a frontal radiograph of the neck, chest, and abdomen.
- Surgical intervention is considered in cases of ingestion of multiple magnets or magnets in combination with other ingested metallic objects.
- While any fracture could be secondary to nonaccidental trauma, classic metaphyseal lesions and rib fractures are more specific for abuse than others.

## Abdominal Emergencies in Young Children

### MALROTATION AND MIDGUT VOLVULUS

#### Epidemiology

Malrotation can be defined as a spectrum of congenital disorders leading to malposition of the bowel in the abdominal cavity due to abnormal rotation of the midgut about the axis of the superior mesenteric artery (SMA). The most acute complication of malrotation is midgut volvulus, a potentially fatal condition that can lead to bowel necrosis and requires immediate intervention. Approximately 75% of patients with symptomatic malrotation/volvulus present until the age of 5 years, with up to 60% of all cases presenting during the first year of life.[1]

#### Clinical Features

In newborns, volvulus usually presents with bilious vomiting, while in older children the clinical symptoms vary widely from intermittent abdominal pain and malabsorption to acute onset of abdominal pain and vigorous vomiting.[2]

#### Diagnostic Investigations

The current reference standard for radiological diagnosis of malrotation is upper gastrointestinal (UGI) series with barium. The preferable mode of administration of contrast is through a nasogastric (NG) tube. Aspiration of the stomach content is recommended prior to contrast administration, as an overdistended stomach may cause displacement of the duodenojejunal junction (DJJ) and obscure the duodenum. It is important to observe the initial passage of barium through the duodenum in real time. When the barium fills the more distal small bowel loops, the duodenum may become obscured, which may limit identification of the course of the duodenum and the position of the DJJ.

Once a small amount of contrast reaches the stomach, the child should be placed in the right decubitus position. This position helps evaluate the normal posterior extension of duodenum to the retroperitoneum. After the proximal duodenum is filled with contrast, the child should be positioned supine to assess the position of the DJJ. On frontal projection, the duodenum should extend leftward, crossing the midline, and the DJJ is normally located leftward of the left pedicle of the vertebra, at least as high as the inferior aspect of the duodenal bulb (Fig. 12.1A).[2,3] Both frontal and true lateral views of the duodenum and DJJ are necessary to assess the rotation. Malrotation is suspected if, on frontal view, the DJJ is positioned medial to the left-sided pedicle (Fig.12.1B) or caudal to the duodenal bulb. On lateral view, a malrotated DJJ is positioned in an intraperitoneal location (more anterior than expected). If the imaging findings are equivocal, follow-through with delayed abdominal radiographs is recommended to identify the position of the cecum. The position of the cecum is not a specific finding and cannot exclude the presence of malrotation.[2–4]

### Midgut Volvulus

In midgut volvulus, the proximal small bowel twists around the superior mesenteric artery and vein. The most typical radiological sign of midgut volvulus is a "corkscrew" appearance of the proximal part of the small bowel (Fig. 12.2A). In patients with severe obstruction, beak-like tapering or abrupt "cutoff" of the duodenum may be identified, with lack of passage of contrast distally (Fig. 12.2B).[2,3]

### Summary

For diagnosis of midgut symptomatic malrotation/ midgut volvulus in emergency settings:

- Use NG tube.
- Aspirate gastric content prior to contrast administration.
- Use small amount of contrast.
- Use right decubitus and true supine position to assess rotation.
- "Corkscrew" appearance or beak-like tapering of the proximal small bowel indicates midgut volvulus. The findings should be immediately reported to the referring service.

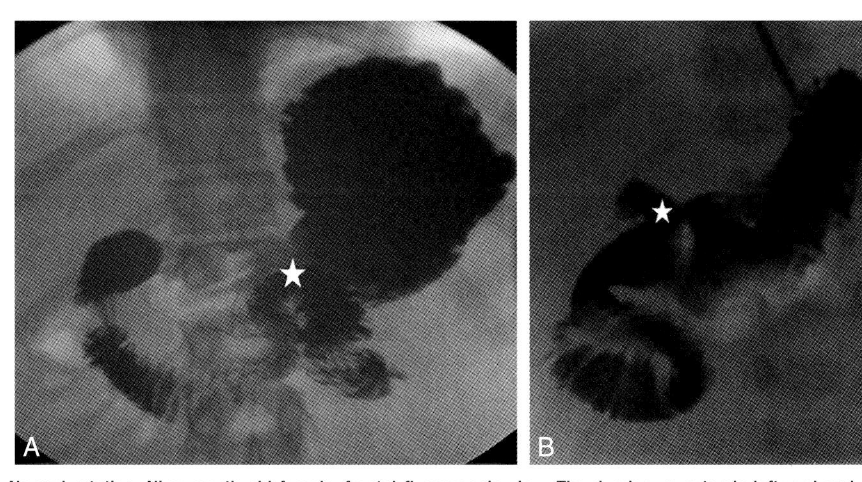


**Fig. 12.1** (A) Normal rotation. Nine-month-old female, frontal fluoroscopic view. The duodenum extends leftward and crosses the midline. The duodenojejunal junction (DJJ; star) is located leftward of the left pedicle of the vertebra as high as the inferior aspect of the duodenal bulb. (B) Malrotation. A 2-month-old male who presented with recurrent vomiting, otherwise healthy. Frontal fluoroscopic view. The duodenum does not cross the midline. The DJJ (star) is medial to the spine.

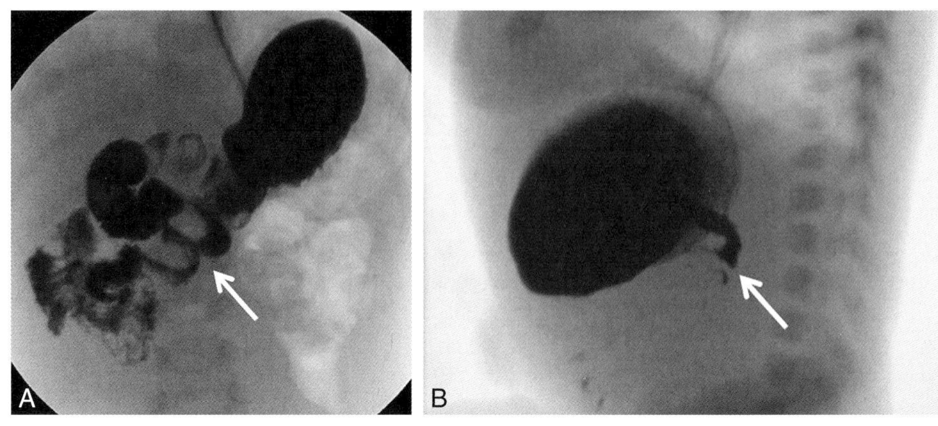


**Fig. 12.2** (A) Midgut volvulus. A 4-month-old male who presented with acute onset of abdominal discomfort and bilious vomiting. Frontal fluoroscopic view. "Corkscrew" appearance of proximal part of the small bowel (arrow), twisted around the superior mesenteric artery and vein. (B) Midgut volvulus. A 3-month-old female who presented with bilious vomiting and electrolyte imbalance. Lateral fluoroscopic view. Cutoff of the duodenum (arrow), with very small amount of contrast distally. Note "corkscrew" appearance and abnormal anterior position of the proximal small bowel.

## INTUSSUSCEPTION

### Epidemiology

Intussusception is an invagination of the proximal segment of bowel (intussusceptum) into the adjacent distal segment (intussuscipiens). In approximately 80% of cases, the intussusception occurs in the ileocolic area when the terminal ileum telescopes into the cecum and ascending colon. Nonreduced intussusception may cause bowel ischemia, necrosis, and perforation.[5] Most cases of intussusception occur between 6 and 9 month of life.

### Clinical Features

The "classic" clinical signs of intussusception are acute colicky abdominal pain, "currant jelly" or bloody stools, palpable abdominal mass, and/or vomiting.[5,6]

### Diagnostic Investigations

Abdominal radiographs cannot be recommended as a screening test for suspected intussusception, due to low sensitivity and specificity. The absence of ascending colon gas or soft tissue opacity within the right upper abdomen raises suspicion for intussusception. Supine and upright or left lateral decubitus views help to exclude free abdominal air in cases of perforation.[5–7]

Abdominal ultrasound (US) serves as a first-line imaging modality in diagnosis of intussusception. It demonstrates 97.9% sensitivity and 97.8% specificity.[5]

The US appearance of intussusception is often described as "target" or "donut" sign, which is related to the appearance of the intussusceptum within the intussuscipiens on transverse view (Fig. 12.3A). On the longitudinal view, intussusception may be reminiscent of kidney ("pseudokidney" sign), which corresponds to the relatively hypoechoic bowel wall surrounding hyperechoic mesenteric fat (Fig. 12.3B). Application of color Doppler contributes to the assessment of intussusception. The absence of blood flow within the wall of intussusceptum and intussuscipiens correlates with bowel ischemia.[5] Other US findings that must be assessed and reported are free abdominal fluid and visualized "lead point" of intussusception, such as a bowel or mesenteric mass or cyst.

It is important to differentiate ileocolic intussusception (ICI) from small bowel-small bowel (SB-SB) intussusception. ICI requires treatment, while SB-SB intussusception is usually transient and in most cases resolves spontaneously. ICI is typically seen within the right abdomen, measuring more than 2.5 cm in diameter, and contains hyperechoic fat and internal mesenteric lymph nodes. Typical SB-SB intussusception with no lead point is usually smaller in diameter, and no internal mesenteric fat or lymph nodes are visualized.[5,6] In most cases of ICI, the initial treatment of choice is nonsurgical reduction with an air or hydrostatic enema.

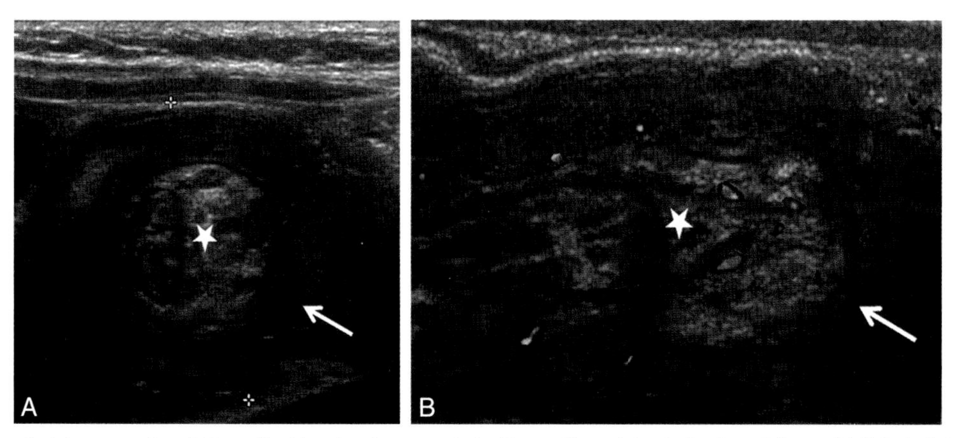


**Fig. 12.3** Ileocolic intussusception. A 7-month-old male who presented with vomiting, abdominal pain and "currant jelly" stool. (A) Transverse greyscale ultrasound (US) image of the right abdomen. "Target" sign, with intussusceptum (star) within the intussuscipiens (arrow). (B) Same patient, longitudinal US image of the right abdomen with color Doppler. "Pseudokidney" sign, hypoechoic bowel wall (arrow) surrounding hyperechoic mesenteric fat (star) within the intussusceptum.

### Summary

- Abdominal US is a first-line imaging modality in the diagnosis of intussusception.
- The presence of mesenteric fat and lymph nodes and the size of the intussusception help differentiate ICI from SB-SB intussusception.

## HYPERTROPHIC PYLORIC STENOSIS

### Epidemiology

Hypertrophic pyloric stenosis is characterized by thickening of the pyloric muscle. It is considered an idiopathic condition and usually occurs in otherwise healthy infants between the third and twelfth weeks of life, most commonly in males and first-born infants.

### Clinical Features

Thickening of the pyloris muscle causes symptoms of gastric outlet obstruction with projectile vomiting after feeds. If diagnosis is delayed, the infant can develop dehydration, weight loss, and electrolyte imbalances. In some cases, there is a palpable mass in the epigastric area known as "pyloric olive."[6,8]

### Diagnostic Investigations

Pyloric US examination is a first-line imaging modality of choice, with almost 100% sensitivity and specificity.[6] US should be obtained with a high-resolution linear transducer (5–12 MHz). Right posterior oblique positioning of the patient helps to visualize the fluid-filled antropyloric region. The US examination is considered positive for pyloric stenosis if it demonstrates thickening of a pyloric muscle of more than 3 mm and a pyloric canal length of more than 15 mm (Fig. 12.4). On the longitudinal view, the appearance of hypertrophic pyloric stenosis has been described as "cervix" sign, resembling the uterine cervix.

In the absence of pyloric stenosis, the visualization of normal pylorus may become challenging. The visualization of opening of the pylorus and passage of the gastric contents through the pyloric canal in real time can help exclude pyloric stenosis.

In infant with vomiting, malrotation and midgut volvulus is the most important differential diagnosis of pyloric stenosis. US examination should include assessment of position and orientation of the SMA and the superior mesenteric vein (SMV). Abnormal SMA/SMV orientation is an indirect sign of malrotation and should be immediately reported to the referring team.

### Summary

- Abdominal US is a modality of choice in the diagnosis of hypertrophic pyloric stenosis.
- SMA/SMV position should be assessed to exclude malrotation as a cause of vomiting.

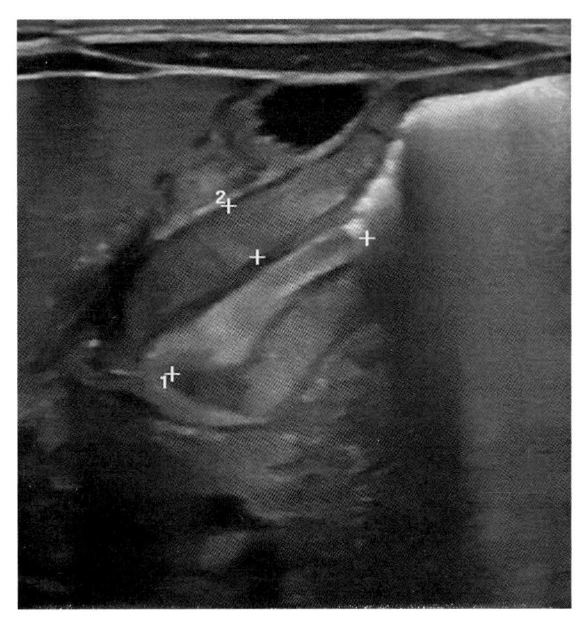


**Fig. 12.4** Hypertrophic pyloric stenosis. A 2-week-old male who presented with projectile nonbilious vomiting and dehydration. Longitudinal greyscale ultrasound image of the pylorus. There is an elongation of the pyloric canal (more than 1.5 cm, measurement 1) and thickening of the pyloric muscle (more than 3 mm, measurement 2).

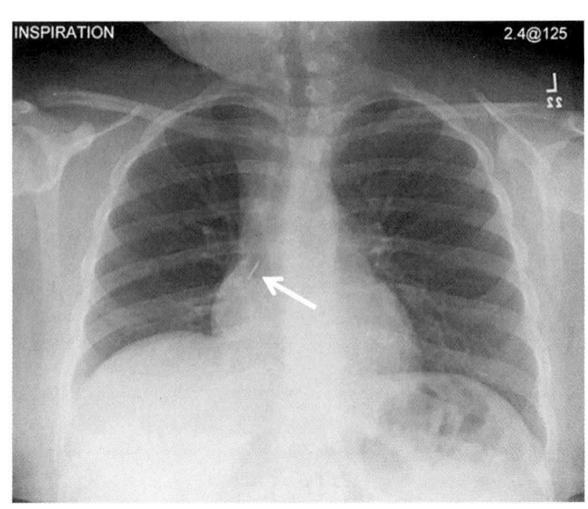


**Fig. 12.5** Foreign body (FB) inhalation. A 14-year-old female who accidentally inhaled a thumbnail. Admitted to the emergency department with vigorous cough, decreased air entrance to the right hemithorax on auscultation. Posteroanterior chest radiograph: there is a radiopaque FB (thumbnail) (arrow), projected over the right main bronchus.

## Foreign Body Inhalation

### Epidemiology

Most cases of foreign body (FB) inhalation occur between the ages of 1 and 3 years.[9] Most aspirated FBs are food particles, small toy parts, and pins. FBs are often located in the trachea at the level of the thoracic inlet, followed by the carina and right bronchus.[9,10]

### Clinical Features

FB aspiration is usually followed by choking, coughing, and wheezing. Dyspnea, stridor, and asymmetrical air entry can also be present.[9,11]

### Diagnostic Investigations

The first imaging modality is a chest and neck radiograph. If the inhaled FB is radiopaque, the radiograph can assess its location, size, shape, and density (Fig. 12.5).

Up to 90% of inhaled FBs cannot be identified on radiograph.[12] The most common sign of a FB aspiration in the lower airways is unilateral lung hyperinflation, best visualized on expiration views. During inspiration, the air bypasses the FB, and during expiration, the bronchus collapses against the FB, causing trapping of the air.[10] On expiration, the normal lung decreases in volume, while the affected lung remains inflated, and thus hyperlucent (Fig. 12.6).[13] Expiratory view in young noncooperating children may be challenging to obtain. The alternative imaging modality is chest fluoroscopy, where the movements of the hemidiaphragms and mediastinum can be assessed in real time.[9] In equivocal cases, nonenhanced chest computed tomography (CT) can be obtained. Negative chest CT helps to avoid unnecessary bronchoscopy.[14] FB aspiration can become a life-threatening emergency. Imaging and treatment are determined by clinical symptoms. Patients with respiratory instability usually undergo emergency bronchoscopy.

### Summary

- Acute onset of cough, wheezing, and/or unilateral lung hyperinflation raises suspicion for FB aspiration.
- The initial examination is frontal neck and chest radiographs.
- Expiratory view or fluoroscopy helps to diagnose air trapping.
- In equivocal cases, chest CT can be used.

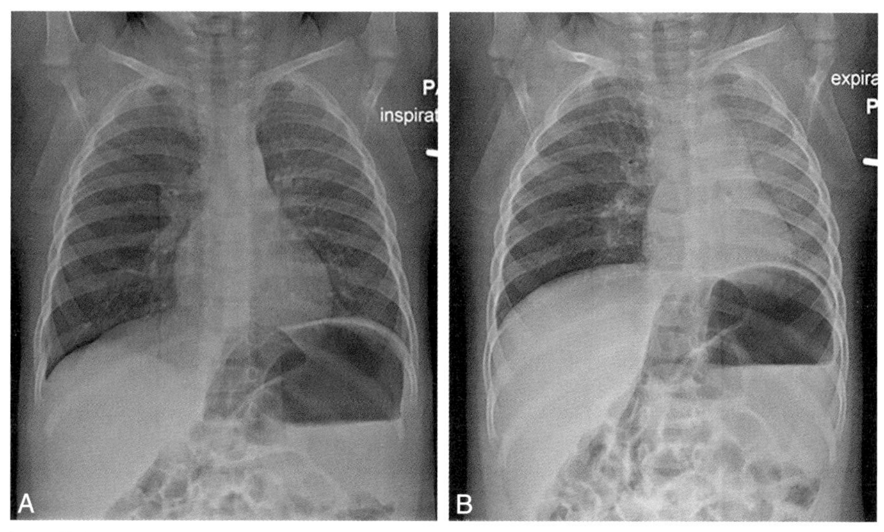


Fig. 12.6 Foreign body (FB) inhalation. A 9-month-old female with history of choking episode, followed by cough and dyspnea. (A) Anteroposterior (AP) chest radiograph in inspiration: no radiopaque FB identified. There is mild hyperlucency of the right hemithorax. (B) AP chest radiograph in expiration: the normal left lung decreases in volume, the right lung remains inflated and hyperlucent. A small piece of carrot within the right main bronchus was revealed on bronchoscopy and removed.

## Foreign Body Ingestion

### Epidemiology

In pediatric patients, the majority of ingested FBs are coins, small toys and crayons, pen caps, and batteries.[12]

### ESOPHAGEAL IMPACTION

#### Clinical Features

Children with esophageal FBs usually present with drooling, refusal to eat, or gagging.

#### Diagnostic Investigations

The first imaging modality is a frontal radiograph of the neck, chest, and abdomen. If the radiographs are negative, fluoroscopy with water-soluble contrast can help exclude esophageal obstruction. CT is the alternative second-line imaging modality of choice.[10,15] If there is a suspicion for complications such as esophageal perforation, mediastinitis, or vascular injury, contrast-enhanced CT is indicated. Esophageal impaction by batteries requires immediate attention, as leakage of the toxic content can cause corrosive injury and esophageal perforation. The radiologist should recognize the radiographic appearance of disc batteries, and not confuse them with coins. Disc batteries demonstrate a double ring, and in profile they have a characteristic beveled edge (Fig. 12.7).[15]

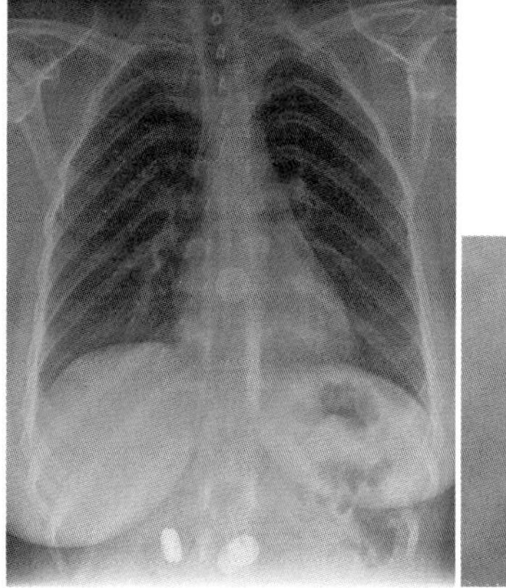

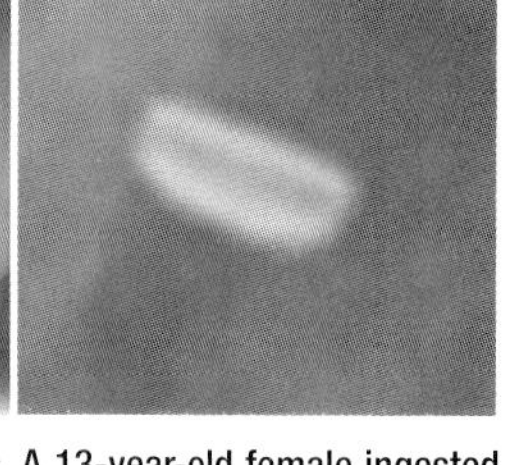

Fig. 12.7 Ingestion of button butteries. A 13-year-old female ingested multiple batteries and presented with gagging and drooling. Posteroanterior chest radiograph: there are multiple batteries. One appears impacted within the distal esophagus, at least four are visualized within the upper abdomen. Note double ring in frontal projection and characteristic beveled edge in profile (small additional image).

### FOREIGN BODY DISTAL TO THE ESOPHAGUS

If a FB reaches the stomach, in the majority of cases (80%–90%) it can pass further through the digestive tract, and rarely requires intervention. Large FBs or FBs with sharp or irregular edges may cause obstruction, especially at sites of anatomic narrowing such as the pylorus, duodenum, ileocecal valve, rectosigmoid colon, and anus.[10,15]

### Clinical Features

Complications of FB impaction in the digestive system include ulceration with risk of perforation and peritonitis, bleeding, infection, or mechanical obstruction.

### Diagnostic Investigations

A frontal radiograph of the neck, chest, and abdomen is the modality of choice. Number, location, and type of radiopaque FBs should be reported. In asymptomatic patients, FBs that do not have worrisome features, and are visualized within the stomach or bowel loops, could be followed up by serial abdominal radiographs. The parents or caregivers are asked to check the stool to ensure rectal passage. Intervention is recommended if the FB fails to pass through the GI tract in 3 to 4 weeks.[10]

## FOREIGN BODIES THAT REQUIRE SPECIAL ATTENTION

### Batteries

Most batteries that pass to the stomach can evacuate spontaneously, and the progress can be monitored by abdominal radiographs. Large batteries that fail to pass through the pylorus, multiple batteries in the GI tract, or signs of perforation should be immediately reported to the referring team. Disc batteries that remain in the stomach for more than 4 days should be removed.[12,15]

### Magnets

Single magnets can be followed up radiographically similarly to other FBs, and are expected to pass spontaneously. Surgical intervention is considered in cases of ingestion of multiple magnets, or magnets in combination with other ingested metallic objects (Fig. 12.8). Attraction of the magnet to metallic objects or other magnets across the bowel wall may cause pressure necrosis and perforation. As the magnets can be similar in appearance to other metallic objects, two or more radiopaque objects adjacent to each other on plain radiographs should raise suspicion and be immediately reported to the referring team.[10,12]

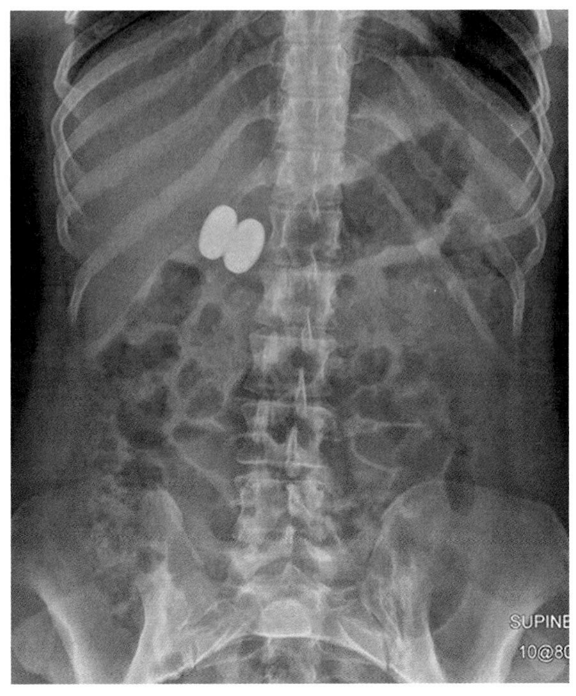


**Fig. 12.8** Ingestion of magnets. A 12-year-old female with abdominal pain. Suspicion for ingestion foreign body (FB). Anteroposterior abdominal radiograph: there are two radiopaque FBs (magnets) adjacent to each other. Immediate attention is required due to high risk of perforation.

### Sharp Objects

Sharp objects within the stomach are usually removed endoscopically. Sharp objects that have passed the pylorus should be monitored radiographically until their passage out of the GI tract. Failure of progression of the sharp object after 3 days raises suspicion for impaction and requires intervention.[10]

### Bezoars

Common types of bezoars in children are trichobezoar (contains hair) and phytobezoar (contains poor digested vegetable matter). Bezoars in the stomach cause delayed gastric emptying and gastric outlet obstruction. Bezoars in the bowel loops can cause partial or complete bowel obstruction. Presence of bezoar can be suspected on plain radiograph. However, abdominal CT is more sensitive and specific, demonstrating intraluminal mass with a "mottled" air pattern[10] (Fig. 12.9).

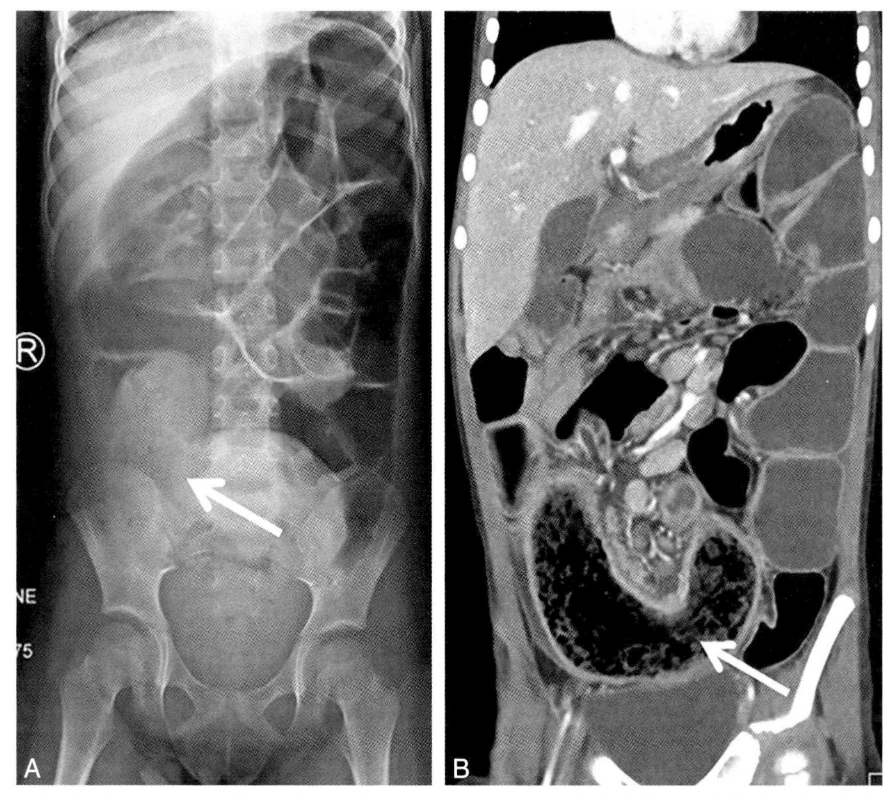


Fig. 12.9 A 7-year-old male who presented with symptoms of bowel obstruction caused by trichobezoar. (A) Supine abdominal radiograph demonstrates heterogeneous "mass-like" elongated opacity (arrow) within the right lower abdomen and dilatation of bowel loops. (B) Coronal reconstruction of contrast-enhanced abdominal computed tomography reveals heterogeneous intraluminal mass with "mottled" air pattern (arrow).

### Summary

- The imaging examination of choice is frontal radiographs of neck, chest, and abdomen.
- Batteries, magnets, or sharp objects require special attention and should be immediately reported to the referring clinical team.

## Pediatric Patients Presenting to the Emergency Department With Malfunctioning Tubes and Lines

### GASTROTOMY AND GASTROJEJUNOSTOMY TUBES

High rates of emergency department (ED) visits have been described in children with gastrostomy tubes (G tubes) and gastrojejunostomy tubes (GJ tubes).[16] These patients typically present due to tube dislodgement, tube malposition, tube obstruction, and skin-related stoma complications.

### Dislodged Tubes

Approximately 4 to 6 weeks after the G/GJ tube insertion, the stoma tract is mature. At this stage, all patients and/or their caregivers are typically instructed to urgently replace completely dislodged tubes with a temporary tube (e.g., Foley catheter that is one size smaller than the dislodged tube) to maintain and protect the stoma tract. If the patient presents to the ED without a temporary tube, the ED physician should attempt to reestablish access to the stoma.

If a temporary tube has been placed due to a dislodged G tube, it is advised to verify that gastric juices are obtained, and the temporary tube can be used for feeding until it is replaced by a G tube at the next available appointment. If there is any doubt about the position of the temporary tube, a small amount of contrast can be injected under fluoroscopy.

If a temporary tube has been placed due to a dislodged GJ tube, feeds should be held until the GJ tube is replaced by interventional radiology. In these cases, the patient may need to be admitted for temporary intravenous (IV) hydration or IV medication, depending on the availability of the interventional radiology team.

If the tract is not mature, a Foley should be gently inserted into the tract in the ED; however, it should not be used until its position within the stomach is confirmed with a contrast study.

### Malpositioned Gastrojejunostomy Tubes

The typical normal appearance of a GJ tube on frontal radiograph is with the tube following the expected course of the duodenum and its tip projecting over the expected location of the proximal jejunum. Patients with GJ tubes that are malpositioned (Fig. 12.10) often present with vomiting of feeds, feeding intolerance, or feeds injected through the jejunostomy port coming out through the stoma or the gastrostomy port.[17] As for completely dislodged GJ tubes, feeds should be held until the GJ tube is reinserted and adequately positioned.

### Tube Obstruction

G tubes and GJ tubes can become clogged with repeated usage or with instillation of material incompatible with the catheter.[17] This will present with resistance to injection of fluids, feeds, or medications. It is advisable to first attempt to flush the tube with warm water, using a back-and-forth motion with the syringe plunger. If unsuccessful, methods of chemical (i.e., enzymes) unclogging should be implemented, and if the obstruction persists, mechanical unclogging by interventional radiology with a wire and/or tube exchange is warranted.

Intussusception can occur in patients with GJ tubes, typically presenting with bilious vomiting, abdominal distension, and pain during feeds. The diagnosis is made by US (Fig. 12.11). Temporary bowel rest is necessary, requiring GJ tube removal and insertion of a temporary G tube that should not be used for feeding. The GJ tube is replaced after 24 to 48 hours of bowel rest.[18] In distinction to ileocolic intussusception, bowel hypoperfusion and perforation is uncommon with GJ tube–associated intussusception.

Skin-related stoma complications include hypergranulation tissue, infection, and gastric leakage.[19] Rarely, patients may develop peristomal abscesses. The presence of drainable abscess can be assessed by US.[20]

## CENTRAL LINES

Patients with port-a-catheters (ports), peripherally inserted central catheters (PICCs), or central venous

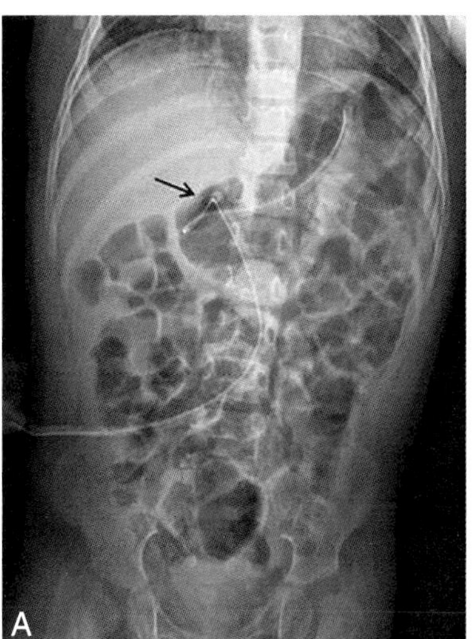


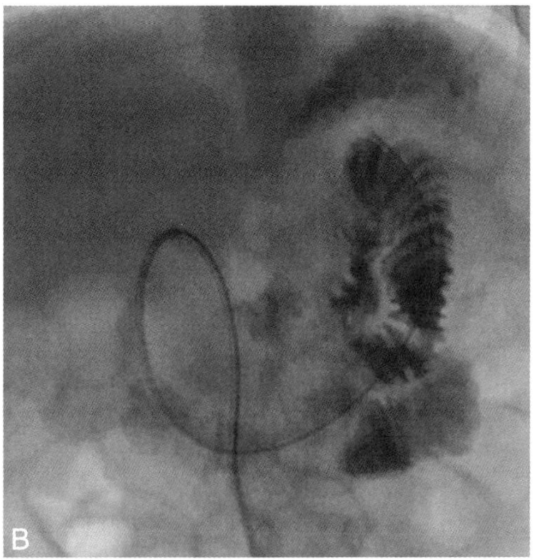


**Fig. 12.10** Abdominal X-ray of a 3-year-old boy presenting with feeding intolerance. (A) Gastrojejunostomy (GJ) tube coiled in the stomach (arrow). (B) The GJ tube was repositioned using fluoroscopy. Normal tip position within the jejunum was confirmed with contrast injection.

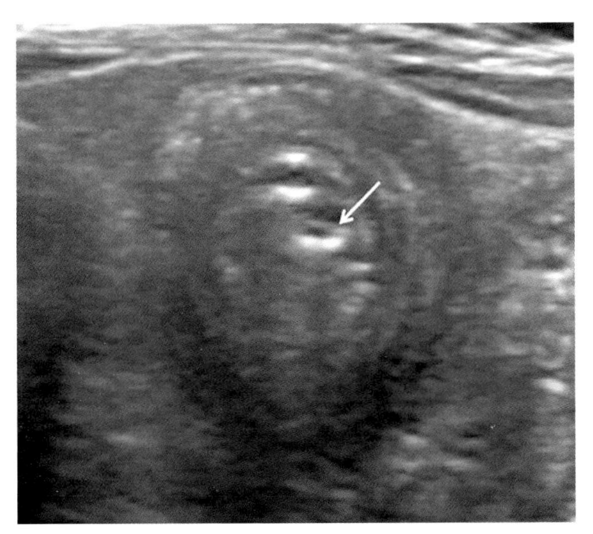

**Fig. 12.11** A 5-year-old girl with a gastrojejunostomy (GJ) tube presented with abdominal pain. Intussusception around the tube (arrow) was noted on ultrasound. The GJ tube was subsequently removed, and a temporary gastrostomy tube was placed.

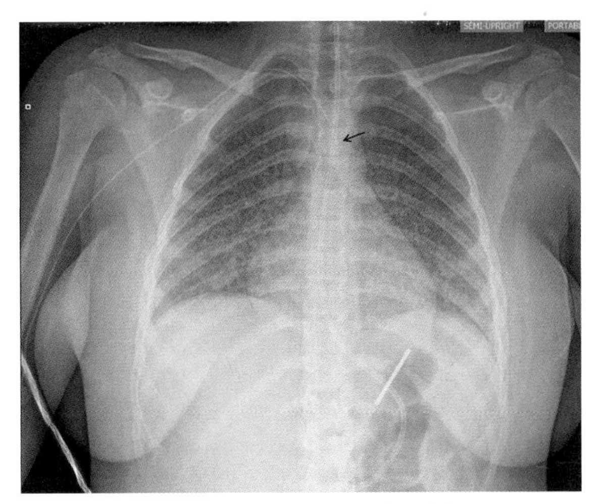

**Fig. 12.12** Chest X-ray of a 12-year-old girl with a right upper extremity peripherally inserted central catheter (PICC) shows the tip projecting over the left aspect of the trachea (arrow), concerning for arterial location (in the absence of persistent left superior vena cava [SVC]). An upper extremity PICC should project over the expected location of the SVC, to the right of the trachea. This incidental finding was confirmed with blood sampling. The tube was immediately removed, and a new venous line was placed.

lines (CVLs) may present to the ED with central line–associated bloodstream infection (CLABSI), mechanical line dysfunction due to blockage, dislodgement, or breakage.

CLABSI is the most common serious complication of central lines, and in the absence of an alternative source of fever, all bloodstream infections in patients with a port, CVL, or PICC are classified as CLABSI.[21] Timely removal of the catheter is indicated if (1) the line is no longer needed; (2) infection is complicated by sepsis, tunnel, or port-a-catheter pocket infection, endocarditis, or suppurative thrombophlebitis; (3) there is relapse of CLABSI with an identical organism; or (4) there is infection with *Staphylococcus aureus*, mycobacteria, fungi such as *Candida, Bacillus cereus*, or some multi-resistant bacteria. After removal of an infected catheter, reinsertion of a new long-term line should ideally be delayed until blood cultures (collected after removal) are negative, to prevent immediate contamination of the new device.[21]

Mechanical line dysfunction may be due to kinking or tip malposition, which can usually be diagnosed on chest X-ray (Fig. 12.12) and requires catheter revision/exchange.[20] Mechanical line dysfunction, however, is more commonly due to a thrombus/clot (Fig. 12.13), in which case the line typically does not draw back or flush forward appropriately,[20] or due to a fibrin sheath enveloping the intravascular portion of the catheter, in which case the central line can be flushed but will not aspirate. The presence of a thrombus can often be assessed by US. If the problem is not resolved with infusion of tissue plasminogen activator, the interventional radiology team should be contacted to attempt catheter rewiring, fibrin stripping, or line exchange/replacement if needed.[22] A line that is partially pulled out is ideally exchanged over a wire. If not feasible and the access site cannot be salvaged, *de novo* placement of a line is warranted.

Line breakage typically presents with local swelling, pain, or skin site leakage on injection (Fig. 12.14). Other signs are resistance to injection, inability to withdraw blood, cough, and chest pain. In these cases, a chest radiograph should be done to identify any migrated broken fragment. Fractured PICC and CVL fragments are retrieved from the heart and pulmonary arteries by using a snare to entrap the fragment, via a femoral, brachial, basilic, cephalic, or jugular approach. A vascular sheath is used to prevent tearing of the vein during the final removal of the fragment.

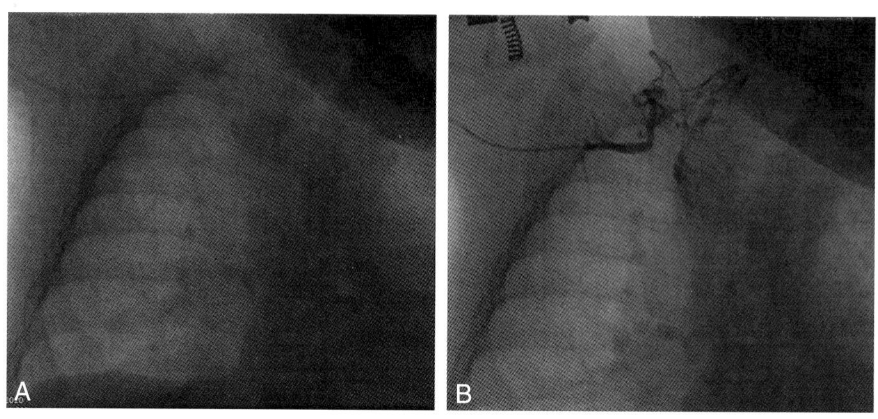


**Fig. 12.13** A 10-month-old female with gastrointestinal failure requiring lifelong total parenteral nutrition presented with malfunction of a right upper extremity peripherally inserted central catheter. (A) A fluoroscopy image shows the tip of the catheter projecting over the expected location of the subclavian vein. In an effort to salvage the access site, multiple attempts to advance a guidewire beyond the level of the catheter tip failed. (B) A venogram was performed that demonstrated chronic vessel occlusion with a conglomerate of small collaterals.

The fragment should be removed sooner rather than later due to the increased risk of cardiac arrhythmia, thrombus formation, and incorporation into the vessel wall.[23]

### NEPHROSTOMY TUBES

Patients with a percutaneous nephrostomy (PCN) tube may present to the ED with infection, obstruction, or catheter dislodgment. Urinary tract infection or tube insertion site infection has been reported to occur in approximately 6% of pediatric nephrostomy tubes, presenting on average 26 days postinsertion (range 2–112 days).[24] Dislodgement of the nephrostomy tube catheter in the pediatric population has been reported in 5% to 14% of patients, and is more common in infants and mostly related to inadequate fixation.[24] In cases of complete dislodgement, an attempt should be made to replace the catheter into the existing tract as soon as possible.[10] If there is concern for partial dislodgment, a catheter check and exchange should be performed under fluoroscopy[25] (Fig. 12.15).

Patients with obstructed PCN tubes will present with one or more of the following: decreased urine output, pericatheter leakage of urine, flank pain, fever, and sepsis. An attempt to exchange an obstructed nephrostomy tube over a wire should be made. If unsuccessful, alternative techniques to salvage the tract such as advancing a peel-away sheath into the collecting system over the obstructed tube, removing the old tube, and inserting a new tube via the peel-away sheath should be taken.[25]

## Imaging of Pediatric Nonaccidental Trauma

### Introduction

Unfortunately, nonaccidental trauma (NAT) is a leading cause of morbidity and mortality in the pediatric population.[26] As such, it is imperative that the radiologist be able to recognize imaging findings suggestive of NAT.

### Epidemiology

Children younger than 3 years of age are most at risk for NAT.[27, 28] Abdominal injury rates are highest in children less than 1 year old.[29]

### Clinical Features

The most common findings of NAT are cutaneous (bruises, skin injury), followed by fractures.[26, 28] Intraabdominal injuries are less common, comprising 2% to 3% of children being investigated for NAT.[27] However, mortality rates due to intraabdominal trauma are reported at 9% to 45%, making it the second highest cause of fatal child abuse behind head injury.[29] Injuries to the bowel and pancreas are more commonly seen in the setting of NAT.[29,30] Clinically, abdominal injuries

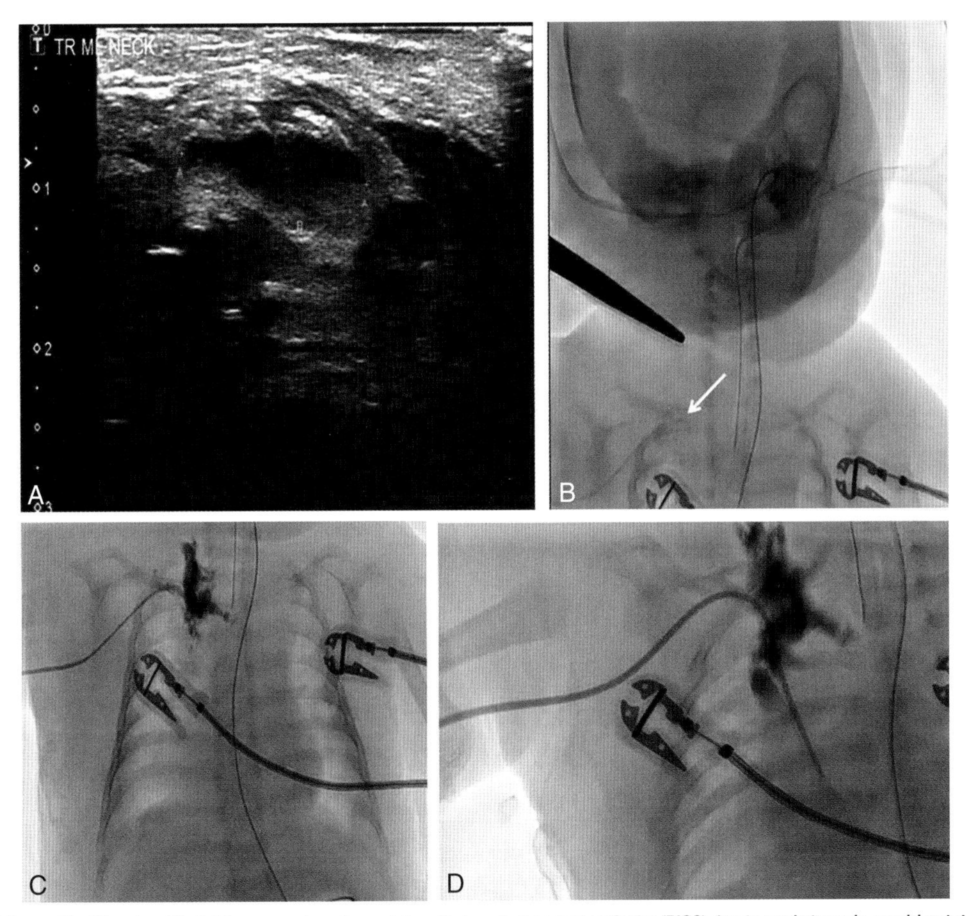


Fig. 12.14 A 2-month-old male with right upper extremity peripherally inserted central catheter (PICC) due to anal stenosis requiring total parenteral nutrition, presented with right neck swelling and cellulitis. (A) An ultrasound study was obtained that showed a fluid collection within the soft tissues at the region of interest. Given concern for extravasation from the PICC, a linogram was obtained. (B) An initial fluoroscopy image showed the tip of the catheter projecting over the subclavian vein (arrow) and a clamp placed at the site of the fluid collection. (C) Contrast injection demonstrated clear extravasation into the collection. (D) The catheter was subsequently exchanged over a wire.

can be occult or demonstrate obvious signs and symptoms. Physical examination and screening laboratory tests (hepatic and pancreatic enzymes) can help determine which patients require imaging.

## FRACTURES

### Imaging Findings

While any fracture could be secondary to NAT, certain types are more specific for abuse than others, as outlined:[31]

High specificity:
- Classic metaphyseal lesions
- Rib (especially posteromedial)
- Scapular
- Spinous process
- Sternal

Moderate specificity:
- Multiple (especially bilateral)
- Various ages
- Epiphyseal separations
- Vertebral body fractures and subluxations
- Digital

Low specificity:
- Subperiosteal new bone formation
- Clavicle
- Long bone shaft

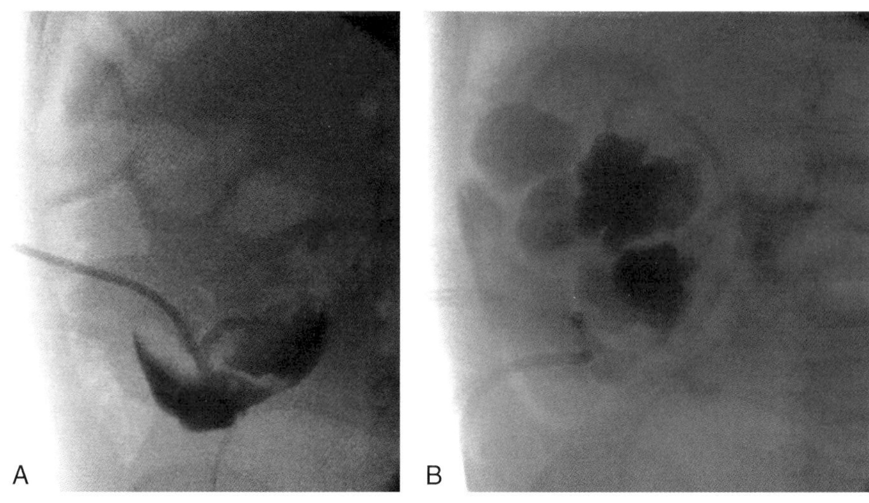


**Fig. 12.15** A 16-month-old male with left-sided ureterovesical junction obstruction and nephrostomy tube presented with absence of drainage. (A) A check of the percutaneous nephrostomy tube under fluoroscopy with contrast injection showed lack of opacification of the collecting system, indication malposition. (B) A new nephrostomy tube was subsequently placed, and adequate tip position was confirmed with contrast injection.

### Classic Metaphyseal Lesions

Also referred to as "bucket handle" or corner fractures. Most commonly seen in the distal femur, proximal and distal tibia/fibula, and proximal humerus. Usually seen in infants. This appearance is nonspecific in children older than 1 year.[32]

These injuries are caused by shearing forces that result in a fracture line that parallels the central physis and then turns to extend below the peripheral aspect of the subperiosteal bone collar[32] (Fig. 12.16).

Most classic metaphyseal lesions (CMLs) heal without the formation of subperiosteal new bone; others can have a variable amount of sclerosis and/or subperiosteal new bone (Fig. 12.17).

CML mimics include metaphyseal injuries from birth trauma or orthopedic manipulation for clubfoot, as well as metabolic bone diseases including rickets, and certain skeletal dysplasias.[32]

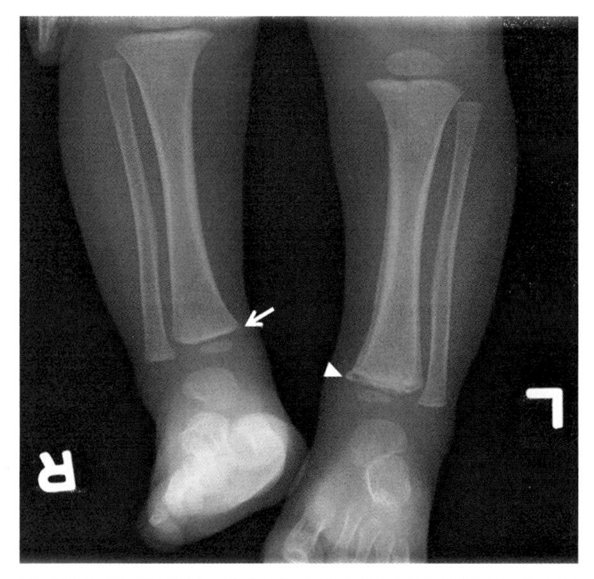


**Fig. 12.16** An 11-month-old female with nonaccidental trauma. Frontal radiograph of the bilateral tibia and fibula demonstrates an acute corner fracture of the medial right distal tibia (arrow) and healing corner fracture of the distal left tibia (arrowhead).

### Rib Fractures

The classic mechanism of injury is anteroposterior compression of the chest, which leads to fractures of the posterior costovertebral junction, lateral ribs, and anterior costochondral junction[28,32] (Fig. 12.18). Rib fractures at other locations are due to other types of chest compression and blunt trauma.

Other causes of rib fractures include difficult or assisted vaginal delivery, as well as metabolic disorders and skeletal dysplasias.[32] While the cardiopulmonary resuscitation technique of encircling the thorax with

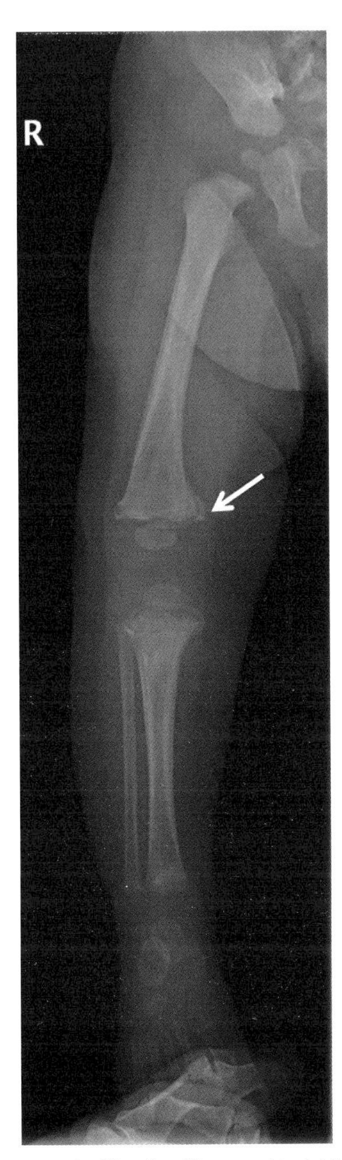


Fig. 12.17 An 8-month-old male with nonaccidental trauma. Frontal radiograph of the right femur, tibia, and fibula demonstrates a healing corner fracture of the distal femur (arrow) and a healing "bucket handle" fracture of the proximal tibia (arrowhead).

both hands has been shown to cause anterior and lateral rib fractures, studies have not found posterior rib fractures in these cases.[28]

Acutely, rib fractures are seen as linear lucencies that are nondisplaced or minimally displaced. As such, detection of acute rib fractures can be quite difficult, because visualization of the lucency depends on

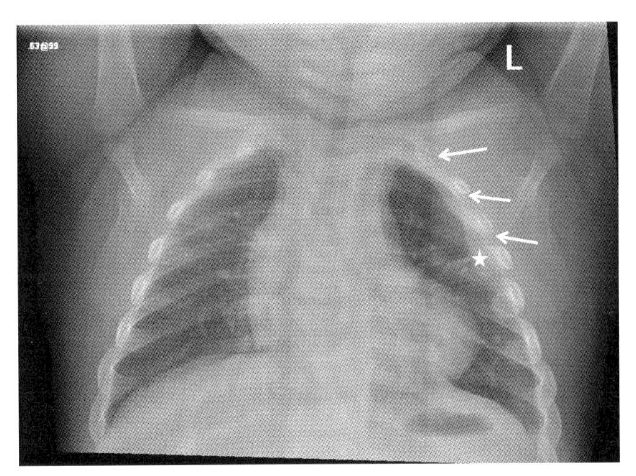


Fig. 12.18 A 5-month-old female with nonaccidental trauma. Frontal chest radiograph shows acute fractures of the left first, second, and third ribs (arrows). There is also a small volume of left pleural fluid (star).

the angle of the fracture in relation to the X-ray beam, as well as the degree of displacement, if present.[33] Therefore, oblique views of the ribs are extremely helpful in diagnosing subtle rib fractures.

During healing, callus formation results in fusiform widening at the fracture site[33] (Fig. 12.19).

### Long Bone Fractures

Diaphyseal fractures in long bones of nonambulatory patients are more suspicious for abuse, whereas these fractures can be accidental in older ambulatory children. These injuries are usually caused by someone grabbing the child's extremity and applying a rotational or bending force that results in an oblique/spiral or transverse fracture[32] (Fig. 12.20). Of these, femoral diaphyseal fractures are the most suspicious for NAT.[28]

### Diagnostic Investigations

#### Radiographic Skeletal Survey

The skeletal survey is the workhorse in the assessment of suspected NAT in patients under 2 years old. In addition to assessing for and dating fractures, it is also used to exclude an underlying metabolic condition or skeletal dysplasia. It should be performed in a standardized way and ideally monitored by the radiologist to assess if additional views are required.

The American College of Radiology and Society for Pediatric Radiology suggest the following views[34]:

- Anteroposterior (AP) humeri
- AP forearms
- Posteroanterior hands
- AP femora

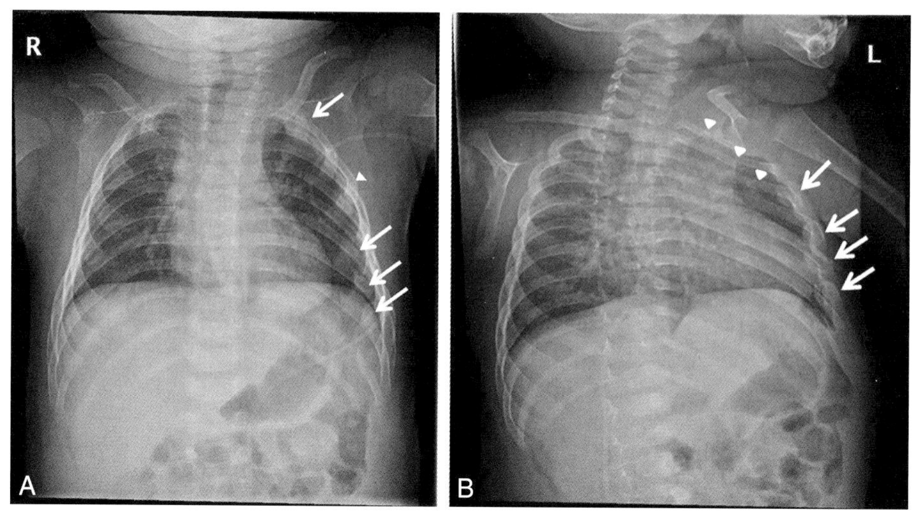


**Fig. 12.19** A 5-month-old female with nonaccidental trauma. (A) Frontal chest radiograph shows multiple healing left rib fractures with callus formation (arrows). There is also a fracture with angulation involving the left third rib (arrowhead). (B) An oblique radiograph of the left ribs shows multiple healing left rib fractures with callus formation (arrows). Acute fractures of the left first, second, and third ribs are also present (arrowheads).

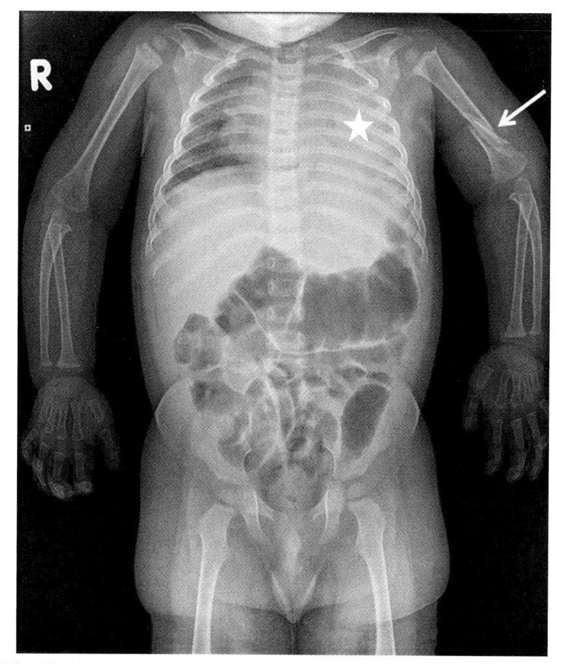


**Fig. 12.20** A 10-month-old male with nonaccidental trauma. Frontal chest and abdominal radiograph with both upper extremities in the field of view shows an acute oblique/spiral fracture of the left mid to distal humeral diaphysis with overlying soft tissue swelling (arrow). There is also diffuse opacification of the left hemithorax, in keeping with pulmonary contusion (star).

- AP lower legs
- AP feet
- AP, lateral, right, and left obliques of the thorax
- AP abdomen, including the pelvis
- Lateral lumbosacral spine
- AP and lateral skull, including the cervical spine

The follow-up skeletal survey obtained 2 weeks after the initial exam provides additional information 12% to 34% of the time.[28] The American Academy of Pediatrics recommends a follow-up study excluding the skull if abuse is strongly suspected clinically or when the initial imaging findings are equivocal or abnormal.[26] The most common new fractures that are seen are those of the ribs, followed by CMLs.

Many studies have shown improvement in detection and decrease in discrepancy with double reading of skeletal surveys; thus, it is recommended to double-read these studies whenever possible.[28]

## Dating Fractures

Dating fractures can be a challenging task. At the very least, healing can usually be determined to be in the early or mature stage (with the exception of CMLs, skull, and spinal fractures).[33] The typical order of healing is as follows: formation of subperiosteal new bone (peak 10–14 days), loss of fracture line and formation of soft callus (both peak at 14–21 days), formation of hard callus (peak 21–24 days), and finally remodeling (peak 1 year).[28]

## INTRAABDOMINAL INJURIES

### Diagnostic Investigations

#### Computed Tomography.

CT of the abdomen and pelvis with IV contrast allows for evaluation of injury to the vasculature and solid organs. In those with genitourinary injury, excretory phase images should also be obtained. Oral contrast is usually not used in the acute trauma setting due to the risk of aspiration, as well as the resultant delay in obtaining the study and potential surgical management. It is important to carefully review the examination in bone window to assess for fractures of the imaged ribs, spine, and pelvis.

#### Ultrasound.

While focused assessment with sonography for trauma can be obtained quickly and easily at the bedside, its sensitivity to detect intraabdominal injury in the pediatric population is relatively low, at 50%.[29] Greyscale US is not sensitive enough to identify solid organ injuries.[27] Contrast-enhanced US has been shown to be 86% to 100% sensitive for identifying solid organ injury compared with contrast-enhanced CT.[27] However, more research is required before this replaces CT as the preferred imaging modality, especially in the emergency setting.

### Imaging Findings

#### Liver and Spleen.

Hepatic injuries are the most common solid organ injury in NAT, with the left lobe most frequently injured.[29, 30] Splenic injuries are less common in NAT, likely because it is relatively protected by the thoracic cage.[29]

The types of hepatic and splenic injuries in NAT are similar to those seen in accidental injury, such as: laceration, fracture, hematoma, and rupture. Hepatic lacerations are the most frequently encountered injury.[29]

Subcapsular hematomas are seen as crescent-shaped regions of low attenuation intimate to and compressing the adjacent liver or spleen.

#### Pancreas.

Pancreatic injury is seen more commonly in NAT compared with other mechanisms.[29] Findings range from pancreatitis to pancreatic laceration or transection.

Because pancreatic and peripancreatic edema from trauma take time to develop, a CT that is acquired soon after the initial injury can demonstrate a false-negative result.[27,29] In the absence of other abdominal injury, any peripancreatic fluid is suggestive of pancreatic injury; most commonly, fluid is seen in the lesser sac.[29] Other findings include enlargement of the gland, ill-defined hypodensity (contusion), and linear hypodensity (laceration or transection).

#### Adrenal and Renal.

Up to 19% of children admitted to hospital with abusive abdominal trauma have renal injuries, usually with multiple other injuries present.[29] As with other solid organ injuries, these include hematomas, contusions, lacerations, and injuries to the vasculature.

Contrast-enhanced CT most commonly depicts adrenal injury as an ovoid lesion with attenuation less than that of the liver and spleen splaying the limbs of the adrenal gland[29] (Fig. 12.21).

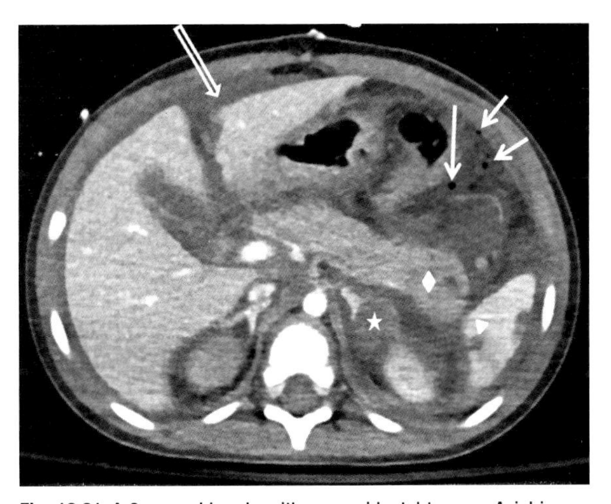

**Fig. 12.21** A 3-year-old male with nonaccidental trauma. Axial image from computed tomography of the abdomen/pelvis with intravenous contrast. There is an ovoid lesion with intermediate attenuation splaying the limbs of the left adrenal gland, concerning for hemorrhage (star). The pancreatic tail is edematous and hypodense, suggestive of contusion, with small focal hypodensity in the pancreatic tail in keeping with laceration (diamond). Small hypodensities in the spleen are concerning for laceration (arrowhead). There is peritoneal free fluid and stranding (hollow arrow), as well as multiple locules of free intraperitoneal air (arrows), which are in keeping with bowel perforation.

**Hollow Viscous.**

Bowel injury (particularly of the duodenum and proximal jejunum) is seen much more commonly in NAT than in accidental trauma.[29] Duodenal hematomas are the most commonly seen bowel injury, with bowel perforation being less common.[30]

CT findings of bowel perforation include pneumoperitoneum, disruption of the bowel wall, and extravasation of oral contrast (if given). Duodenal hematoma is suspected on CT when there is intraperitoneal fluid, focal mesenteric fluid, and duodenal wall thickening with or without a focal mass.[30]

## Conclusion

While any injury to a child could be accidental, it is important to recognize that certain injuries are more commonly seen in the setting of NAT, such as CMLs, posteromedial rib fractures, pancreatic, and hollow viscous injuries. The radiologist should be able to recognize patterns that are suggestive of NAT using various modalities, most frequently the radiographic skeletal survey and CT.

In conclusion, every emergency and trauma radiologist should be familiar with most common pediatric emergences and their imaging presentations. Prompt and accurate diagnosis is essential to provide the best treatment strategies for young patients, and to prevent life-threatening complications.

## REFERENCES


1. Aboagye J, Goldstein SD, Salazar JH, et al. Age at presentation of common pediatric surgical conditions: Reexamining dogma. *J Pediatr Surg*. 2014;49(6):995–999.
2. Applegate KE, Anderson JM, Klatte EC. Intestinal malrotation in children: a problem-solving approach to the upper gastrointestinal series. *Radiographics*. 2006;26(5):1485–1500.
3. Kumbhar SS, Qi J. Fluoroscopic diagnosis of malrotation: technique, challenges, and trouble shooting. *Curr Probl Diagn Radiol*. 2020;49(6):476–488.
4. Strouse PJ. Disorders of intestinal rotation and fixation ("malrotation"). *Pediatr Radiol*. 2004;34:837–851.
5. Edwards EA, Pigg N, Courtier J, Zapala MA, MacKenzie JD, Phelps AS. Intussusception: past, present and future. *Pediatr Radiol*. 2017;47(9):1101–1108.
6. Cogley JR, O'Connor SC, Houshyar R, Al Dulaimy K. Emergent pediatric US: what every radiologist should know. *Radiographics*. 2012;32(3):651–665.
7. Carroll AG, Kavanagh RG, Ni Leidhin C, Cullinan NM, Lavelle LP, Malone DE. Comparative effectiveness of imaging modalities for the diagnosis and treatment of intussusception: a critically appraised topic. *Acad Radiol*. 2017;24(5):521–529.
8. Esposito F, Di Serafino M, Mercogliano C, et al. The pediatric gastrointestinal tract: ultrasound findings in acute diseases. *J Ultrasound*. 2019;22(4):409–422.
9. Sahin A, Meteroglu F, Eren S, Celik Y. Inhalation of foreign bodies in children: experience of 22 years. *J Trauma Acute Care Surg*. 2013;74(2):658–663.
10. Pugmire BS, Lim R, Avery LL. Review of ingested and aspirated foreign bodies in children and their clinical significance for radiologists. *Radiographics*. 2015;35(5):1528–1538.
11. Johnson K, Linnaus M, Notrica D. Airway foreign bodies in pediatric patients: anatomic location of foreign body affects complications and outcomes. *Pediatr Surg Int*. 2017;33(1):59–64.
12. Laya BF, Restrepo R, Lee EY. Practical imaging evaluation of foreign bodies in children: an update. *Radiol Clin North Am*. 2017;55(4):845–867.
13. Brown JC, Chapman T, Klein EJ, et al. The utility of adding expiratory or decubitus chest radiographs to the radiographic evaluation of suspected pediatric airway foreign bodies. *Ann Emerg Med*. 2013;61(1):19–26.
14. Ahmed OG, Guillerman RP, Giannoni CM. Protocol incorporating airway CT decreases negative bronchoscopy rates for suspected foreign bodies in pediatric patients. *Int J Pediatr Otorhinolaryngol*. 2018;109:133–137.
15. Kramer RE, Lerner DG, Lin T, et al. Management of ingested foreign bodies in children: a clinical report of the NASPGHAN Endoscopy Committee. *J Pediatr Gastroenterol Nutr*. 2015;60(4):562–574.
16. Berman L, Hronek C, Raval MV, et al. Pediatric gastrostomy tube placement: lessons learned from high-performing institutions through structured interviews. *Pediatr Qual Saf*. 2017;2(2):e016 23.
17. Kumbhar SS, Plunk MR, Nikam R, Boyd KP, Thakrar PD. Complications of percutaneous gastrostomy and gastrojejunostomy tubes in children. *Pediatr Radiol*. 2020;50(3):404–414.
18. Temple M, Marshalleck FE Pediatric Interventional Radiology. 2014;318.
19. Farrelly JS, Stitelman DH. Complications in pediatric enteral and vascular access. *Semin Pediatr Surg*. 2016;25(6):371–379.
20. Townley A, Wincentak J, Krog K, Schippke J, Kingsnorth S. Paediatric gastrostomy stoma complications and treatments: A rapid scoping review. *J Clin Nurs*. 2018;27(7-8):1369–1380.
21. Wolf J, Curtis N, Worth LJ, Flynn PM. Central line-associated bloodstream infection in children: an update on treatment. *Pediatr Infect Dis J*. 2013;32(8):905–910.
22. Nayeemuddin M, Pherwani AD, Asquith JR. Imaging and management of complications of central venous catheters. *Clin Radiol*. 2013;68(5):529–544.
23. Chait PG, Temple M, Connolly B, John P, Restrepo R, Amaral JG. Pediatric interventional venous access. *Tech Vasc Interv Radiol*. 2002;5(2):95–102.
24. Shellikeri S, Daulton R, Sertic M, et al. Pediatric percutaneous nephrostomy: a multicenter experience. *J Vasc Interv Radiol*. 2018;29(3):328–334.
25. Huang SY, Engstrom BI, Lungren MP, Kim CY. Management of dysfunctional catheters and tubes inserted by interventional radiology. *Semin Intervent Radiol*. 2015;32(2):67–77.
26. Nguyen A, Hart R. Imaging of non-accidental injury; what is clinical best practice? *J Med Radiat Sci*. 2018;65(2):123–130.
27. Henry MK, Bennett CE, Wood JN, Servaes S. Evaluation of the abdomen in the setting of suspected child abuse. *Pediatr Radiol*. 2021;51(6):1044–1050.
28. Marine MB, Forbes-Amrhein MM. Fractures of child abuse. *Pediatr Radiol*. 2021;51(6):1003–1013.

29. Sheybani EF, Gonzalez-Araiza G, Kousari YM, Hulett RL, Menias CO. Pediatric nonaccidental abdominal trauma: what the radiologist should know. *Radiographics*. 2014;34(1):139–153.
30. Malik A, Faerber EN. Pediatric abdominal and pelvic imaging in non-accidental trauma. *Appl Radiology*. 2018;47(4):16–21.
31. O'Connor JF, Cohen J. Dating fractures. In: Kleinman PK, ed. *Diagnostic imaging of child abuse*. 2nd ed. St. Louis: Mosby; 1998:168–177.
32. Offiah A, van Rijn RR, Perez-Rossello JM, Kleinman PK. Skeletal imaging of child abuse (non-accidental injury). *Pediatr Radiol*. 2009;39(5):461–470.
33. Dwek JR. The radiographic approach to child abuse. *Clin Orthop Relat Res*. 2011;469(3):776–789.
34. American College of Radiology *ACR–SPR practice parameter for the performance and interpretation of skeletal surveys in children*. Reston: American College of Radiology; 2016:1–9.

# Index

Page numbers followed by 'f' indicate figures and 't' indicate tables.

C

D

R



S